To Professor Hitchings
with kind regards from
Christian Jansen-Cuypers
May 2000

Atlas of Ophthalmology

Springer

Berlin
Heidelberg
New York
Barcelona
Hong Kong
London
Milan
Paris
Singapore
Tokyo

G. K. Krieglstein · C. P. Jonescu-Cuypers
M. Severin · M. A. Vobig

Atlas of Ophthalmology

With 771 Colored Figures

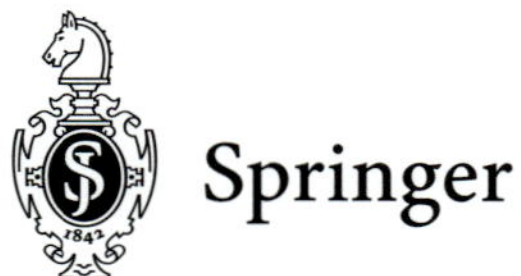

Springer

Professor Dr. Günter K. Krieglstein
Dr. Christian P. Jonescu-Cuypers
Dr. Maria Severin
Dr. Michael A. Vobig

Zentrum für Augenheilkunde, Universität Köln
Joseph-Stelzmann-Straße 9, 50931 Köln, Germany

ISBN 3-540-64454-7
Springer-Verlag Berlin Heidelberg New York

Library of Congress Cataloging-in-Publication Data
Atlas of ophthalmology / G.K. Krieglstein...[et al.]. p.; cm. Includes bibliographical
references and index.
ISBN 3-540-64454-7 (alk. paper)
1. Eye-Diseases-Atlases. I. Krieglstein, G.K.
[DNLM: 1. Eye Diseases-Atlases. WW 17 A8818 2000]
RE71.A856 2000 617.7'0022'2 - dc21

Springer-Verlag is a company in the specialist publishing group of BertelsmannSpringer
© Springer-Verlag Berlin Heidelberg 2000
Printed in Germany.

Cover-Design: de'blik, Berlin
Typesetting: Data conversion by Springer-Verlag, Heidelberg
Printing and bookbinding: Triltsch, Würzburg

SPIN: 10678732   15/3135 ih - 5 4 3 2 1 0
Printed on acid-free paper

Preface

This atlas provides a comprehensive introduction into the field of ophthalmology. It is intended primarily for medical students, nevertheless it makes an excellent reference work for clinicians and practitioners.
It is not meant to the replace the classical textbook, but rather to complement it. In this particular field of medicine, in which photographic documentation of the majority of disorders is feasible, an atlas is of extraordinary didactic importance.

The authors wish to express their appreciation and thankfulness to the many collaborators. The cooperation with the team at Springer editorials was remarkably constructive. Special credit is given to the staff in the photographic department of the clinic for their habitual eagerness and their friendly support during the collection of photographic material.

Cologne, autumn of 1999

G.K. Krieglstein   C.P. Jonescu-Cuypers   M. Severin   M. A. Vobig

Contents

1 Eyelids 1

2 Lacrimal System 29

3 Conjunctiva 41

4 Cornea 65

5 Sclera 113

6 Lens 123

7 Uvea 145

8 Pupil 171

9 Glaucoma 181

10 Vitreous 221

11 Retina 233

12 Optic Nerve 287

13 Visual Pathways 305

14 Orbit 315

15 Optics and Refraction 335

16 Ocular Motility 351

17 Ocular Symptoms 365

18 Trauma 371

19 Tropical Eye Diseases 399

Subject Index 407

Eyelids

1

1.1 Applied anatomy and examination techniques

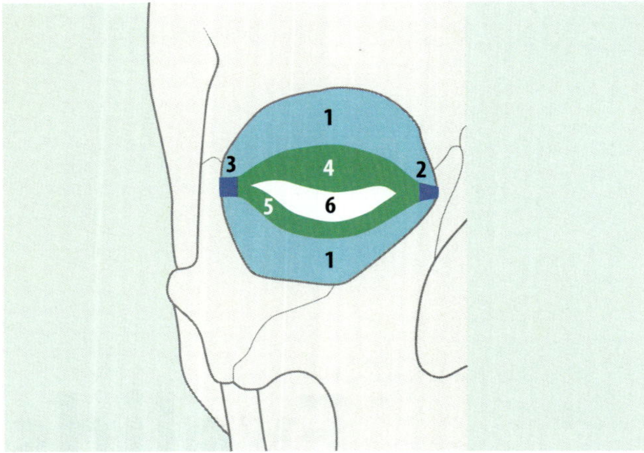

Figure 1.1 Connective tissue fascia and ligaments at the anterior opening plane of the right orbit, schematic drawing: (1) superior and inferior orbital septum; (2) medial canthal tendon; (3) lateral canthal tendon; (4) superior tarsal plate, (5) inferior tarsal plate; (6) palpebral fissure.

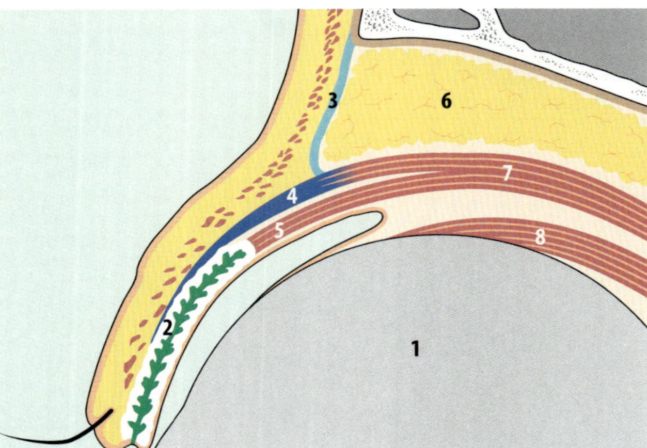

Figure 1.2 Cross-section through the upper eyelid in the midline. (1) globe; (2) tarsal plate; (3) orbital septum; (4) aponeurosis of the levator palpebrae muscle; (5) Müller´s muscle; (6) orbital fat; (7) levator palpebrae muscle; (8) superior rectus muscle.

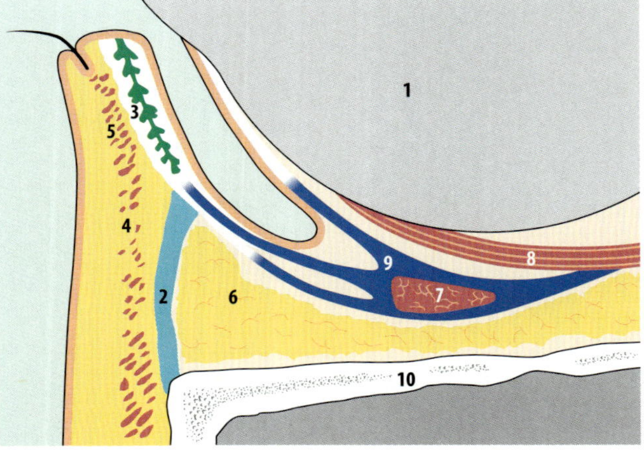

Figure 1.3 Cross section through the lower eyelid in the midline. (1) globe; (2) orbital septum; (3) tarsal plate; (4) preseptal portion of the orbicularis oculi muscle; (5) pretarsal portion of the orbicularis oculi muscle; (6) orbital fat; (7) inferior oblique muscle; (9) Lockwood´s ligament; (10) inferior bony orbital wall.

Figure 1.4 Lower eyelid eversion for the inspection of the tarsal conjunctiva, the inferior fornix and the bulbar conjunctiva.

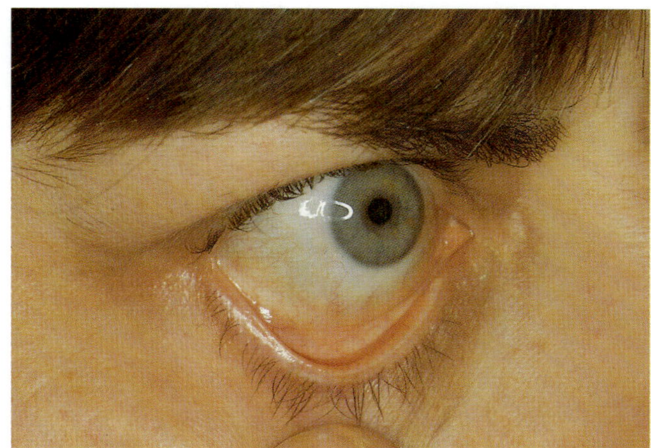

Figure 1.5 Upper eyelid eversion for inspection of the superior tarsal conjunctiva and the tarsal sulcus. The lashes of the upper eyelid are gently grasped, pulled downwards while pressure is exerted posteriorly and medially at the upper tarsal border with a cotton applicator.

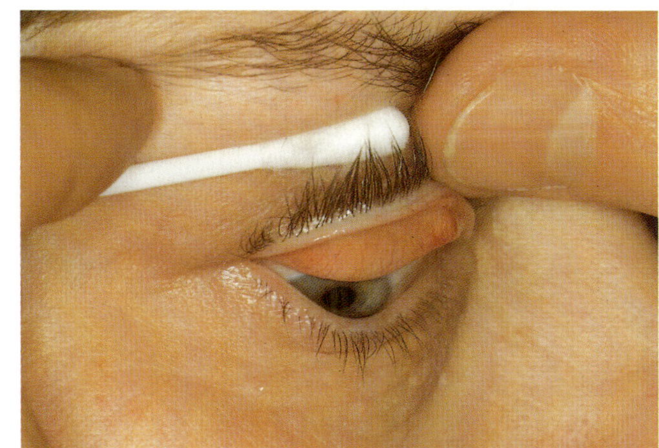

Figure 1.6 Double eversion of the upper eyelid for inspection of the superior conjunctival fornix. The superior eyelid is doubled over a Desmarres retractor and turned outwards so the superior fornix can be inspected.

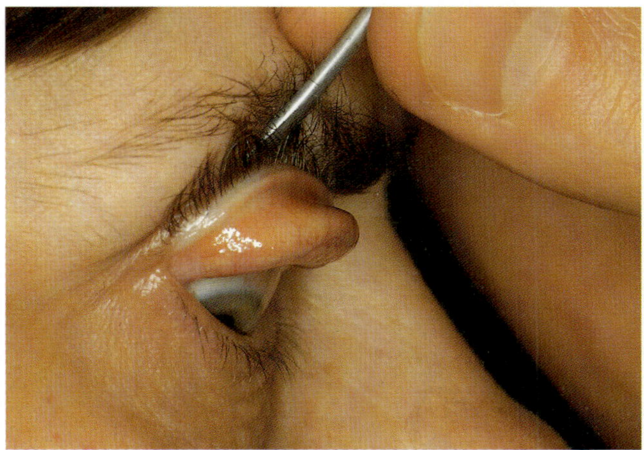

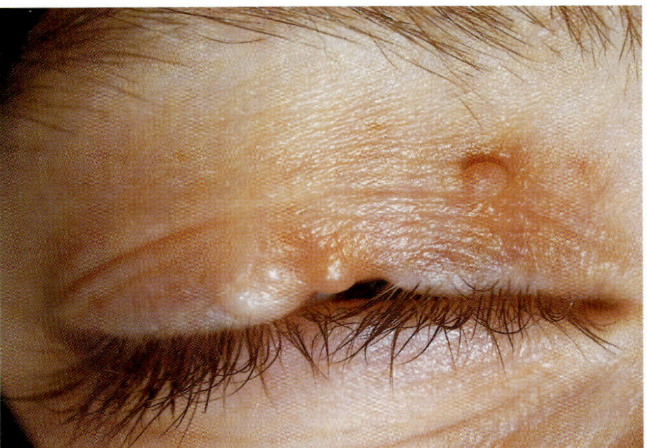

Figure 1.7 Coloboma in the upper eyelid. The condition is characterized by a notch in the upper eyelid margin. In this area, the upper tarsal plate as well as the lashes are missing. This reduction deformity may be associated with syndromes and other ocular deformities. Surgical repair should be conducted in large colobomas.

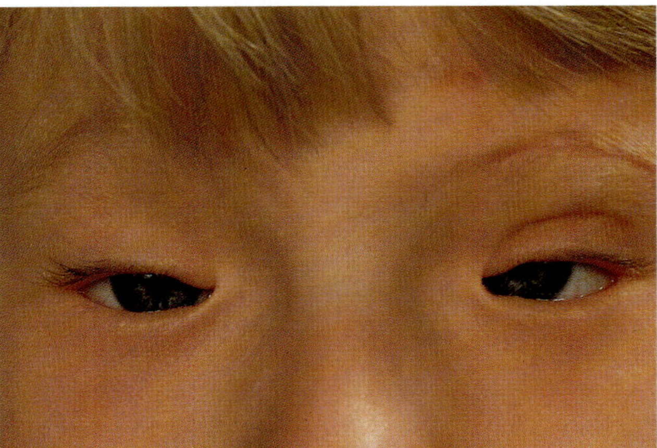

Figure 1.8 Epicanthus in an infant. Epicanthus is characterized by vertical folds of skin covering the nasal canthus. The lacrimal caruncle and the plica semilunaris are not visible. A physiologic epicanthus is present to some degree in most children and gradually decreases. Marked, pathologic epicanthus should be surgically corrected.

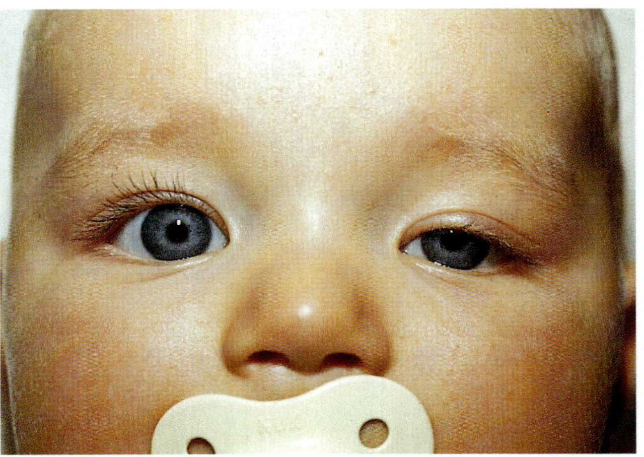

Figure 1.9 Left sided congenital ptosis in an infant. In the left, ptotic eye the upper eyelid margin covers the superior portion of the pupil, while in the unaffected eye the superior portion of the iris is visible. The condition is caused by a congenital impairment of the levator muscle.

Figure 1.10 Congenital entropion. The figure shows a congenital entropion of the left lower eyelid in a 1 year old infant with marked trichiasis (contact of eyelashes with cornea and conjunctiva). The eyelashes are very soft and flexible at this age, so trichiasis seldomly causes keratitis. Surgical repair is necessary in some cases, spontaneous resolution is frequent.

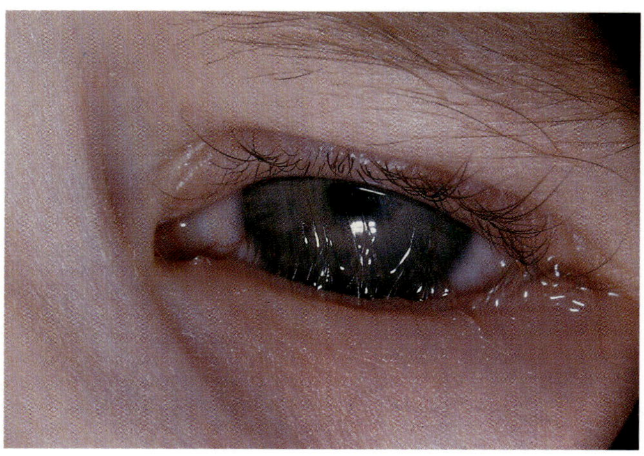

Figure 1.11 Bilateral blepharophimosis in an infant. The palpebral fissure is reduced in size horizontally and vertically. This feature may be associated with ptosis or epicanthus. A characteristic viewing posture is usually assumed. Surgical repair of the eyelids is needed in order to prevent muscular contractions and cervical deformities resulting from the viewing posture.

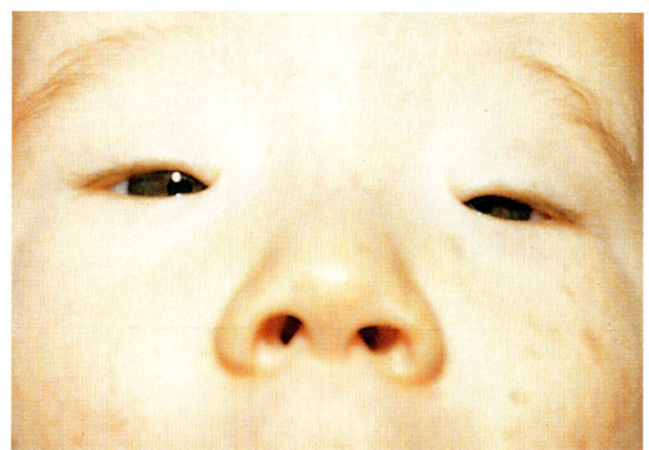

Figure 1.12 Bilateral congenital ptosis in a 4 year old child. A minor opening of the palpebral fissure can only be achieved by innervation of the frontal muscle. A suspension procedure is indicated in order to prevent the sequelae of the assumed viewing posture.

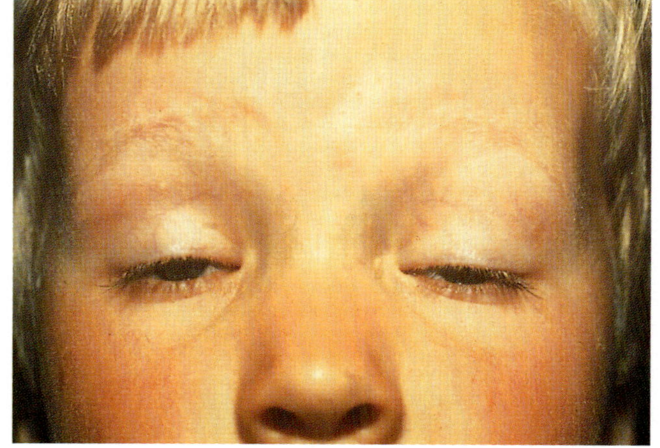

1.3 Eyelid malpositions

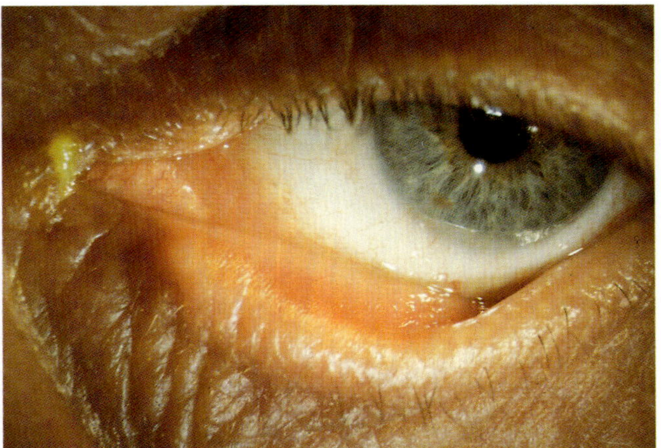

Figure 1.13 Involutional ectropion in advanced age. The inferior eyelid margin is everted away from the globe. The lower punctum is not exposed to the lacrimal lake, resulting in epiphora. The predisposing factors are laxity of the palpebral skin, horizontal laxity of the eyelid, weakness of the fascia and elongation of the medial and lateral canthal tendon.

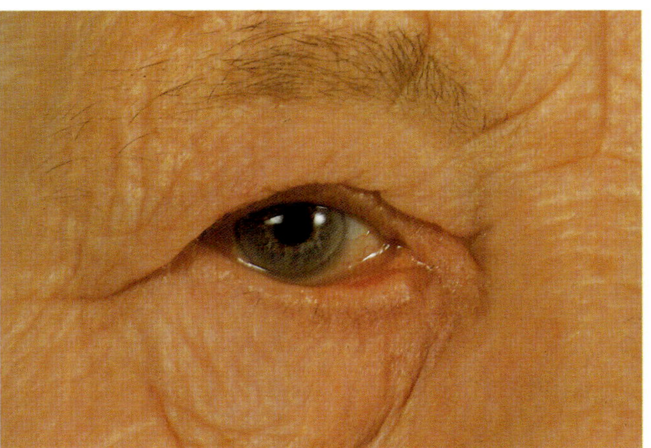

Figure 1.14 Medial ectropion of the right lower eyelid in advanced age. Owing to laxity of the medial canthal tendon, the medial portion of the lower eyelid with the lower punctum is everted. The consequences are epiphora as well as dermatitis of the lower eyelid due to permanent moisture of the skin and irritation by frequent rubbing. An inversion of the eyelid to the appropiate position can be achieved by surgical tightening of the medial canthal tendon.

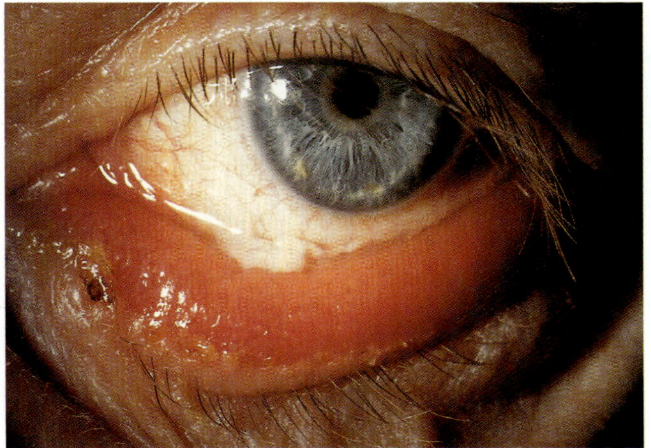

Figure 1.15 Paralytic ectropion in facial nerve palsy. The entire lower eyelid is everted away from the globe due to the atony of the orbicularis muscle. The tarsal conjunctiva is edematous and hyperemic, a reflectory watery-mucous conjunctival secretion develops.

Figure 1.16 Mechanical ectropion due to a fibroma in the lower eyelid of a patient suffering from neurofibromatosis type 1. The fibroma causes a gravitational eversion of the lower eyelid.

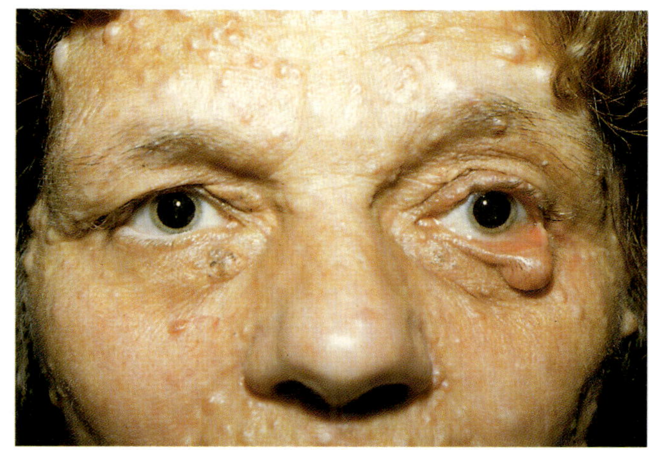

Figure 1.17 Surgical technique used for the repair of involutional ectropion, schematic drawing. The lower eyelid is shortened by an excision of a full-thickness wedge, compensating for the laxity of the medial and lateral canthal tendon. The eyelid margin, the tarsal plate (1) and the muscle layer (2) are sutured with different material after removal of the wedge.

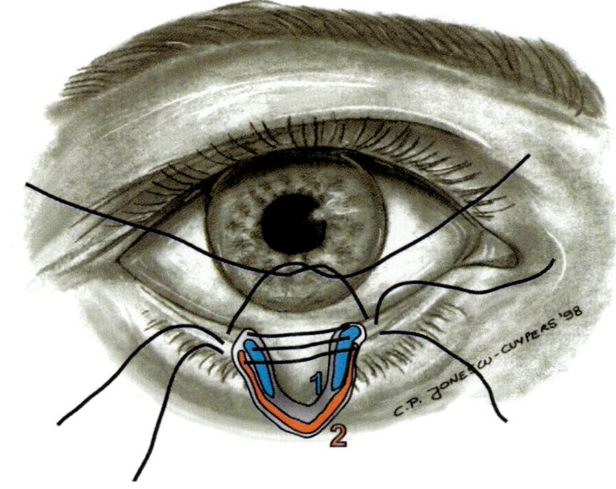

Figure 1.18 Various surgical approaches used for the repair of involutional ectropion, schematic drawing (right eye). The surgical approach is to be directed towards the underlying etiologic factors of the ectropion: (1) mobilization of a triangular skin flap with temporal shift and excision of skin; (2) shortening of the medial and lateral canthal tendon at their bony insertion; (3) wedge-excision; same surgical approach as in figure 1.17.

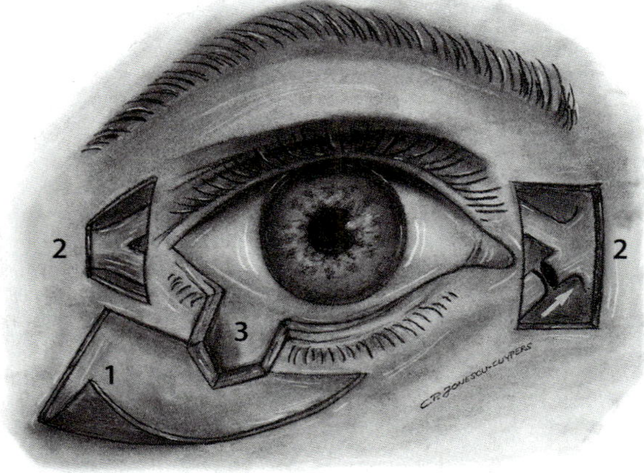

1.3 Eyelid malpositions

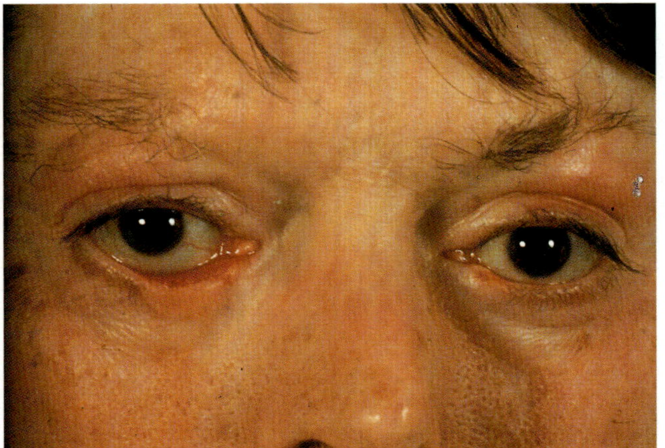

Figure 1.19 Cicatricial ectropion in the right eye after severe facial burn. Vertical shortening of the skin in the nasolabial region by scarring results in tension on the lower eyelid margin, which is everted away from the globe. The lower punctum is everted, causing epiphora.

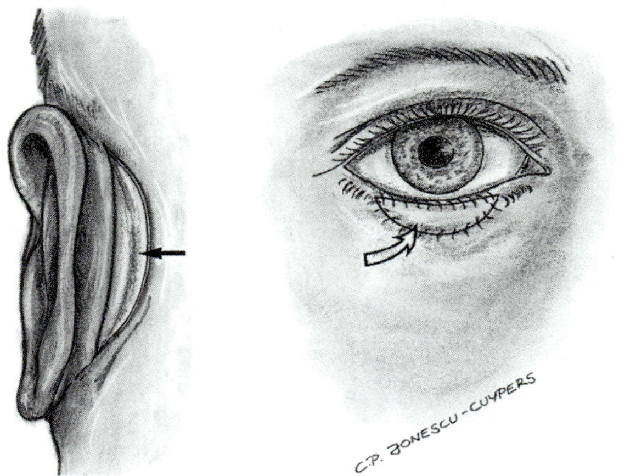

Figure 1.20 Surgical approach for the correction of cicatricial ectropion, schematic drawing. An elliptic full-thickness skin graft is taken from the retroauricular crease (*black arrow*), after thinning of the posterior surface, the graft is positioned in the lower eyelid in order to release cicatricial tension to the eyelid margin *(white arrow)*.

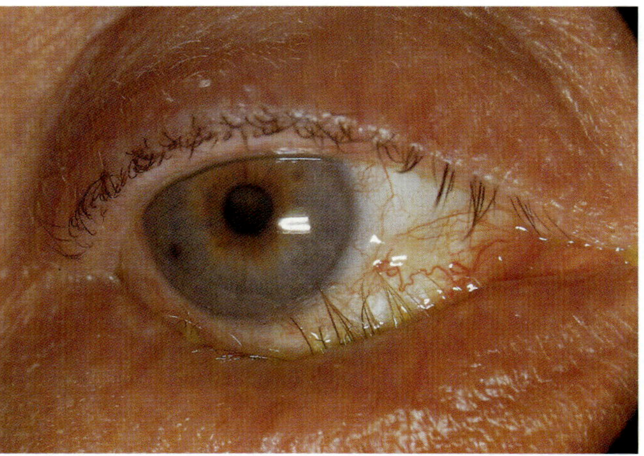

Figure 1.21 Involutional, senile entropion. With eyelid laxity, the preseptal orbicularis muscle overrides the tarsus, resulting in an inward turning of the eyelid and contact of eyelashes with cornea and conjunctiva (trichiasis).

Figure 1.22 Surgical approach for the correction of involutional entropion, schematic drawing. A piece of skin with adjacent orbicularis oculi muscle is resected. The sutures are placed through cutis and subcutis (1), the muscle-layer (2), the lower margin of the tarsal plate (3), the orbital septum (4) and back anteriorly through subcutis and cutis. Tightening the knots of the sutures has an everting effect on the lower eyelid, resulting in correction of the ectropion.

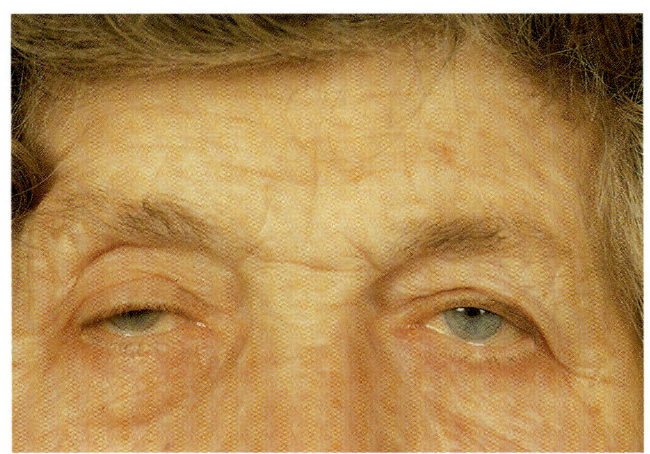

Figure 1.23 Aponeurotic ptosis in advanced age. In advanced age, a disinsertion of the aponeurosis of the levator muscle may occur, resulting in acquired ptosis. The aponeurotic ptosis is more pronounced in the right eye, the pupil is completely covered, resulting in a lack of binocular vision.

Figure 1.24 Myogenic ptosis in myasthenia gravis. To compensate for the reduced opening of the palpabral fissure, the patient activates the frontalis muscle and assumes a characteristic viewing posture of backward angulation of the head.

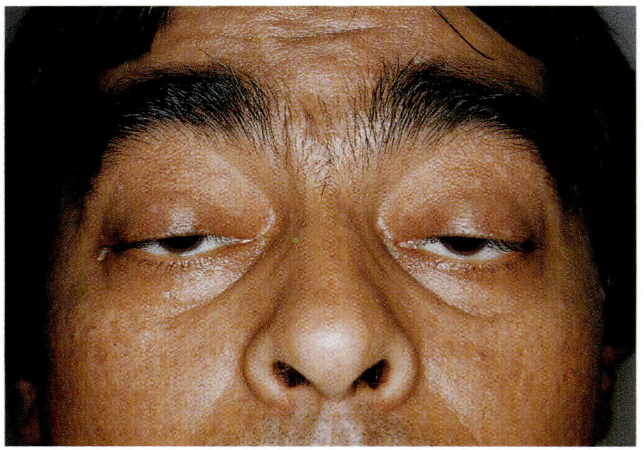

1.3 Eyelid malpositions

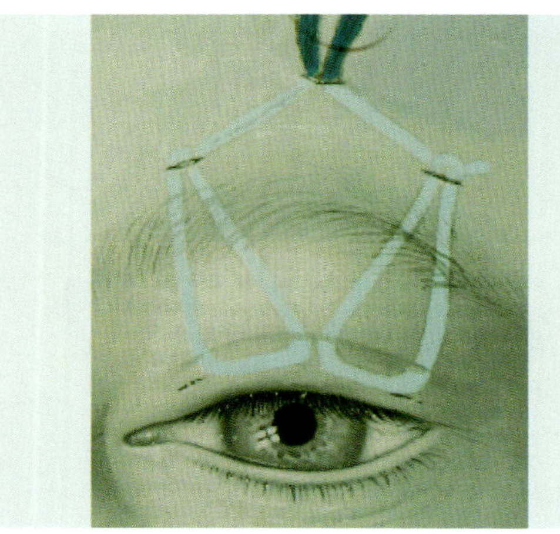

Figure 1.25 Surgical approach for the correction of ptosis with either none or deficient function of the levator muscle, schematic drawing. Two slings of autologous fascia lata or "goretex" are passed from the frontalis muscle through the orbicularis to the upper eyelid margin and tied 1 cm above the eyebrows. Lifting of the eyebrow (innervation of the frontalis muscle) results in lifting of the upper eyelid.

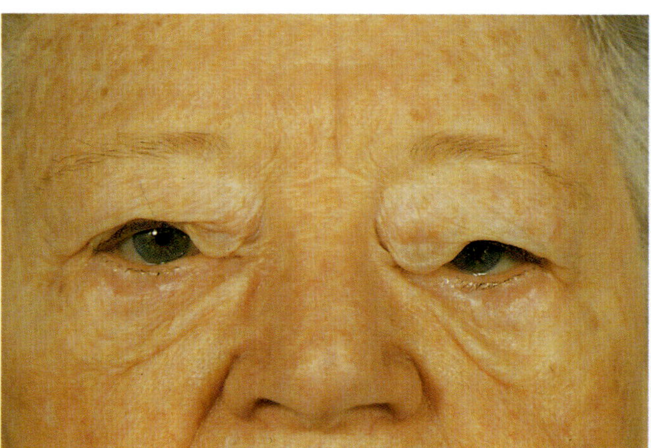

Figure 1.26 Dermatochalasis in advanced age. Laxity of the eyelid skin leads to redundancy of skin. The condition may resemble ptosis.

Figure 1.27   Contact dermatitis after application of wet compresses with camomile preparation. Contact dermatitis is characterized by severe itching, erythema and edema of the eyelid skin. Blisters may develop. The changes are usually restricted to the area of contact between skin and the noxious agent.

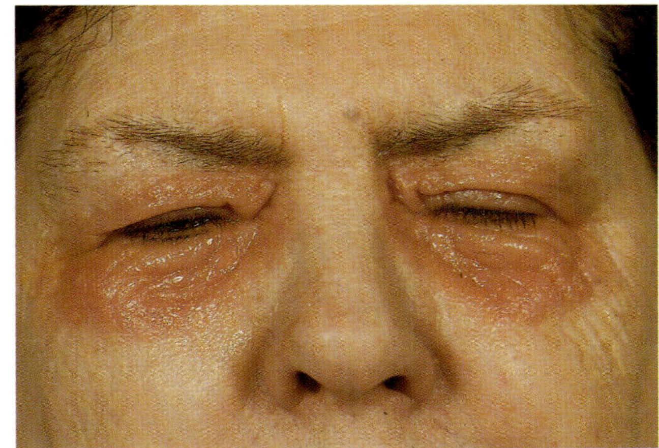

Figure 1.28   Acute allergic periocular dermatitis with marked eyelid edema, suppurative urticaria and muco-serous secretion in the palpebral fissure after application of antibiotic ointment. In severe cases, the dermatitis may spread.

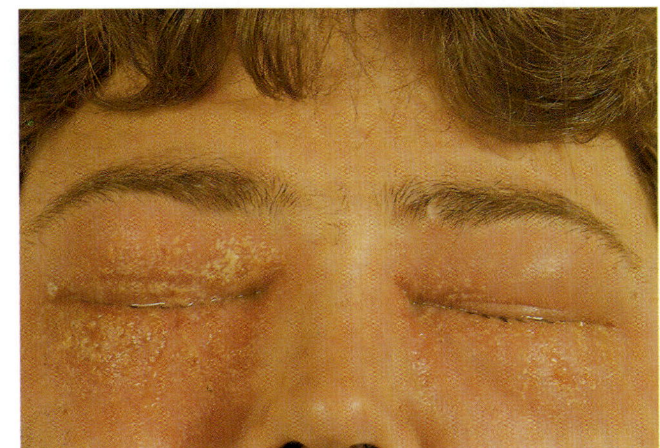

Figure 1.29   Atopic dermatitis of the eyelids with severly itching eczematous skin lesions at the eyelid margins. Marked skin folds.

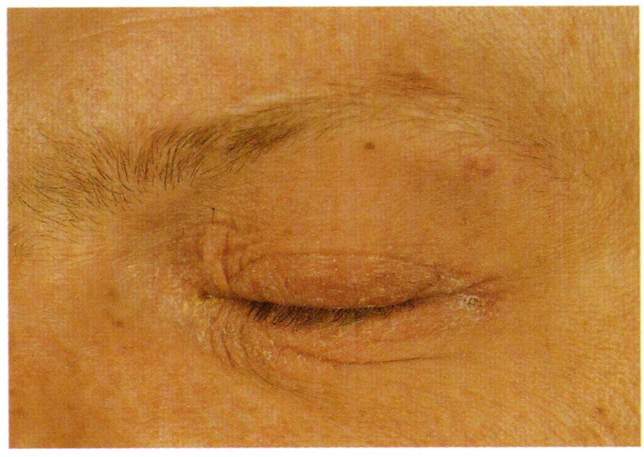

1.4 Disorders of the eyelid skin

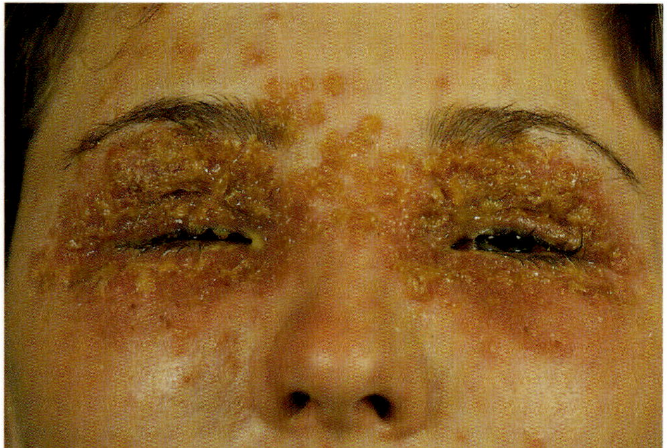

Figure 1.30 Impetigo. Bilateral eyelid pyodermia with putrid crusts.

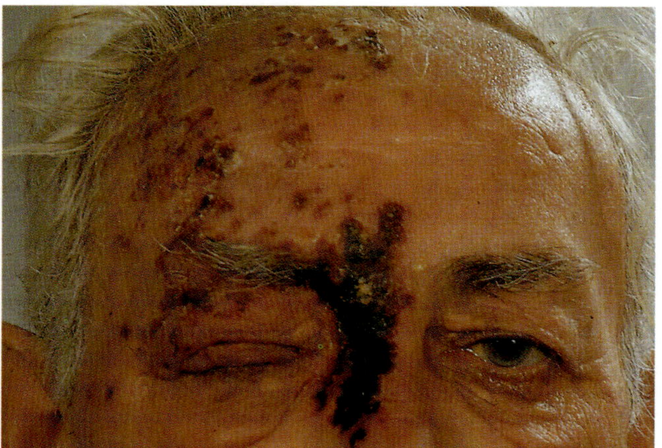

Figure 1.31 Herpes zoster in the eyelid region. The segmental arrangement of the skin lesions follows the first division of the trigeminal nerve, an involvement of the nasociliary nerve indicates ocular involvement.

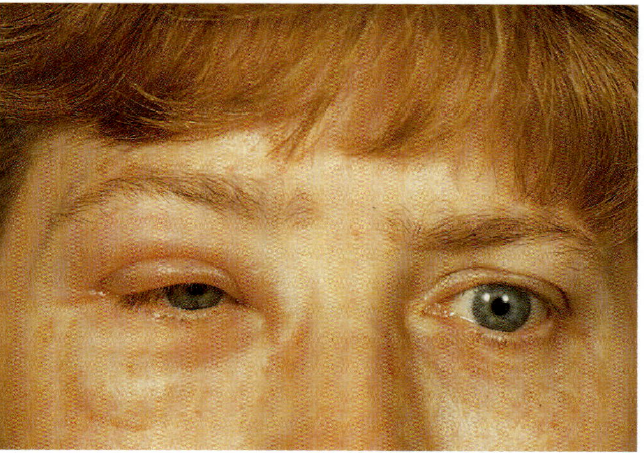

Figure 1.32 Allergic edema of the right upper and lower eyelids following an insect bite. Note the redness and swelling of the eyelids with marked narrowing of the palpebral fissure.

Figure 1.33 Status post severe facial burn with ulceration in the eyebrow region and the eyelid margins and formation of contractures, keloids and trichiasis of the upper eyelids.

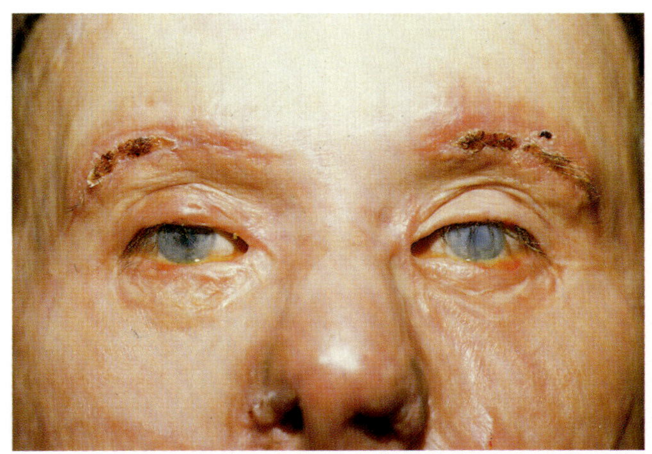

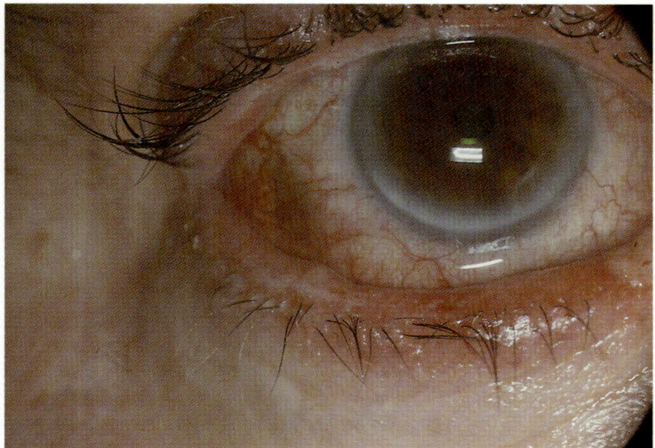

Figure 1.34 Chronic blepharitis with hyperemia, swelling and rounding of the eyelid margin. Various causes: skin disorders, metabolic disorders, staphylococcal infection.

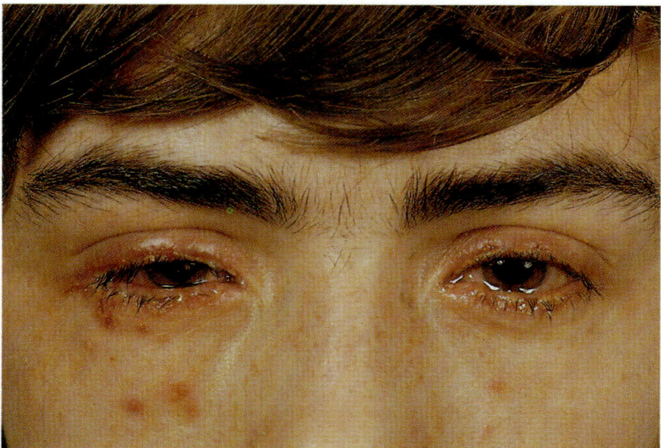

Figure 1.35 Bilateral blepharitis in the upper and lower eyelids in herpes simplex virus infection in a 28 year old patient.

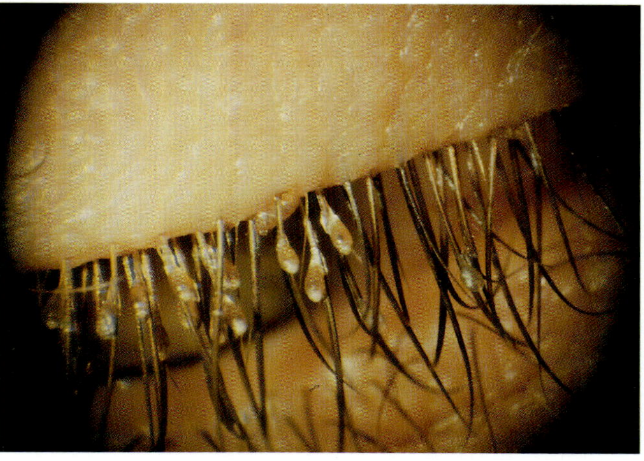

Figure 1.36 Blepharitis caused by Phthirus pubis (crab louse). Deposition of egg cases (nits) on the hair shafts of the lashes.

Figure 1.37 Molluscum contagiosum in the upper eyelid. The inflammatory tumor, located within the row of lashes, shows a typical central umbilication. Spontaneous resolution is frequent.

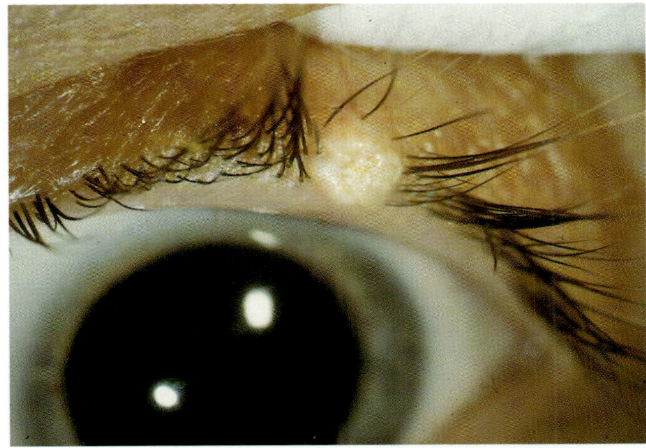

Figure 1.38 Distichiasis. An additional row of eyelashes emanates proximally to the original lashes and rubs the cornea (trichiasis).

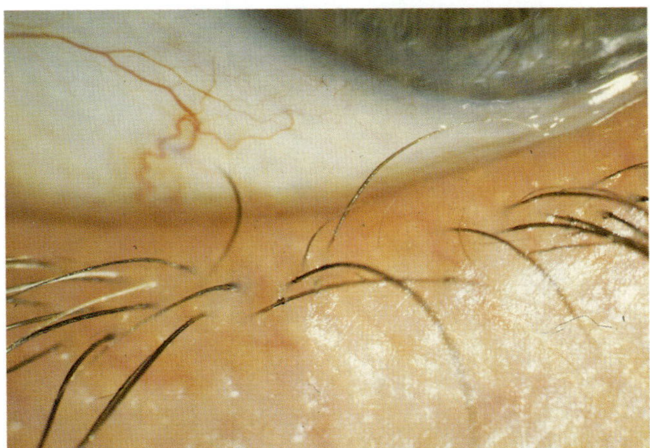

1.6 Disorders of the eyelid glands

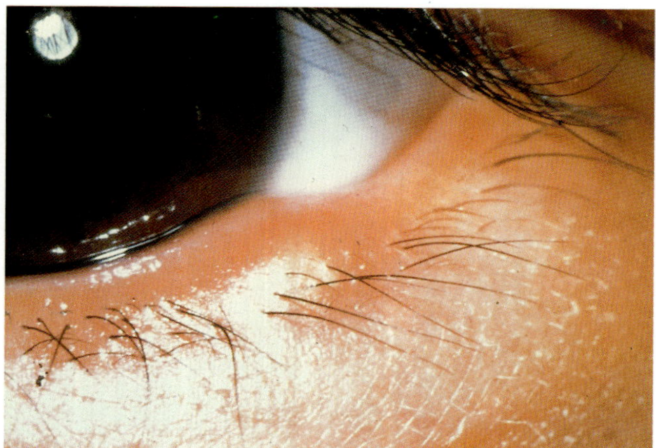

Figure 1.39 External hordeolum (stye): acute inflammation of the sebaceous gland (gland of Zeis). Most frequently caused by Staphylococci. Recurrence may occur. Systemic disorders, e.g. diabetes mellitus should be ruled out.

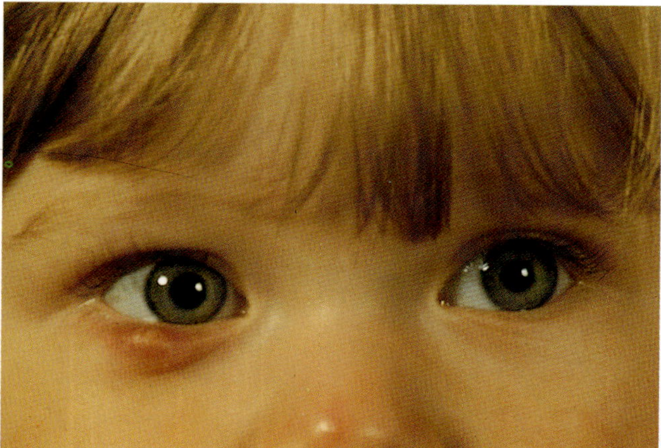

Figure 1.40 External hordeolum in the right lower eyelid of a 4 year-old girl. Note the marked swelling of the infected Meibomian gland in the midline of the lower eyelid with concomitant erythema.

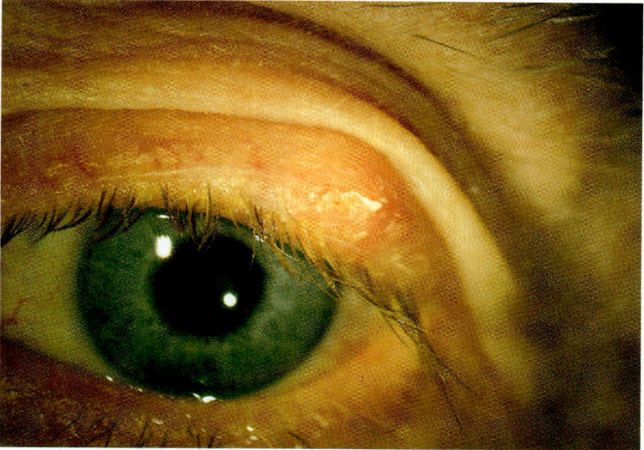

Figure 1.41 Meibomian gland cyst in the upper eyelid (chalazion). Chronic granulomatous inflammation caused by build-up of secretions. Treatment: excision.

Figure 1.42 Retention cyst of a gland of Moll in the lower eyelid (apocrine gland with transparent secretion).

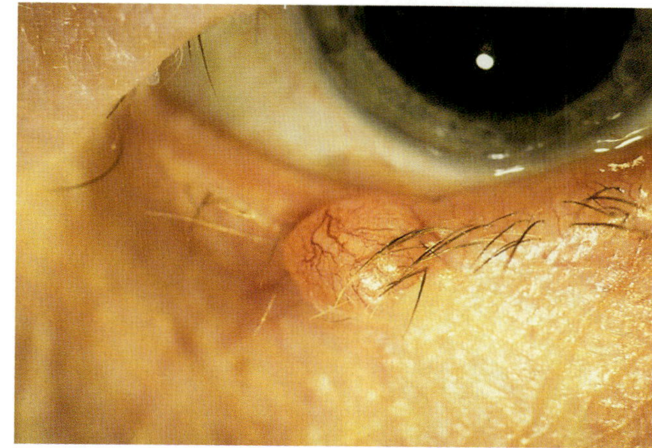

Figure 1.43 Retention cyst of a gland of Zeis in the medial portion of the lower eyelid (sebaceous gland with intransparent secretion).

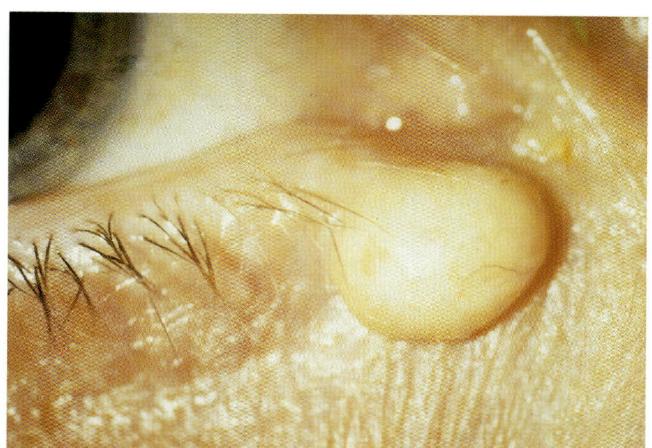

Figure 1.44 Retention cyst of a gland of Zeis with doughy content within the row of lashes of the lower eyelid.

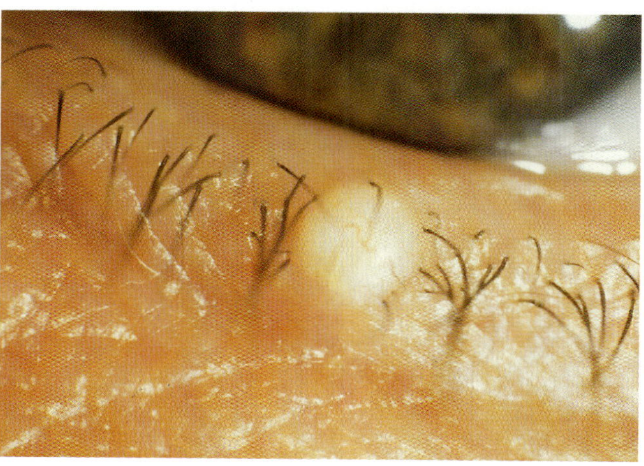

1.6 Disorders of the eyelid glands

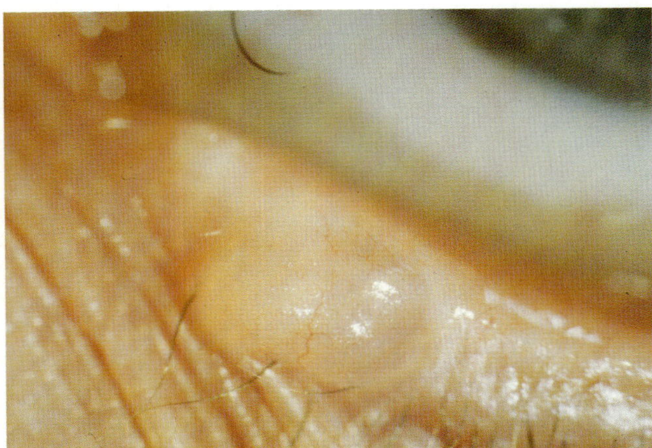

Figure 1.45 Retention cyst of a gland of Moll in the lower eyelid with intransparent content.

Figure 1.46   Xanthelasmas in the upper eyelids and medial canthus. The lesions respresent depositions of lipid. Levels of plasma cholesterol should be checked and diabetes mellitus ruled out.

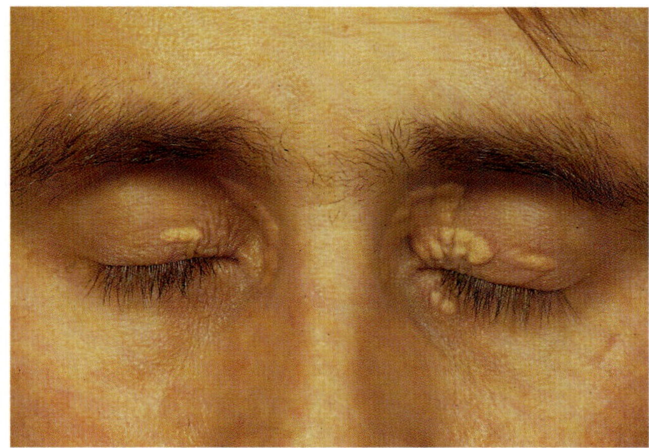

Figure 1.47   Dermoid cyst in the lateral upper eyelid in an infant. Benign tumor with sebum-like content as well as epidermal tissue. Slow growth. Treatment consists of complete excision.

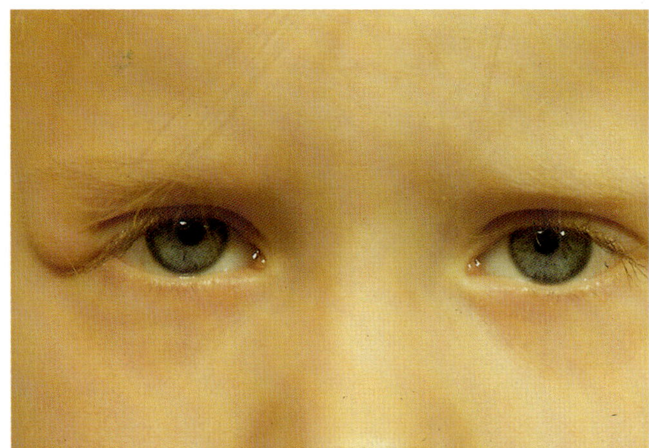

Figure 1.48   Seborrheic keratosis in the lower eyelid.

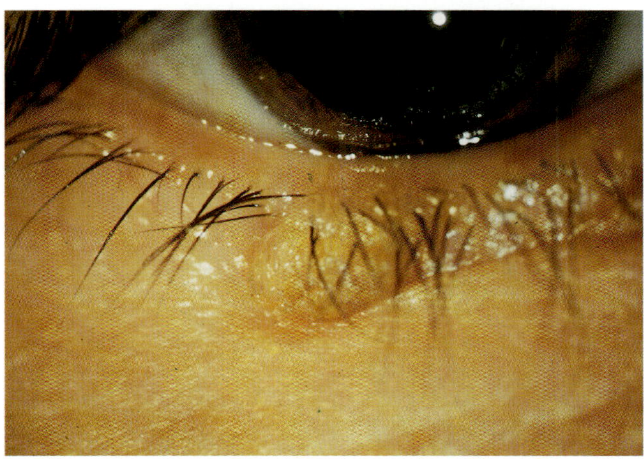

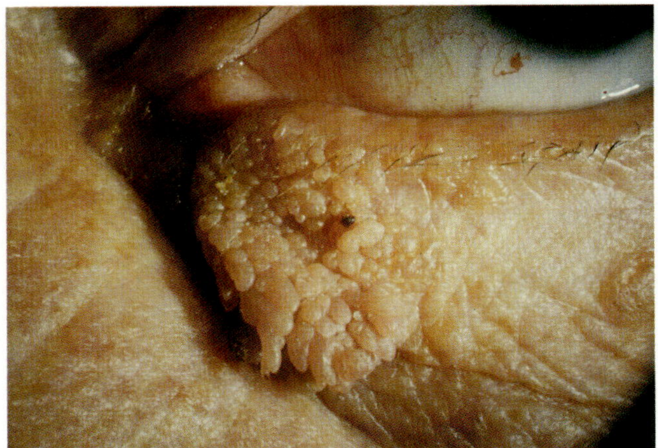

Figure 1.49 Seborrheic keratosis, large lesion in the medial lower eyelid in a 74 year-old patient.

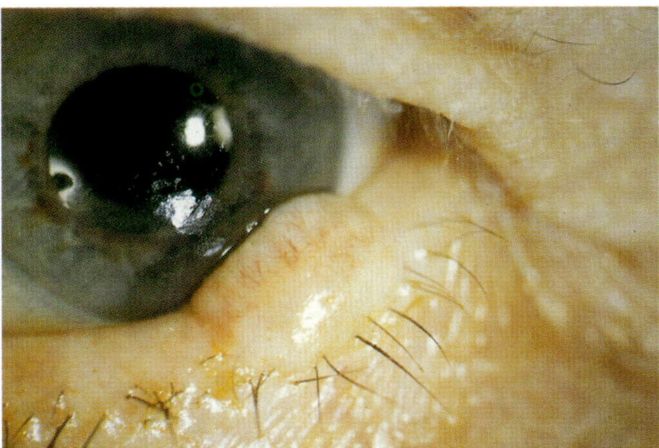

Figure 1.50 Papilloma in the lower eyelid margin of a 60 year-old patient.

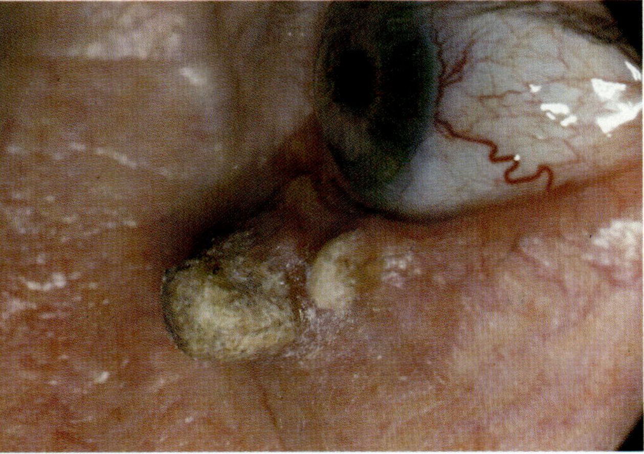

Figure 1.51 Cornu cutaneum (cutaneous horn) in the lower eyelid of an older patient. The lesion represents an extreme hyperkeratosis.

Figure 1.52 Cavernous hemangioma in the lower eyelid and lateral canthus of the right eye in an infant. Spontaneous resolution is possible. Surgical removal only if amblyopia is to be prevented.

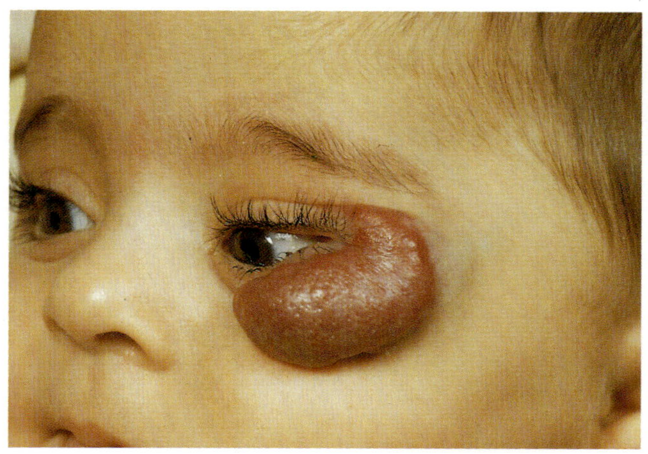

Figure 1.53 Large periocular hemangioma following the first division of the left trigeminal nerve in a 60 year-old patient with Sturge-Weber syndrome.

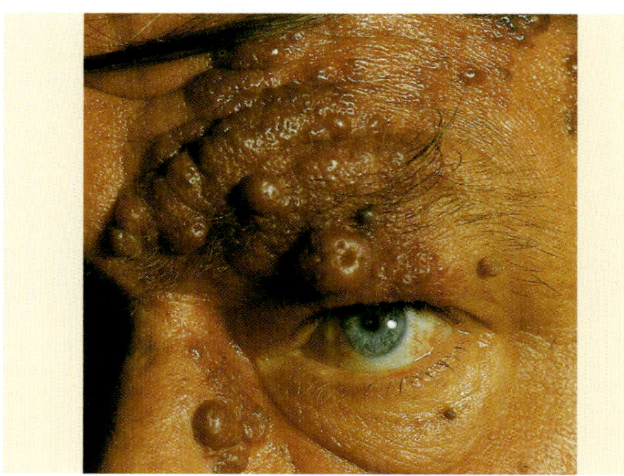

Figure 1.54 Nevus in the lower eyelid of a juvenile.

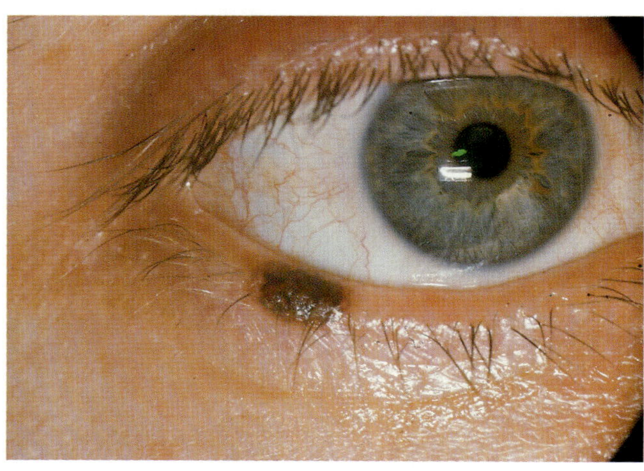

1.7 Benign eyelid tumors

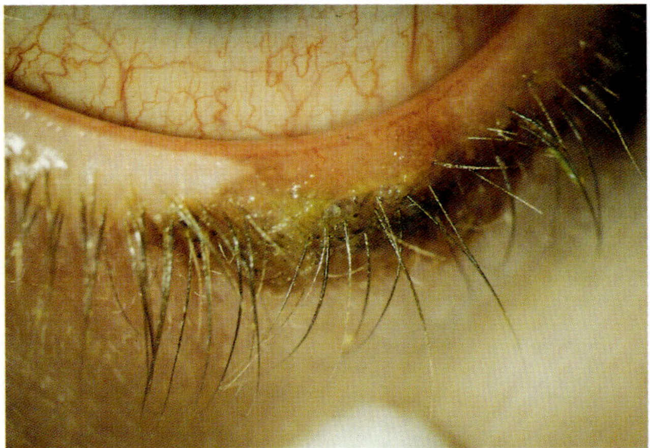

Figure 1.55 Nevus in the lower eyelid margin, including the row of lashes of a 50 year-old patient. The lesion is suspect of melanoma.

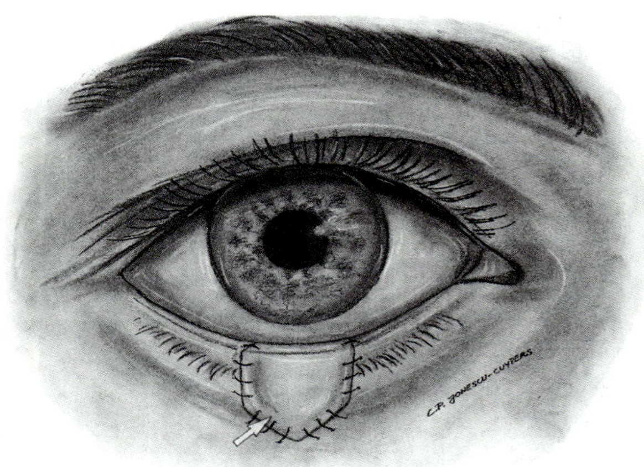

Figure 1.56 Schema of the surgical approach used for the resection of the lesion shown in figure 1.55 with broad excision of the lower eyelid and closure of the resulting defect with an eyelid graft taken from the contralateral eye. Tarsal, muscle and skin sutures are applied for the insertion of the full-thickness graft.

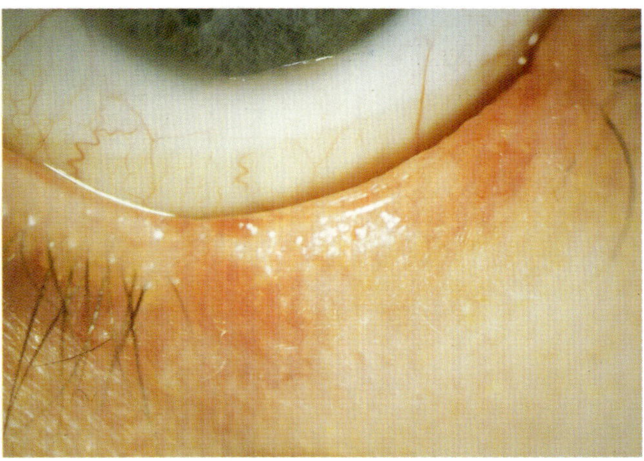

Figure 1.57 Same patient as in figure 1.55 three months after resection of the pigmented skin tumor and defect closure with a full-thickness eyelid graft from the contralateral eye. The graft has healed, however, the row of lashes could not be preserved.

Figure 1.58 Nodular basal cell carcinoma in the lower eyelid of an older patient. Basal cell carcinoma is the most frequent malignant tumor of the eyelids.

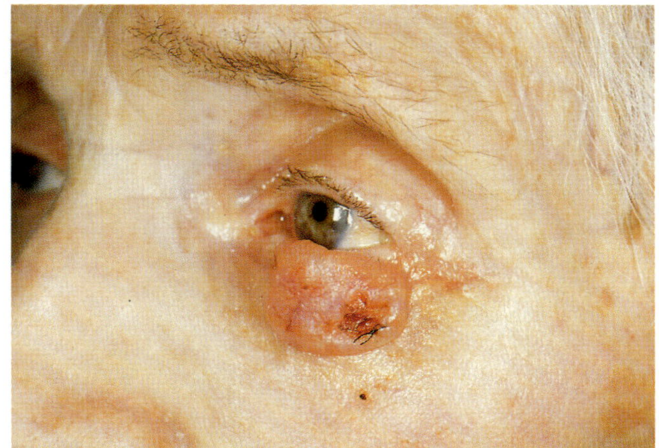

Figure 1.59 Nodular basal cell carcinoma in the medial canthus. The rolled borders are an important diagnostic feature.

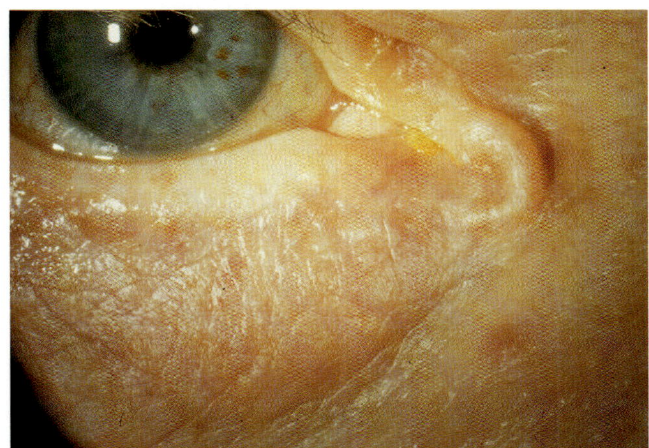

Figure 1.60 Nodular basal cell carcinoma in the lower eyelid margin with central ulceration and notching of the eyelid margin.

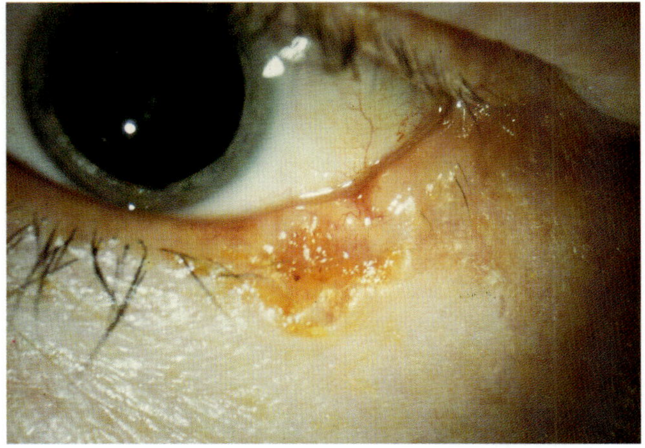

1.8 Malignant eyelid tumors

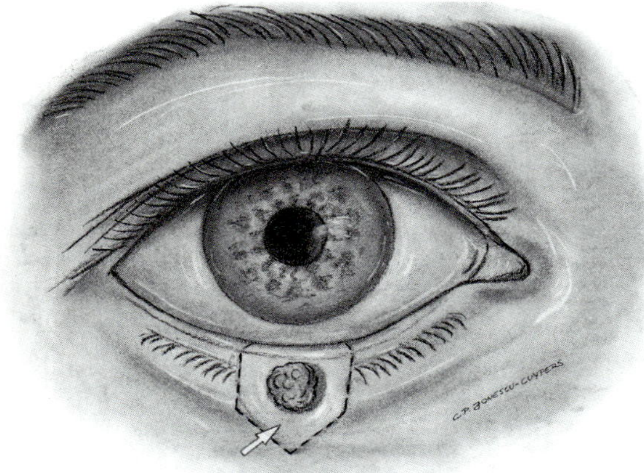

Figure 1.61 Schema of the surgical excision of a tumor in the lower eyelid margin. Rhomboid excision of the tumor with defined margin of clinically normal tissue *(white arrow)*. Lamellar or full-thickness resection of the eyelid depending on the clinical aspect.

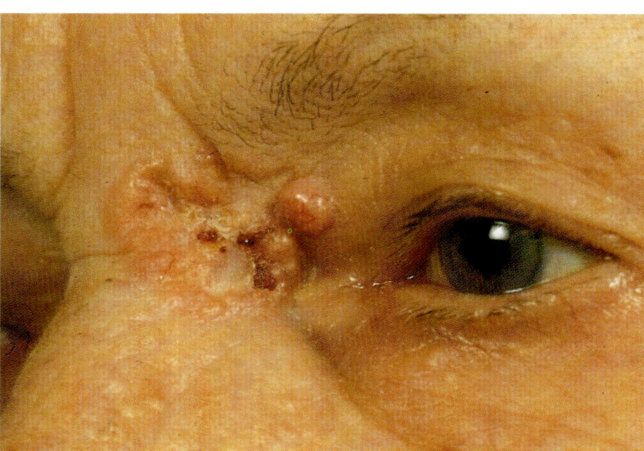

Figure 1.62 Large basal cell carcinoma in the medial canthus and nose bridge of a 68 year-old patient.

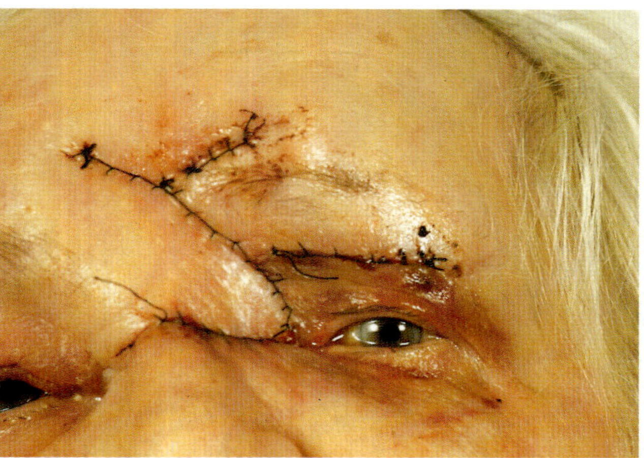

Figure 1.63 Same patient as in figure 1.62 on the second postoperative day following excision of the tumor in the medial canthus and nose brige and defect closure with a rotation flap sutured in place using 6-0 silk.

Figure 1.64 Schema of the surgical approach used for closure of a skin defect resulting from the excision of a basal cell carcinoma in the medial canthus of the right eye. *Top* excision site and dimensions of rotation flap. *Bottom* closure of skin defect in the medial canthus with a rotation flap.

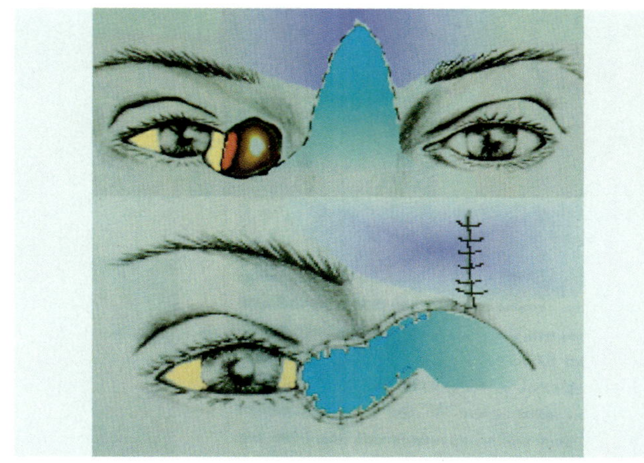

Figure 1.65 Excision of a tumor in lower eyelid and closure of the resulting skin defect with a rotation flap. *Left* excision site of the tumor inferiorly to the medial canthus and two triangular skin excisions for the creation of a rotational flap. *Right* partial rotation of the skin flap.

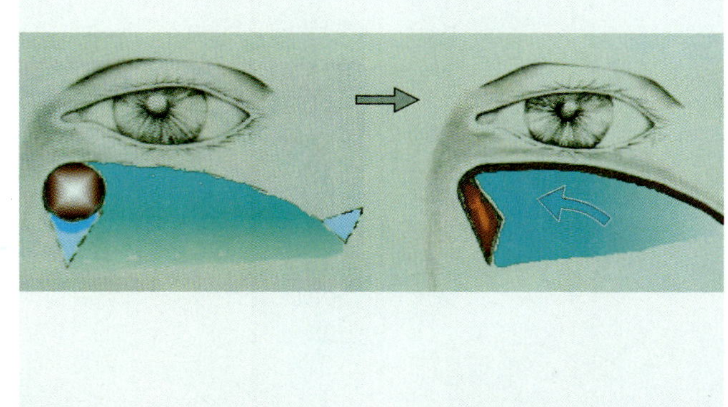

Figure 1.66 Squamous cell carcinoma in the lower eyelid. Unlike basal cell carcinoma, squamous cell carcinoma may metastasize.

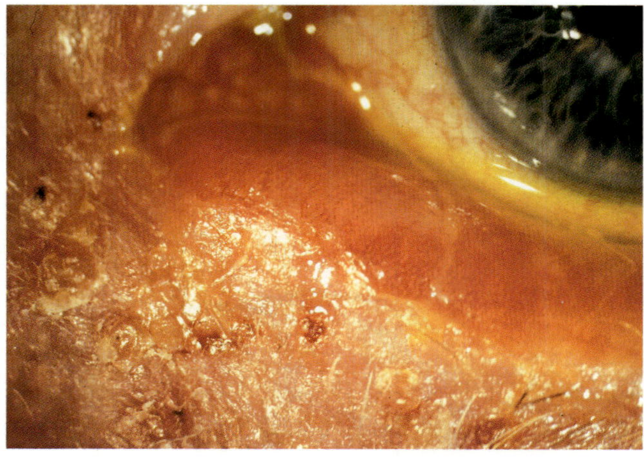

1.8 Malignant eyelid tumors

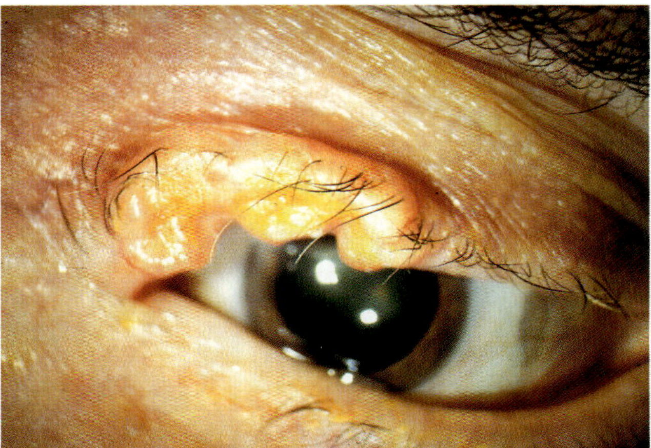

Figure 1.67 Sebaceous gland carcinoma in the upper eyelid.

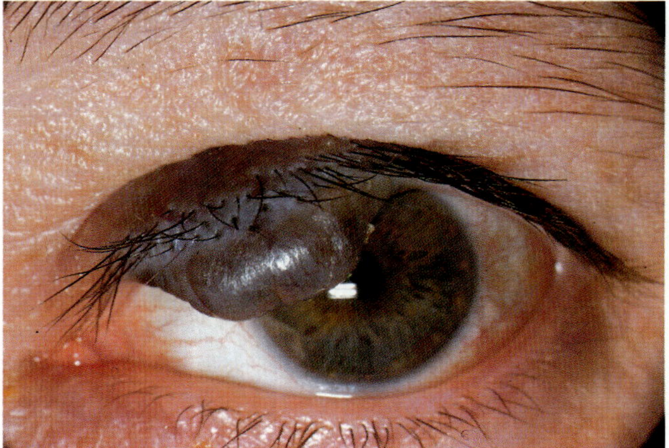

Figure 1.68 Mailgnant melanoma in the upper eyelid. Rare tumor, which may show a malignant course. Invasion of the surrounding tissue, early lymph node involvement and metastases.

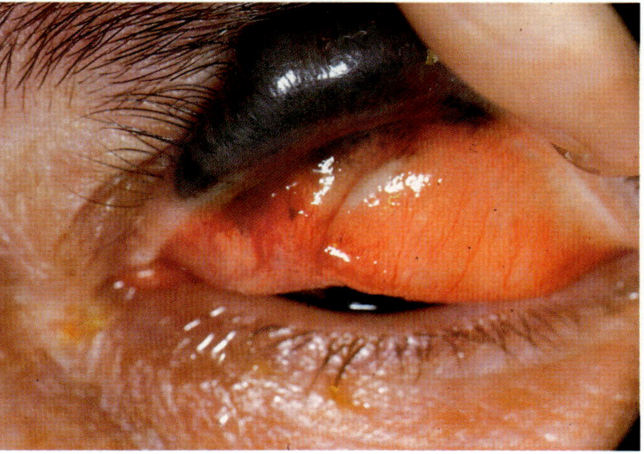

Figure 1.69 Same patient as in figure 1.68. The invasion of the tarsal conjunctiva by the malignant melanoma becomes visible after eversion of the upper eyelid.

Figure 1.70   Kaposi´s sarcoma in the upper eyelid of a 40 year-old patient with HIV infection. The oblong purple skin tumor is located in the upper eyelid crease. The skin at the temple shows additional lesions. The vascular tumor can affect various tissues, it is mostly found in association with HIV infection.

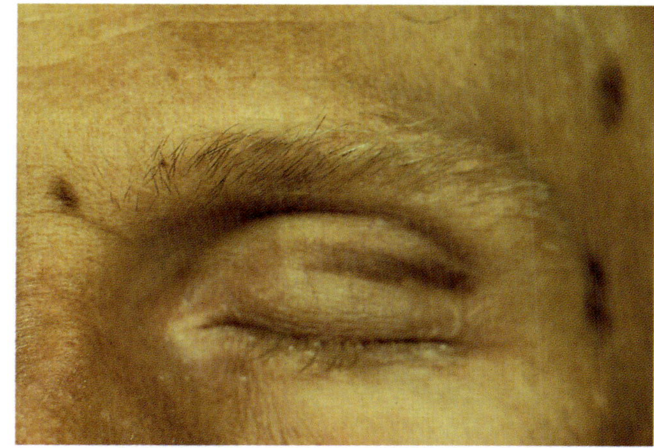

Figure 1.71   Periocular involvement in T-cell lymphoma in a 68 year-old patient. The right upper eyelid is affected by the tumor as well as the contralateral cheek.

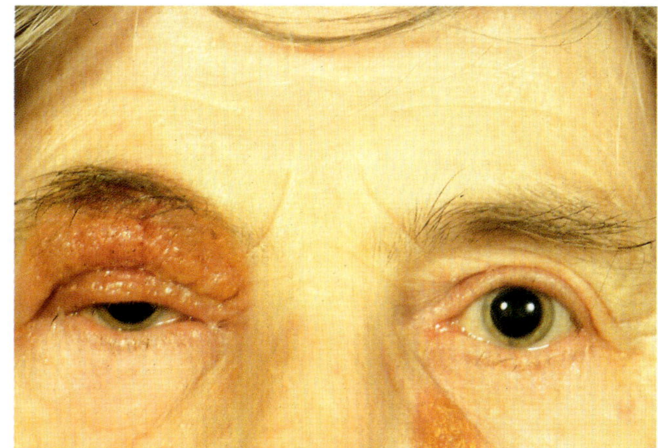

Lacrimal system

2.1 Applied anatomy and examination techniques

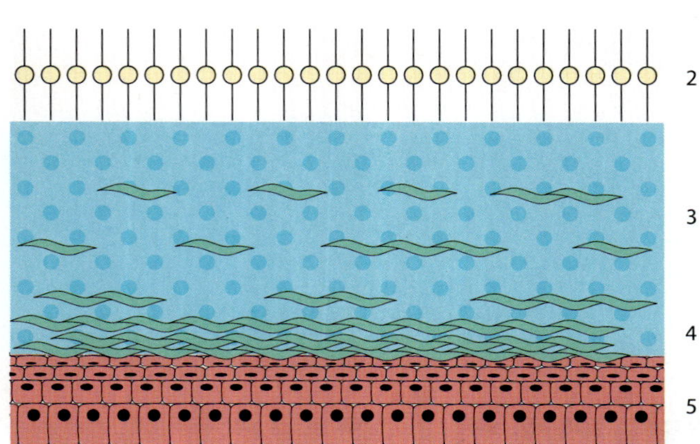

Figure 2.1 Schema of the composition of the precorneal tear film. (1) air; (2) superficial oily layer, interface to air; (3) aqueous layer with diluted mucin; (4) mucoid layer; (5) corneal epithelium. The superficial oily layer is produced by the meibomian glands. It prevents evaporation of the underlying aqueous layer. The aqueous layer is produced by the main lacrimal gland and the accessory lacrimal glands. The tear film contains antimicrobial substances and electrolytes. The mucoid layer connects the corneal epithelium with the aqueous layer.

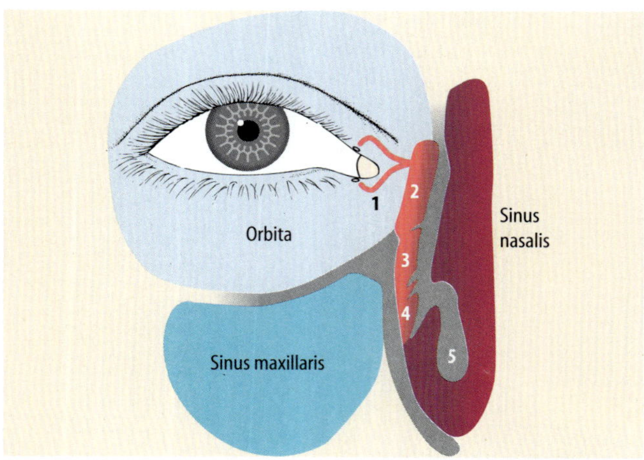

Figure 2.2 Schema of the lacrimal drainage sytem *(light red)* with the nasal sinus *(dark red)* and surrounding structures: (1) lacrimal canaliculi; (2) lacrimal sac; (3) nasolacrimal duct with valves of Krause, Hyrtl and Taillefer; (4) valve of Hasner at the end of the nasolacrimal duct; (5) inferior turbinate (concha nasalis inferior).

Figure 2.3 Inspection of the palpebral portion of the lacrimal gland. Underneath the everted upper eyelid the palpebral portion of the lacrimal gland can be herniated into view.

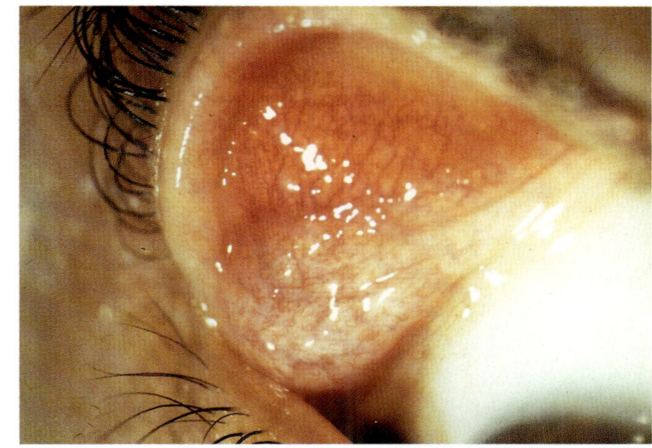

Figure 2.4 Schirmer´s test: two special filter paper strips are inserted in the lower fornix and the amount of wetting is measured. A result of less than 1 mm/minute is considered pathologic.

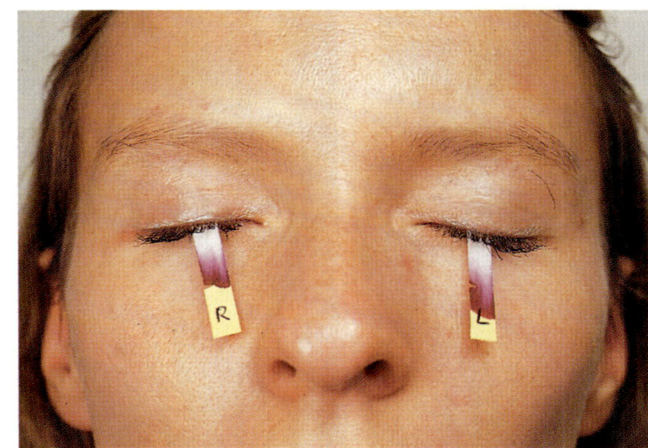

Figure 2.5 Rose bengal staining: rose bengal dye stains devitalized epithelial cells and mucus in the temporal inferior palpebral fissure.

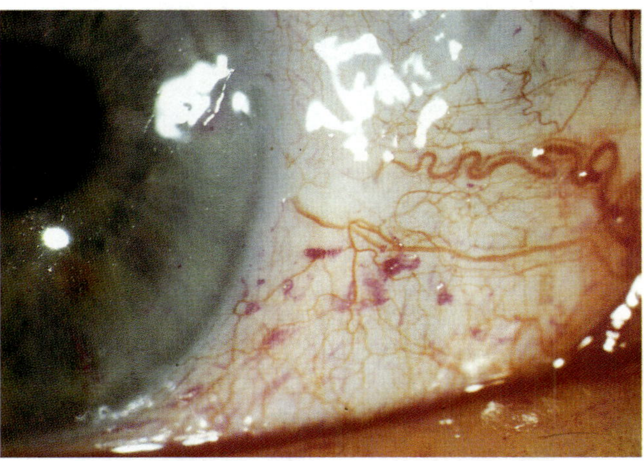

2.1 Applied anatomy and examination techniques

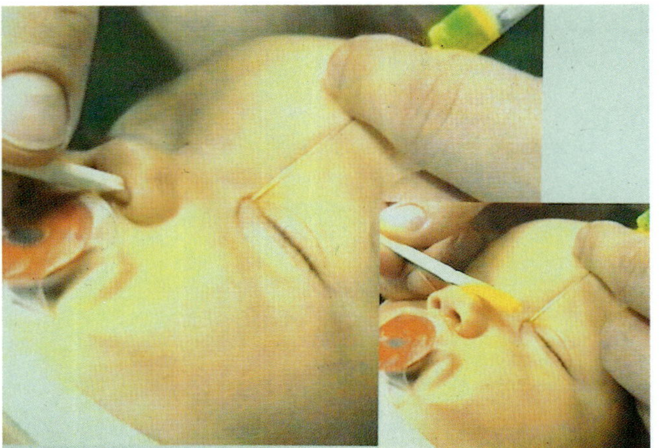

Figure 2.6 Irrigation of the lacrimal drainage system in an infant: a straight lacrimal cannula is inserted into the nasolacrimal duct via the inferior punctum, the inferior canaliculus and the lacrimal sac. The irrigation solution contains fluorescein dye. A cotton swab is placed under the inferior nasal turbinate in order to absorb the irrigation solution. If the drainage system is patent, fluorescein dye is recovered from the nose *(bottom right)*.

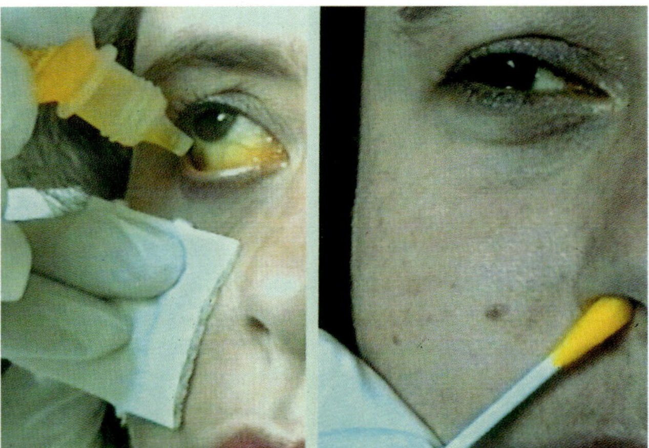

Figure 2.7 Fluorescein dye test: fluoresein drops are instilled into the conjunctival sac *(left)*, if the drainage system is patent, the puncta are in normal position and the lacrimal pump mechanism is intact, the fluorescein dye can be recovered from the nose a few seconds later *(right)*.

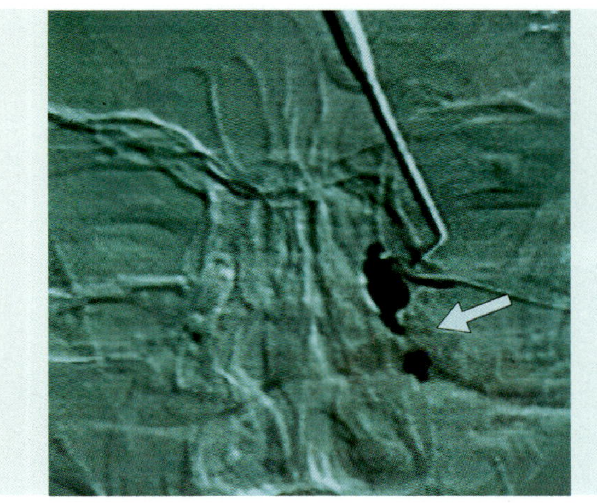

Figure 2.8 Digital subtraction dacryocystography: an angulated lacrimal cannula is inserted into the inferior canaliculus via the inferior punctum. The lacrimal sac is filled with contrast medium *(appears black)*. With increased irrigation pressure the dye passes to the nasolacrimal duct indicating an infrasaccal stenosis.

Figure 2.9   Dacryocystogram, x-ray of the lacrimal sac and naso-lacrimal duct with contrast dye. The upper punctum is blocked with a conical probe. The contrast dye has been injected through the inferior canaliculus. Filling of the lacrimal sac and partial filling of the nasolacrimal duct can be seen. The passage to the nose is blocked.

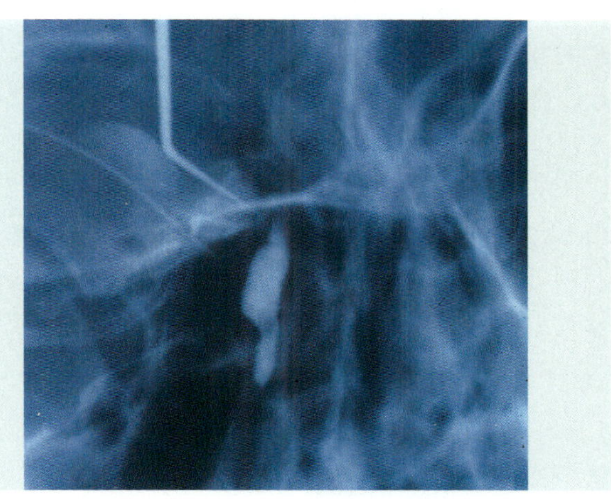

2 Lacrimal system

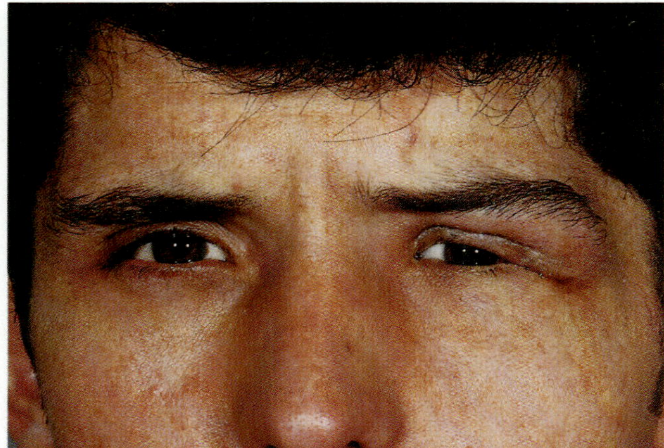

Figure 2.10 Acute dacryoadenitis: superior lateral eyelid swelling with "S"-shaped curve of the upper eyelid margin. The condition can result from bacterial and viral infections. In children, an association with mumps, measels or infectious mononucleosis may exist. Complications are rare.

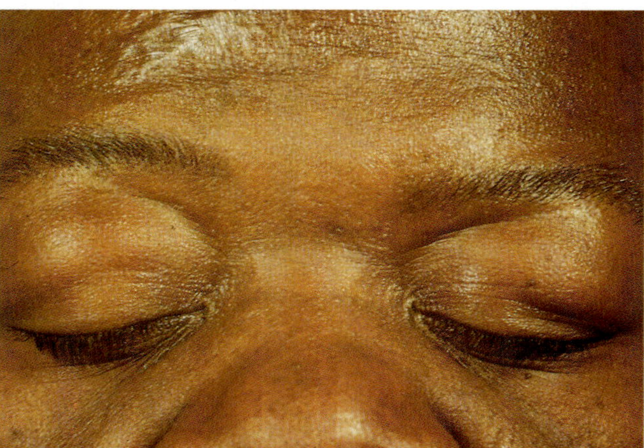

Figure 2.11 Chronic dacryoadenitis: bilateral non-tender superior lateral eyelid swelling in sarcoidosis. Systemic disease, such as tuberculosis, lues, leukaemia and lymphogranulomatosis need to be ruled out.

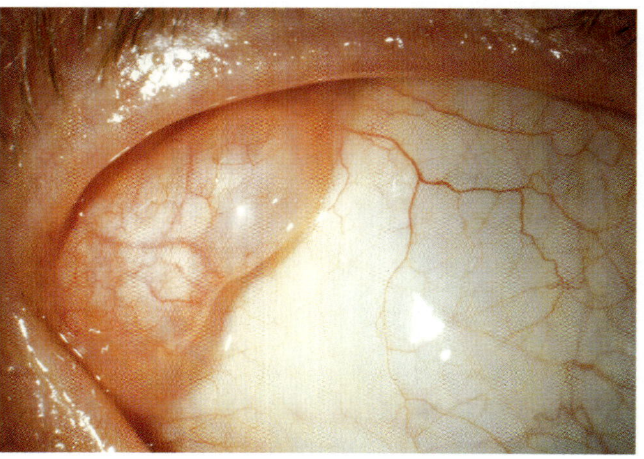

Figure 2.12 Tumor of the lacrimal gland: solid, partly cystic enlargement of the palpebral lacrimal gland, which becomes visible upon retraction of the upper eyelid. Mixed-cell tumors are benign, treatment consists of complete surgical excision. Adenoid cystic carcinoma is a highly malignant neoplasm, orbital exenteration has to be considered.

Figure 2.13 Lacrimal gland tumor, appearance on CT. The axial CT shows an ill-defined lesion in the superior lateral aspect of the orbit *(square mark)* between the globe and the zygomatic bone. The globe is displaced nasally, the sclera is indented and cannot be clearly differentiated from the tumor.

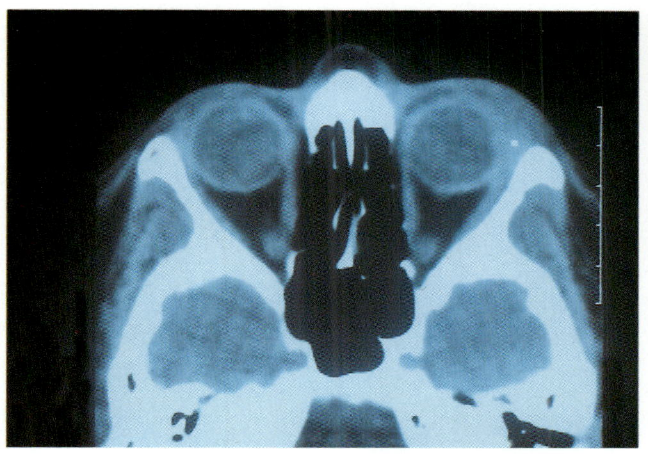

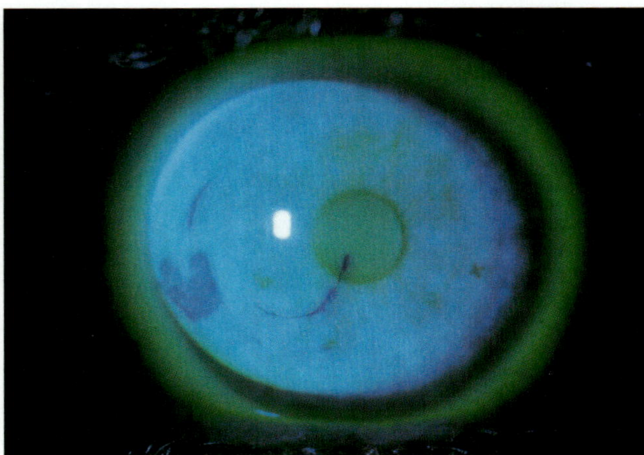

Figure 2.14 Tear film break-up: the *dark blue* regions (comma-shaped paracentrally, fleck at the limbus at 8 o'clock position) are holes in the precorneal tear film (fluorescein stained tear film in blue light). The appearance of such holes shortly after blinking indicates an instability of the tear film.

Figure 2.15   Chronic dacyostenosis in an infant: crusts on the eyelid margins result from dried tears with blockage of the nasolacrimal duct at the valve of Hasner.

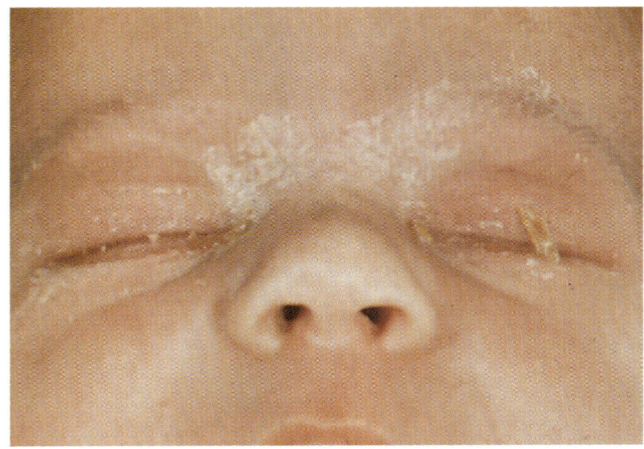

Figure 2.16   Trauma to the inferior canaliculus: the inferior canaliculus is lacerated between the punctum and the medial canthus.

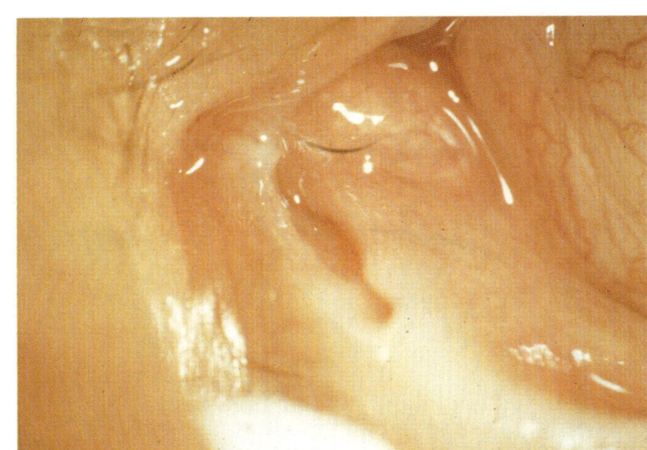

Figure 2.17   Intubation of the lacrimal canaliculi with a silicone tube serving as a bridge for lacerated canaliculi.

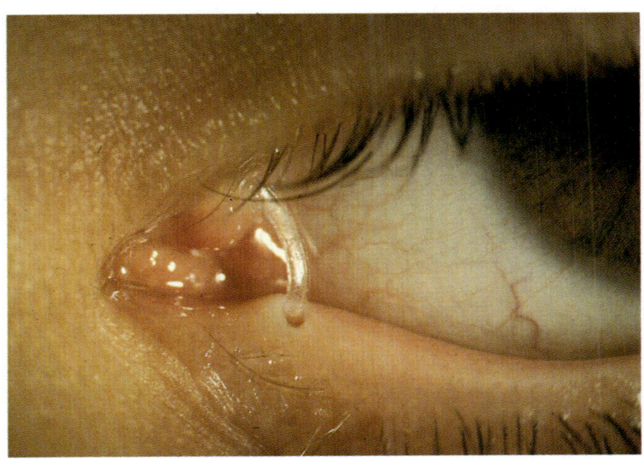

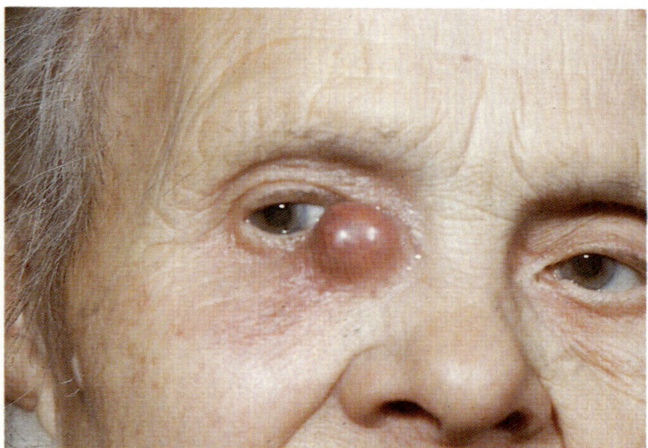

Figure 2.18 Acute dacryocystitis: the painful, fluctuant inflammatory tumor in the medial canthus corresponds to an empyema of the lacrimal sac. The condition is caused by a bacterial infection with stenosis of the nasolacrimal duct.

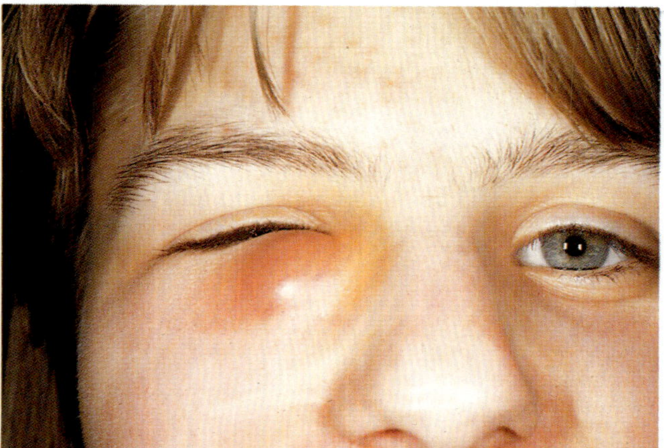

Figure 2.19 Acute dacryocystitis in a child. In contrast to the acute dacryocystitis in the older patient (figure 2.18) the surrounding tissue is markedly affected showing erythema and edema. Venous spreading of the infection can result in cavernous sinus thrombosis and sepsis.

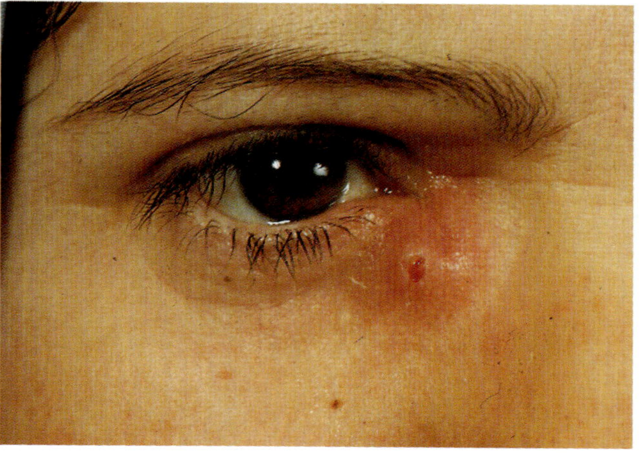

Figure 2.20 Acute dacryocystitis in an adult with spontaneous anterior dischargement. The perforation is located at the most elevated part of the inflammatory tumor. Surgical repair of the obstructed lacrimal drainage systems must include careful excision of the perforation in order to prevent the formation of a fistula.

Figure 2.21 Severe acute dacryocystitis spreading to the inferior eyelid. Systemic antibiotic treatment has to be started immediately in order to prevent complications. After the inflammation subsides, the underlying obstruction of the lacrimal drainage system must be surgically repaired.

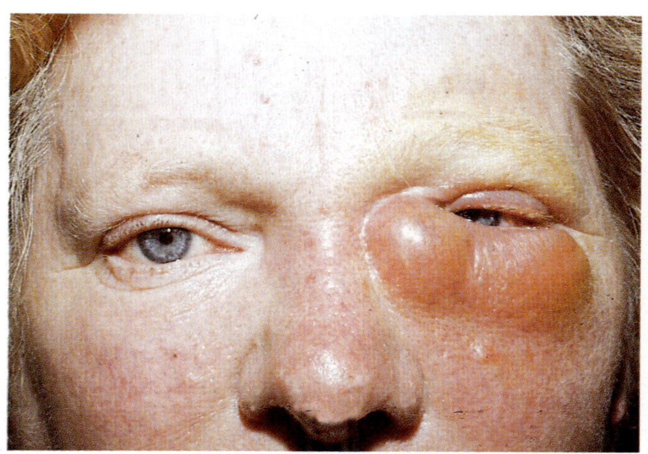

Figure 2.22 Technique of dacryocystorhinostomy (DCR). *Left frame:* top view, after exposure of the lacrimal sac (1) and trephination of the bone superiorly to the lacrimal crest, the nasal mucosa (2) becomes visible. The anterior portion of the lacrimal sac is opened, anterior and posterior flaps are created and anastomosed with the nasal mucosa. *Right frame:* cross-section, the created anastomosis between the opened lacrimal sac (1) and the nasal cavity (2).

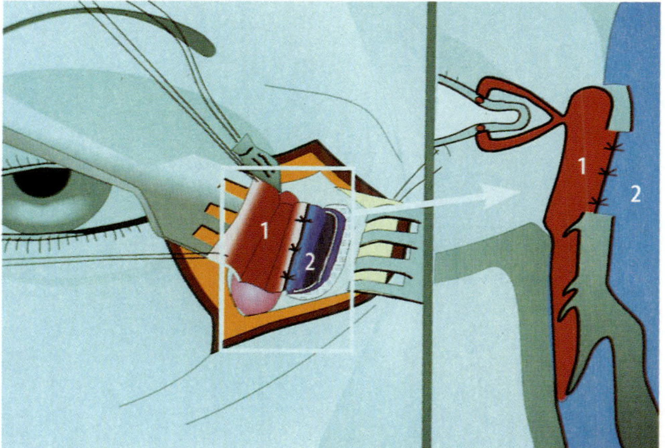

Conjunctiva

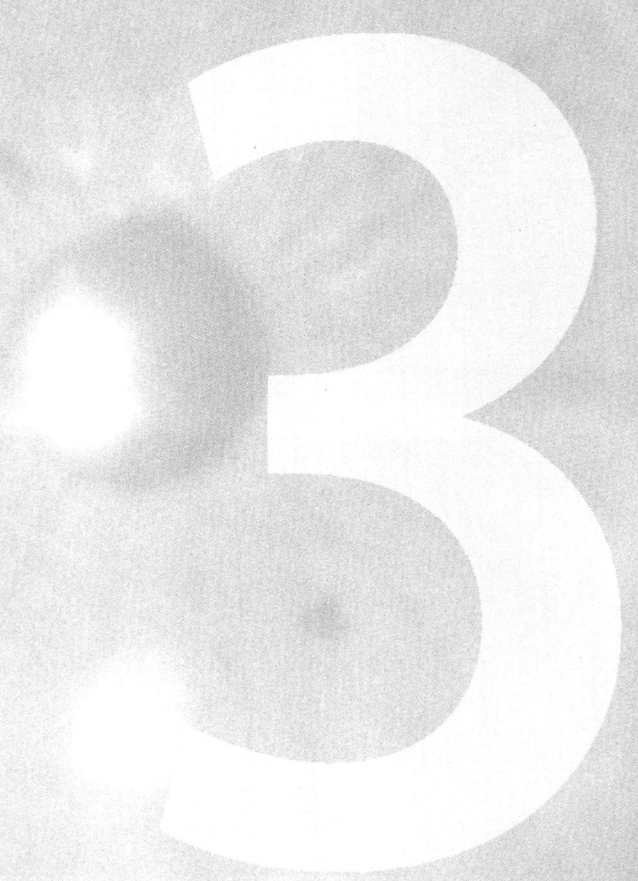

3.1 Applied anatomy, examination techniques and frequent findings

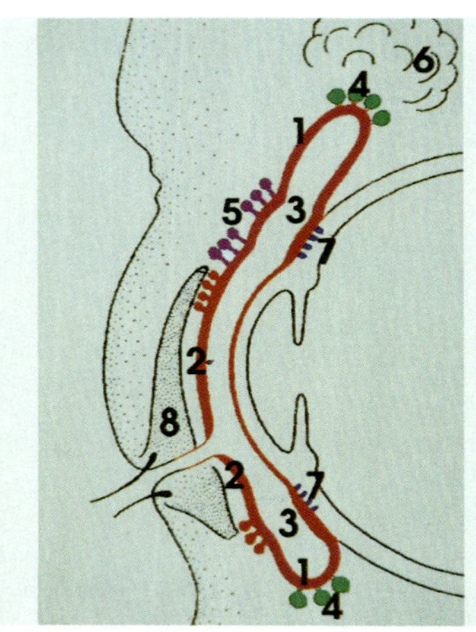

Figure 3.1 Schematic diagram of the topography of the conjunctiva and the adnexes: (1) inferior and superior fornix; (2) inferior and superior tarsal conjunctiva; (3) pseudoglands of Henle (crypt-like infoldings of the epithelium with goblet cells); (4) glands of Krause (accessory lacrimal glands); (5) glands of Wolfring (accessory lacrimal glands); (6) lacrimal gland; (7) glands of Manz; (8) superior tarsus.

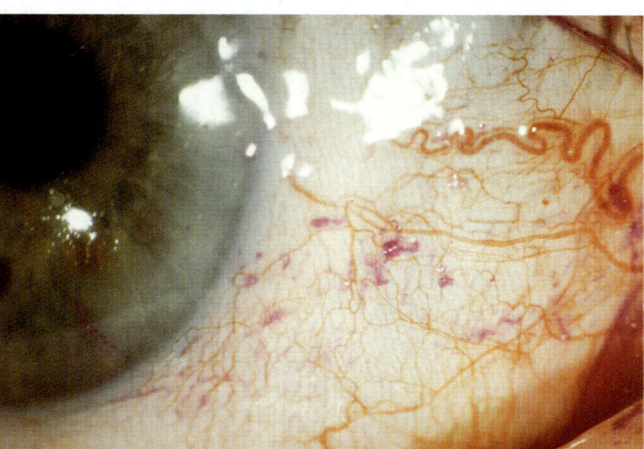

Figure 3.2 Staining of desquamated epithelial cells with rose bengal vital dye. Rose bengal dye stains devitalized epithelial cells as well as intact epithelial cells with lacking mucoid layer. Used for the diagnosis of keratoconjunctivitis sicca (dry eye syndrome).

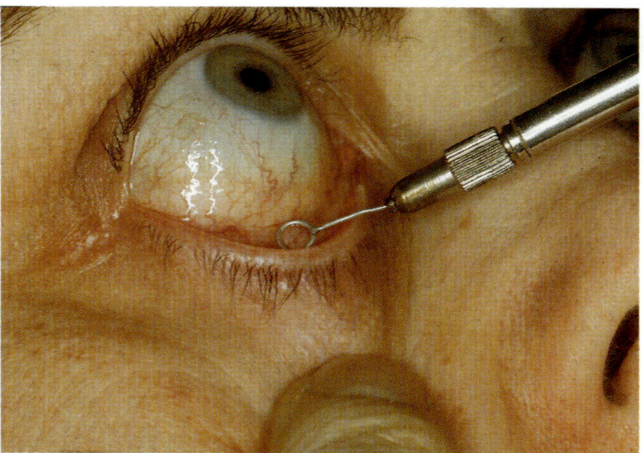

Figure 3.3 Conjunctival smear. A specimen, which is taken by stroking the conjunctival sac with a sterile platinum loop, is transferred to an agar plate for microbial culture and microbial sensitivity testing.

Figure 3.4 Bacteria in a conjunctival smear. In the light areas of the conjunctival smear (stained with methylene blue), the bacteria appear as small round and rod-shaped condensations (enlarged 250 fold).

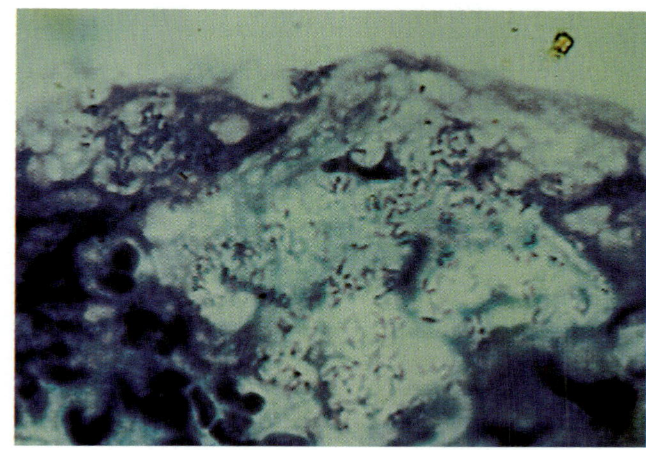

Figure 3.5 Detection of fungi in a conjunctival smear. The fungal mycelium becomes visible after staining of the smear.

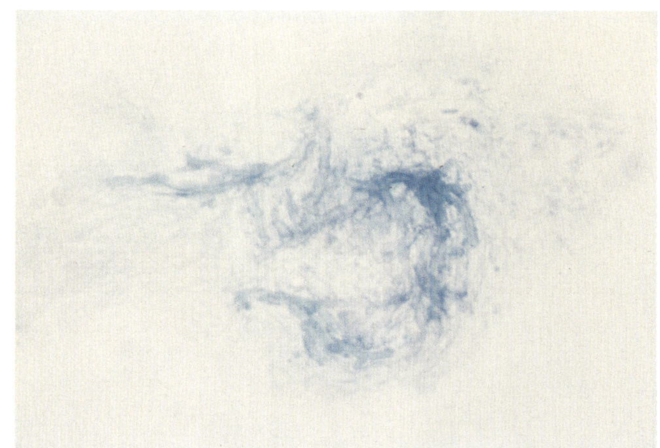

Figure 3.6 Leucocytes in a conjunctival smear (Giemsa stain, enlarged 250 fold).

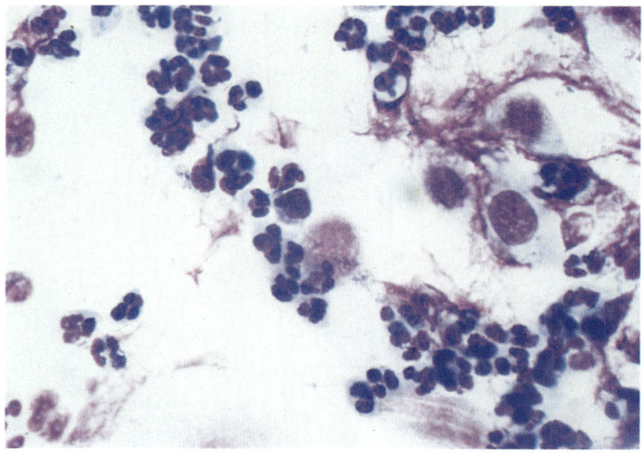

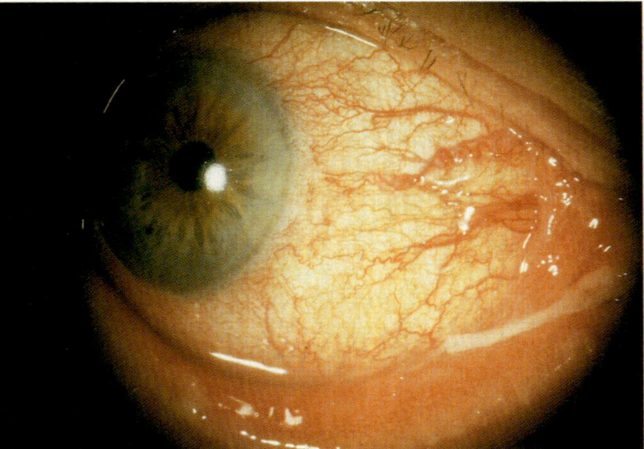

Figure 3.7 Conjuntivitis with mucopurulent discharge in the inferior fornix. Hyperemia of the bulbar and tarsal conjunctiva.

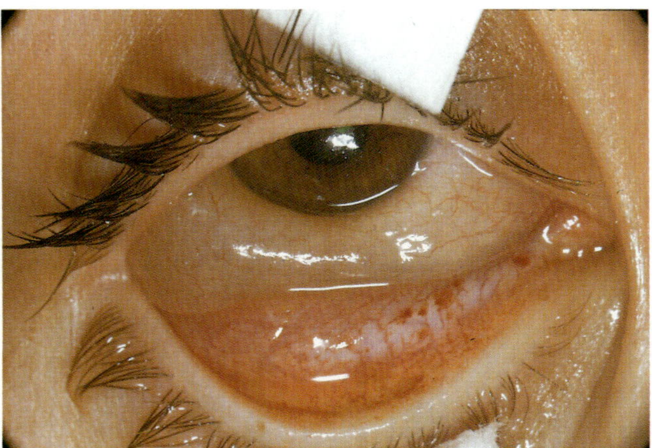

Figure 3.8 Conjunctival chemosis. Marked chemosis occurs in allergic reactions and due to mechanical obstruction to drainage.

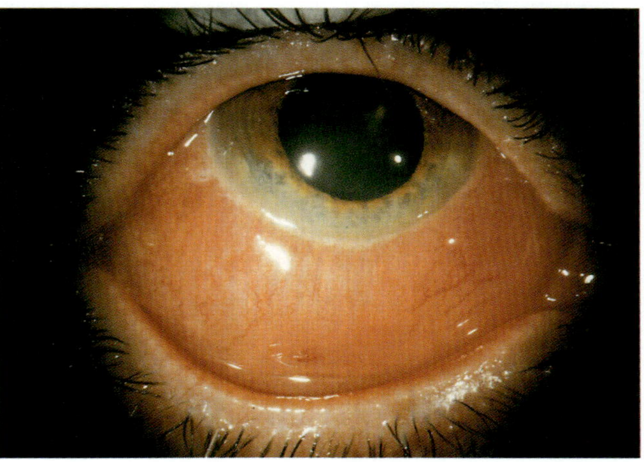

Figure 3.9 Chemosis of the bulbar conjunctiva with hyperemia. The conjunctiva shows edematous swelling (chemosis) and marked hyperemia. The combination of chemosis and hyperemia indicates an inflamatory process.

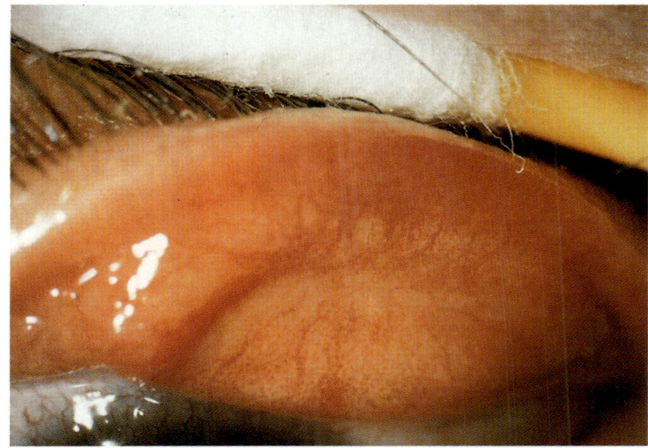

Figure 3.10 Conjunctivitis of the tarsal conjunctiva, view after eversion of the upper eyelid. The tarsal conjunctiva is injected and edematous.

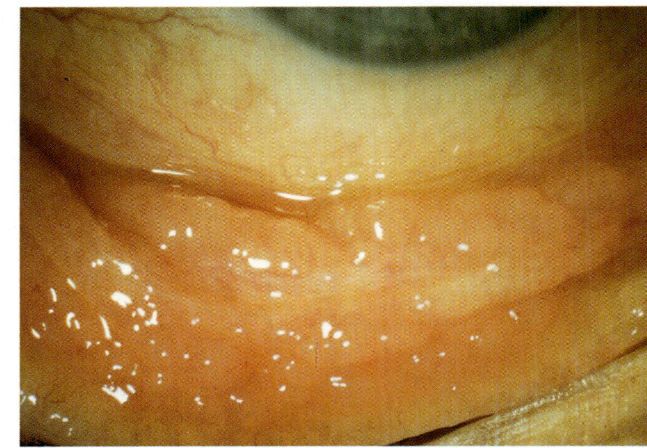

Figure 3.11 Follicular conjunctival reaction in the inferior fornix. The inferior conjunctival fornix shows massive hypertrophy of lymphatic tissue, so-called conjunctival follicles, which are characteristic for allergic and viral conjunctivitis.

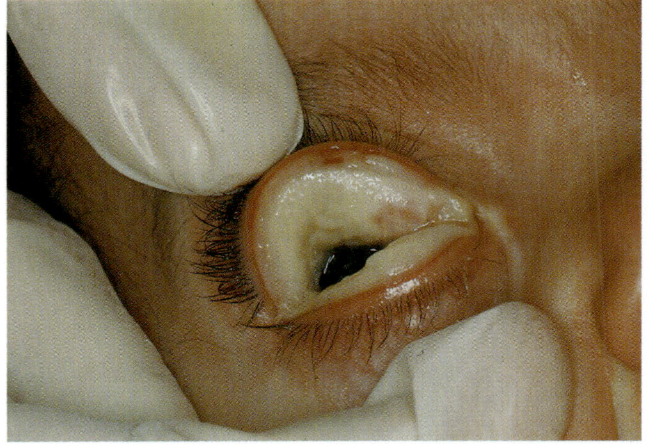

Figure 3.12 Membranous conjunctivitis in an infant. Upon eversion of the upper and lower eyelid, the tarsal conjunctiva shows an apposition of whitish membranes. Pseudomembranes (easily removable without tissue damage) can form in conjunctivitis of various origins. "True" membranes (firmly attached to the underlying conjunctiva) form in severe inflammations, such as diphteria and gonococcal conjunctivitis.

3.1 Applied anatomy, examination techniques and frequent findings

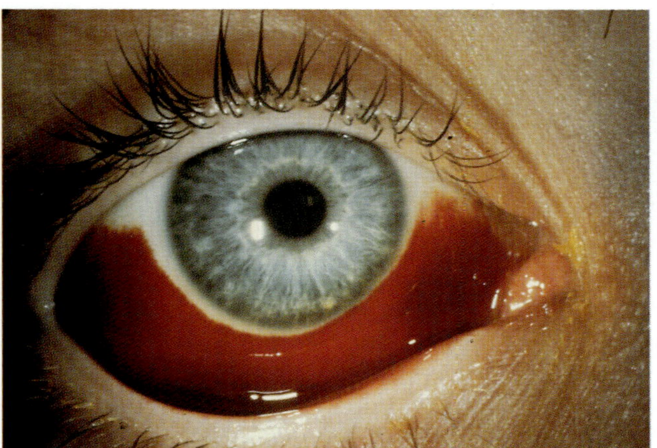

Figure 3.13 Subconjunctival hemorrhage. The figure shows an extensive subconjunctival hemorrhage. The condition can be associated with trauma or systemic disorders, such as diabetes mellitus, hypertension and coagulopathies. Spontaneous resorption occurs.

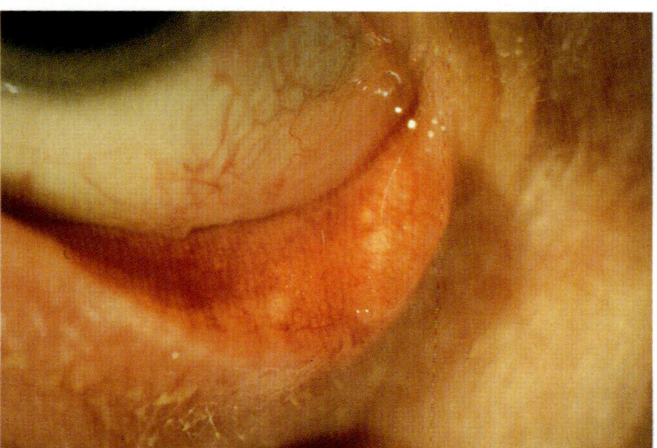

Figure 3.14 Inspissated meibomian glands in the tarsal conjunctiva. Inadequate secretion leads to inspissation and calcification of the meibomian glands, appearing as elevated inclusions of the tarsal conjunctiva associated with hyperaemia.

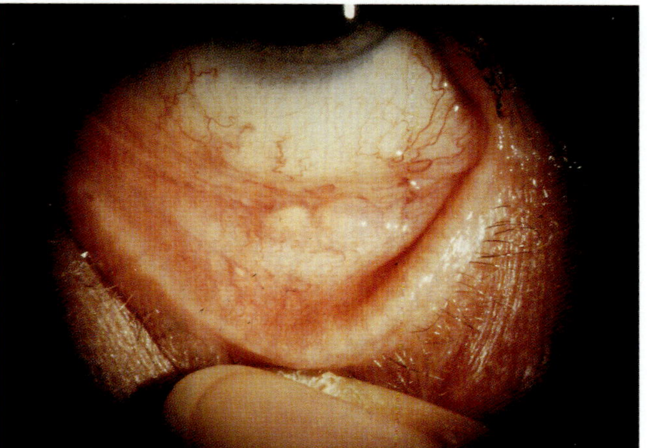

Figure 3.15 Conjunctival cysts in the inferior fornix.

Figure 3.16 Conjunctival cysts at the limbus.

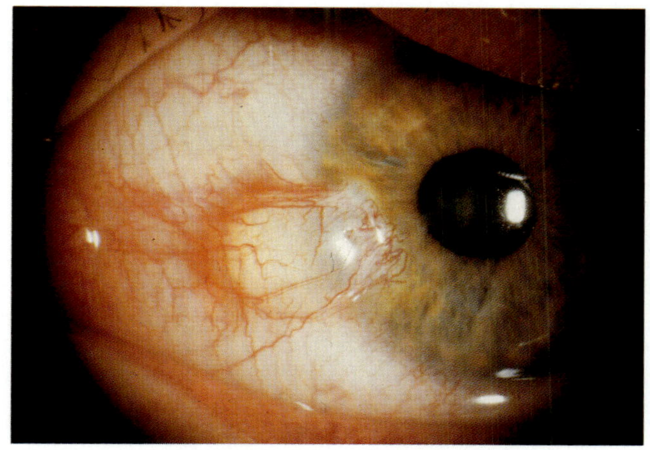

Figure 3.17 Trachoma, stage II. Follicles of the tarsal conjunctiva and incipient scarring.

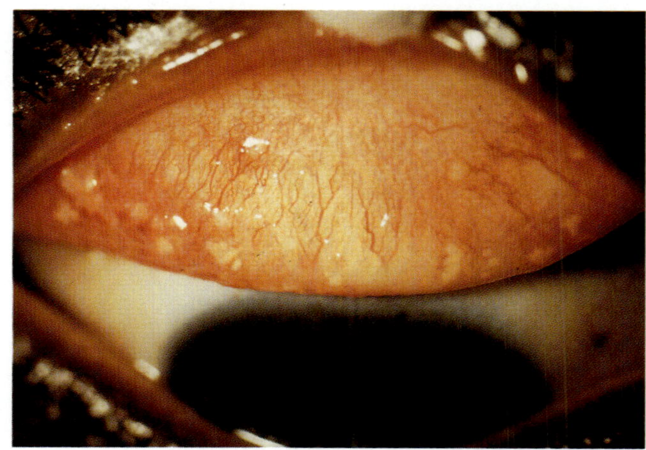

Figure 3.18 Sludge phenomenon in conjunctival vessels. There is a visible granularity to the blood-column, which is caused by an increased bood-viscosity. A medical examinaton should be conducted.

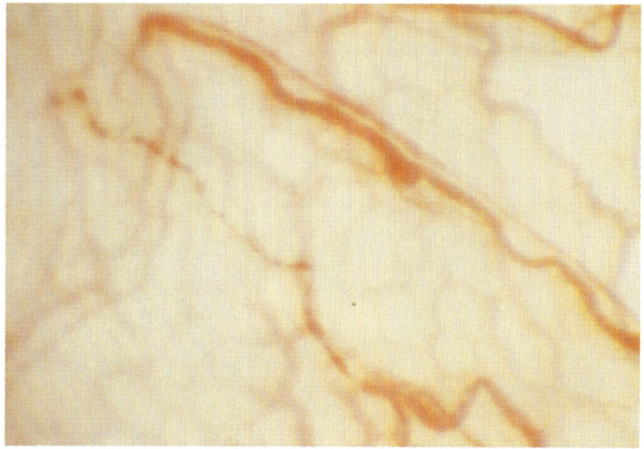

3.2 Degenerative changes of the conjunctiva

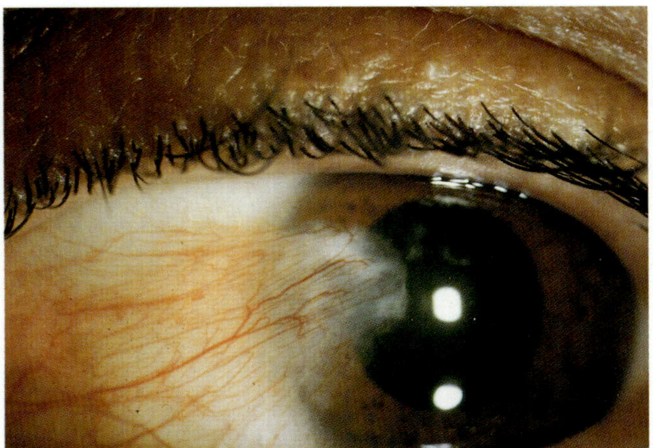

Figure 3.19 Pterygium in the nasal aspect of the palpebral fissure of the right eye. The conjunctiva has grown horizontally over the limbus and invaded the cornea, the so-called apex extends as far as 3 mm centrally to the limbus. Pterygium is a degenerative lesion of unknown etiology, characterized by growth towards the center of the cornea.

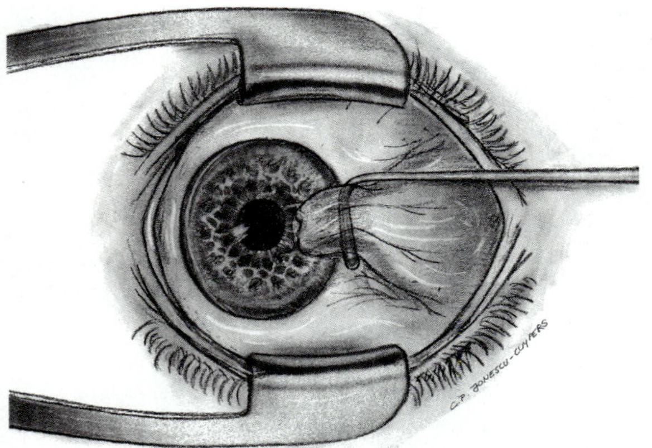

Figure 3.20 Surgical technique for removal of a pterygium. The cap of the pterygium is prosected and undermined with a blunt instrument.

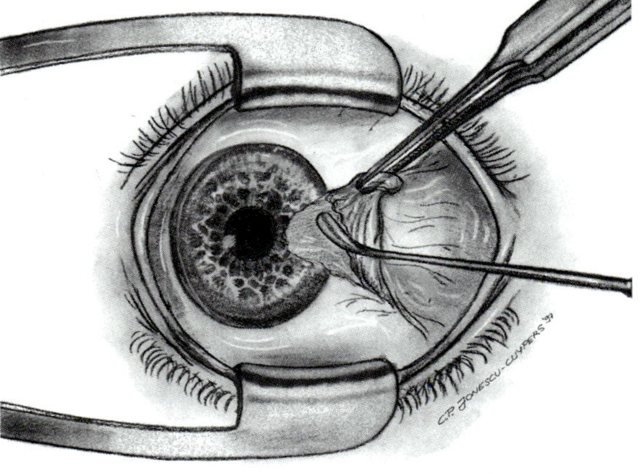

Figure 3.21 Sharp dissection of the apex from the cornea and removal of metaplastic epithelium with a scraping instrument. Excision of pterygium and affected conjunctiva. High risk of recurrence despite complete excision.

Figure 3.22 Recurrence of a pterygium on the nasal interpalpebral bulbar conjunctiva with broad apex, reaching almost to the center of the cornea. Complications: impaired vision, astigmatism, restricted motility.

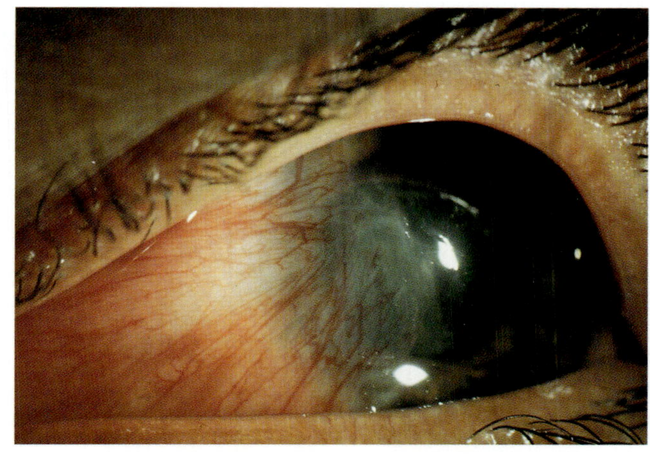

Figure 3.23 Status post surgical removal of the pterygium shown in figure 3.22 with lamellar keratoplasty. The pterygium was excised and the resulting corneal defect was filled with a lamellar corneal button sutured in place with interrupted 10-0 nylon.

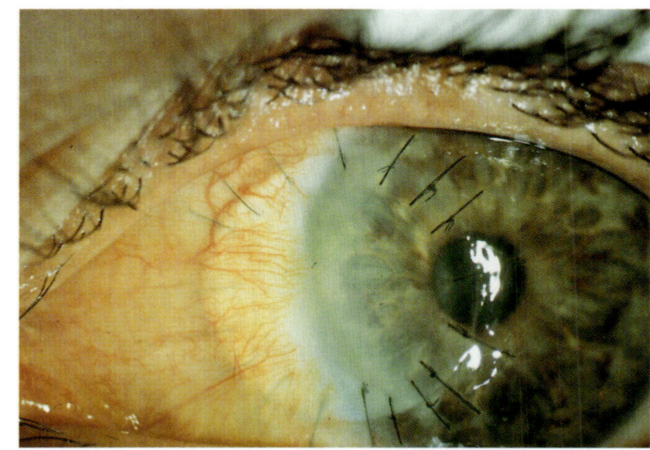

Figure 3.24 Pinguecula. Slight elevation of the conjunctiva caused by degenerative changes with inclusion of hyalin and occasionally lipid. The lesions are essentially harmless, treatment is not required.

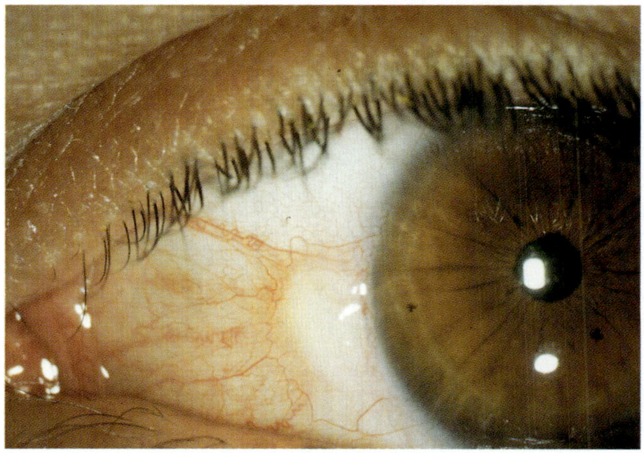

3.2 Degenerative changes of the conjunctiva

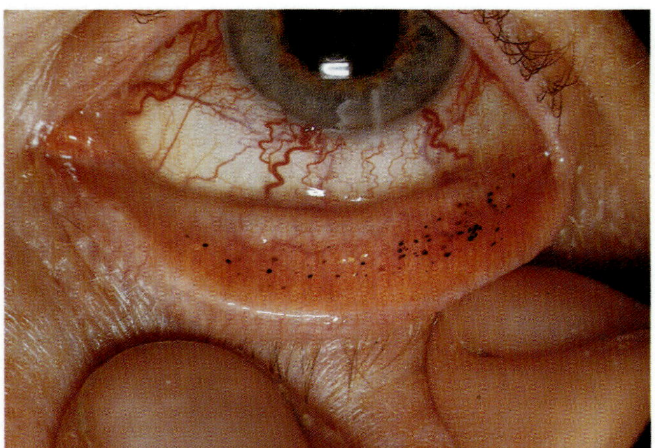

Figure 3.25 Pigmented deposits in the bulbar conjunctiva after longstanding epinephrine therapy. Epinephrine (topical medication to lower intraocular pressure in glaucoma) is oxidized to dark colored adrenochrome, which is deposited in the conjunctiva.

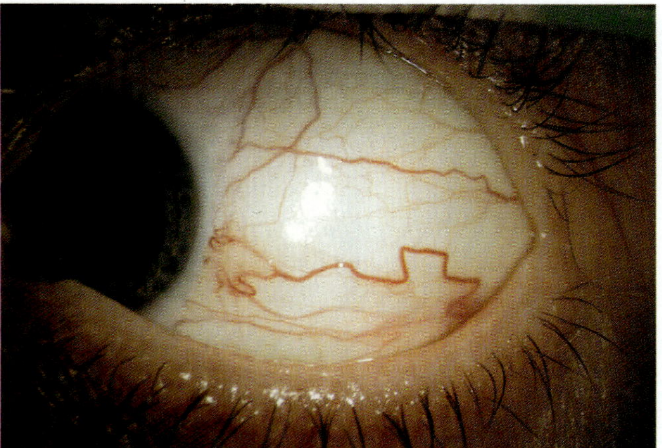

Figure 3.26 Idiopathic dilatation of the epibulbar conjunctival veins. The differential diagnosis includes orbital processes, arterio-venous fistulas, obstruction of venous drainage and phakomatoses, such as Sturge-Weber syndrome.

Figure 3.27 Gonococcal conjunctivitis in a newborn. Characteristic clinical presentation with severe eyelid edema and copious purulent discharge from the closed palpebral fissure. There is risk for the development of corneal perforation. If gonococcal conjunctivitis is suspected, antimicrobial therapy has to be initiated immediately.

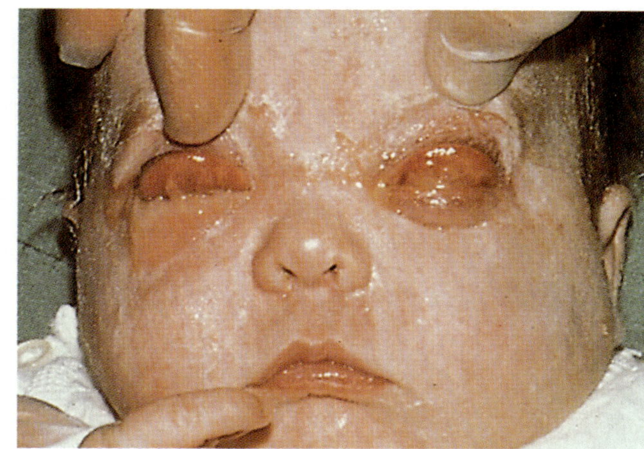

Figure 3.28 Membranous conjuncivitis caused by C. diphtheriae. The tarsal conjunctiva is covered by a whitish "true" conjunctival membrane. "True" conjunctival membranes occur also in gonococcal conjunctivitis. Removal of such membranes causes bleeding and pain.

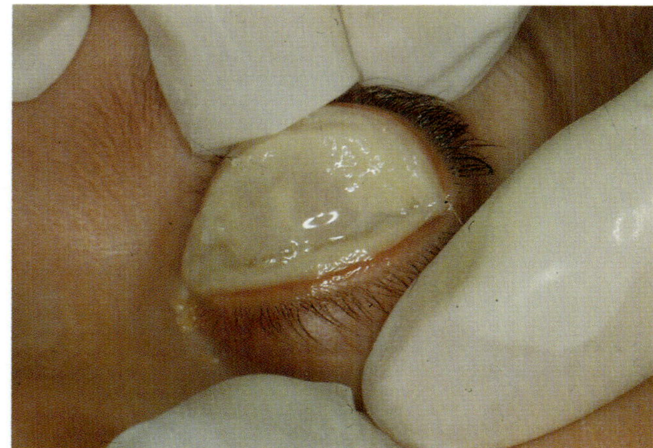

Figure 3.29 Epidemic keratoconjunctivitis (EKC), clinical picture with conjunctival hyperemia and muco-serous discharge. Highly contagious viral infection with adenovirus type 8 or 19. Associated with lymph node swelling. Risk of corneal involvement with development of subepithelial opacities.

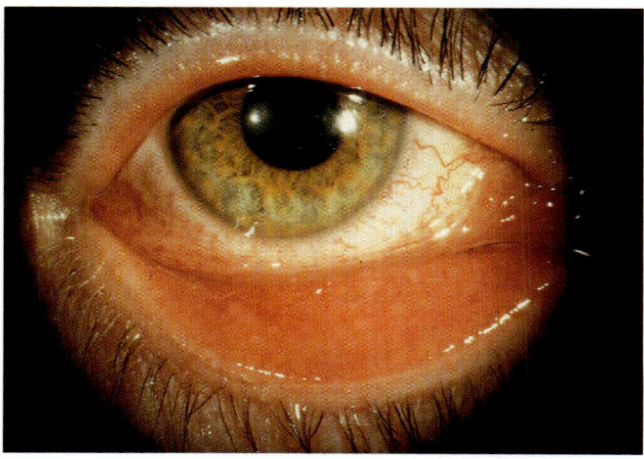

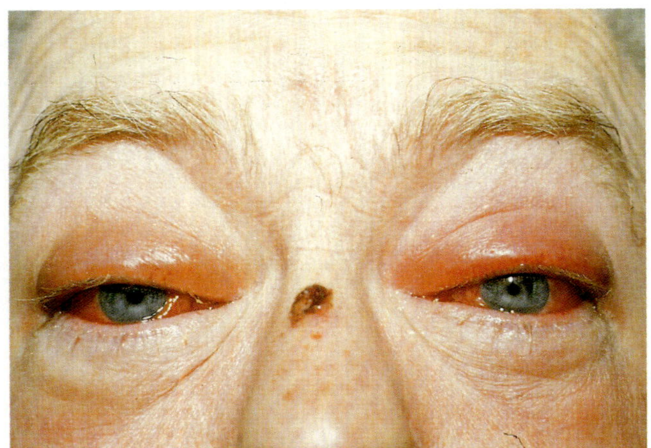

Figure 3.30 Severe epidemic keratoconjunctivitis (EKC), clinical picture with marked bilateral erythema and swelling of the eyelids.

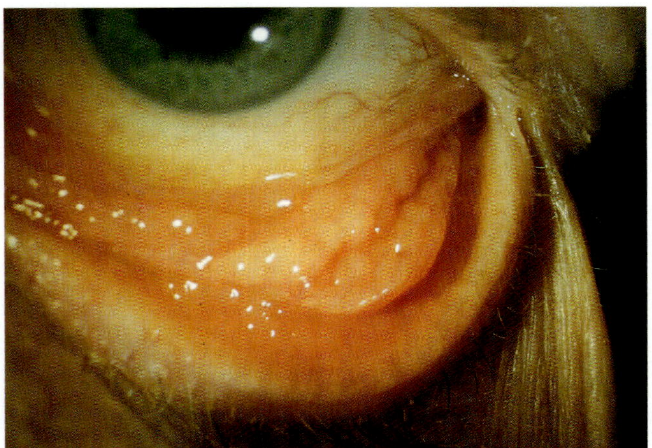

Figure 3.31 Follicular conjunctival reaction in the inferior fornix caused by Chlamydia infection. Similar finding in viral infections.

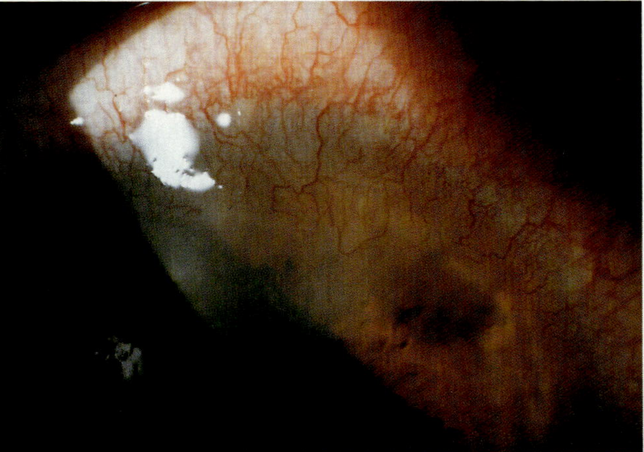

Figure 3.32 Perilimbal vascular pannus in trachoma. Corneal involvement occurs in form of marginal corneal infiltration with formation of fibrovascular pannus and dellen.

Figure 3.33 Trachoma stage III: advanced scarring of the tarsal conjunctiva. Mostly horizontal linear scars.

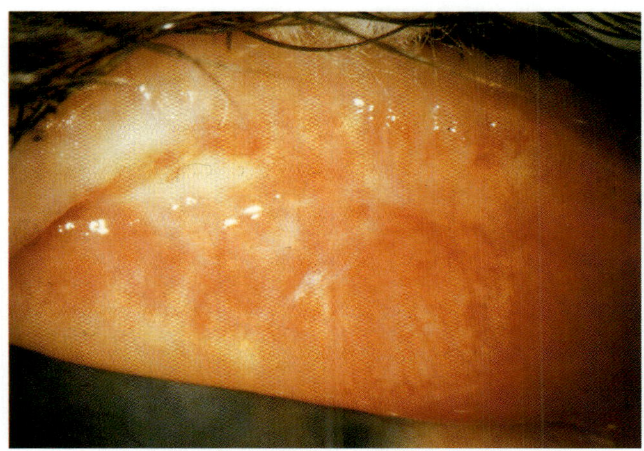

3.4 Allergic disorders of the conjunctiva

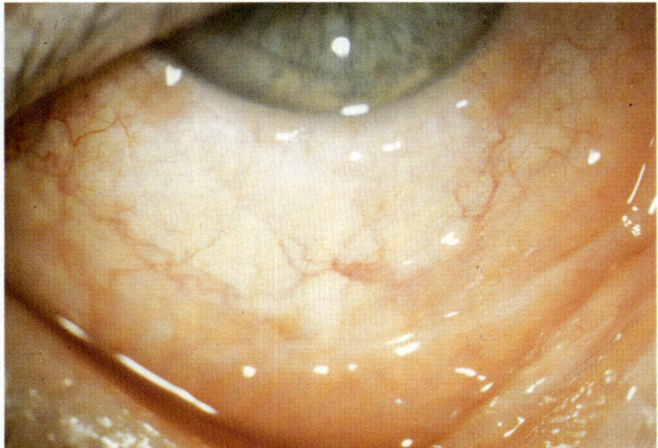

Figure 3.34　Chemosis of the bulbar conjunctiva, follicles in the inferior fornix in allergic conjunctivitis.

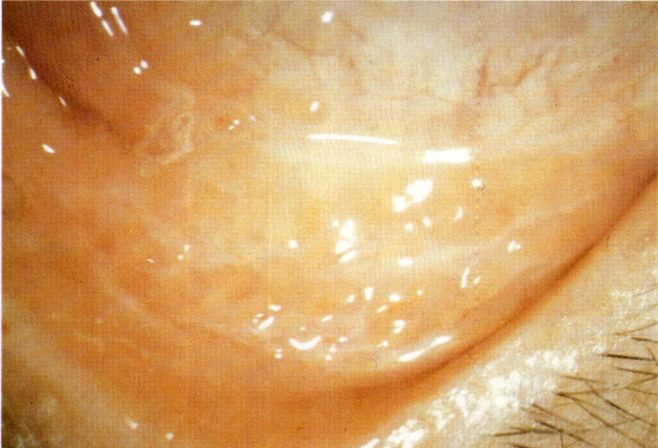

Figure 3.35　Mucous discharge in the inferior fornix in allergic conjunctivitis.

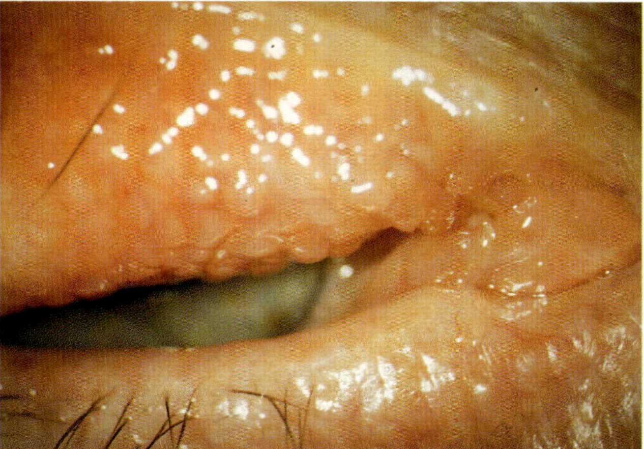

Figure 3.36　Follicular reaction of the superior tarsal conjunctiva in allergic conjunctivitis associated with atopia.

Figure 3.37 Giant papillary conjunctivitis after contact-lens wear for many years.

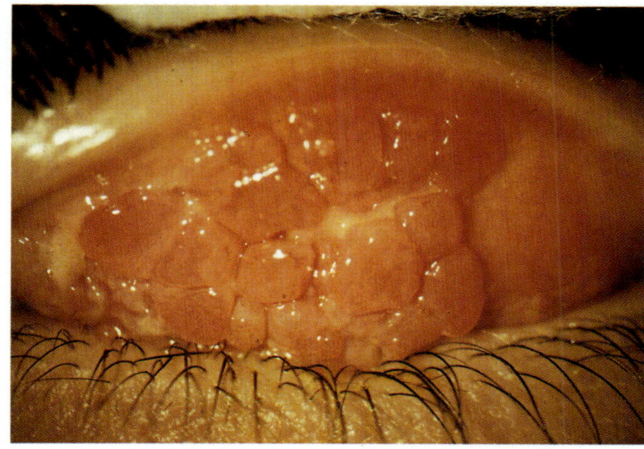

Figure 3.38 Allergic edema and erythema of the upper and lower lid in severe unilateral allergic conjunctivitis.

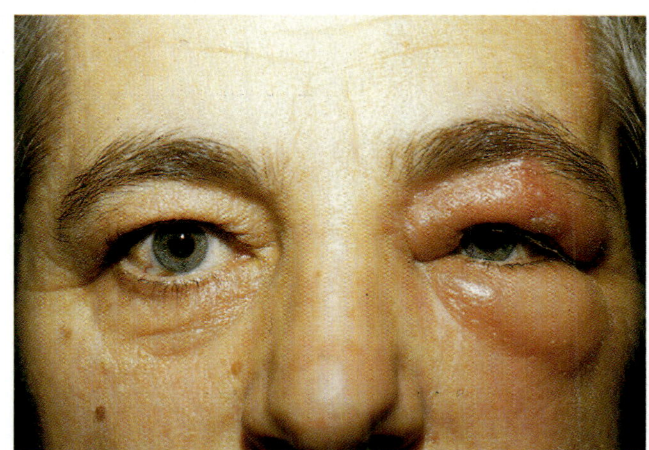

Figure 3.39 Severe conjunctivitis with formation of pseudomembranes and symblephara in Stevens-Johnson syndrome. The conjunctival changes include loss of golblet cells, atresia of the lacrimal excretory ducts and formation of symblephara.

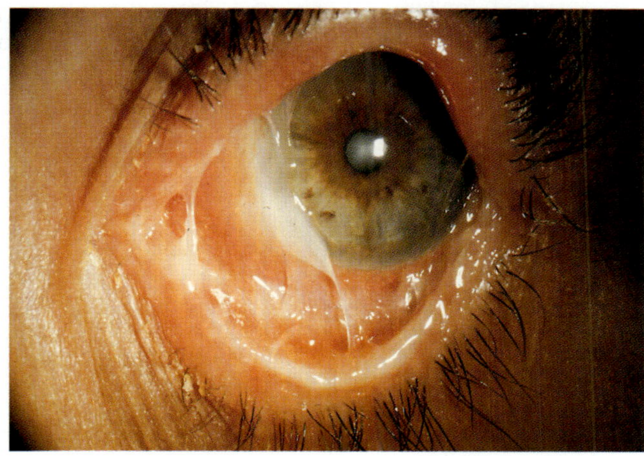

3.4 Allergic disorders of the conjunctiva

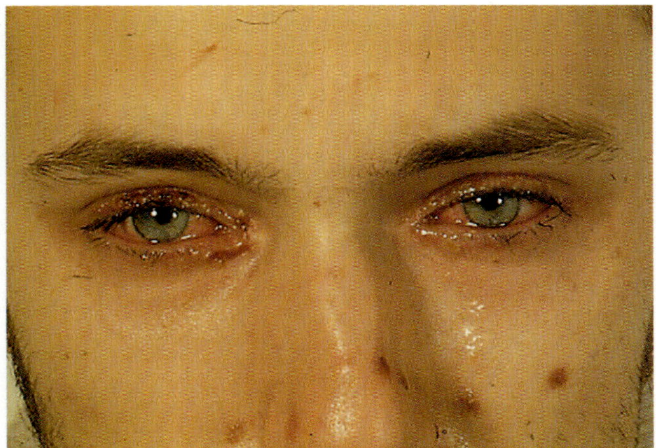

Figure 3.40 Eyelid involvement in Stevens-Johnson syndrome.

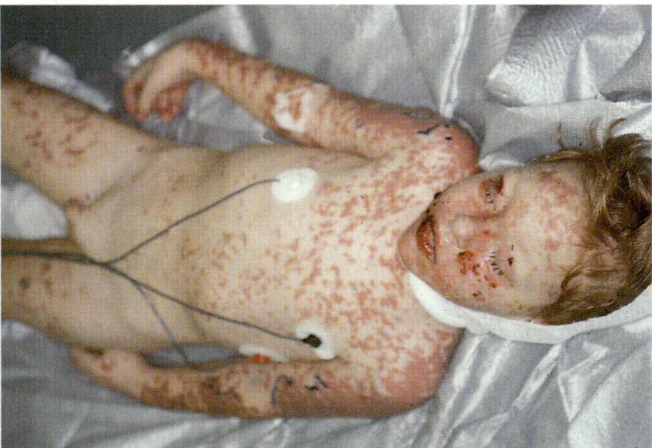

Figure 3.41 Lyell syndrome, severe involvement of the entire integumentum in an infant.

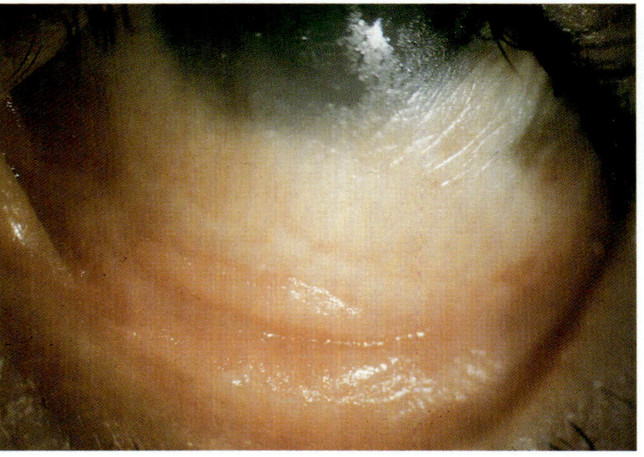

Figure 3.42 Severe xerosis of the conjunctiva with metaplasia. Complete loss of goblet cells. The cornea is dry, ulceration and perforation may occur. The changes are often consequent to vitamin A deficiency.

Figure 3.43 Pseudopemphigoid of the conjunctiva induced by topical medication, mostly antiglaucomatous drops. The conjunctival changes with formation of symblephara, loss of goblet cells and atresia of the lacrimal excretory tracts resemble ocular pemphigoid.

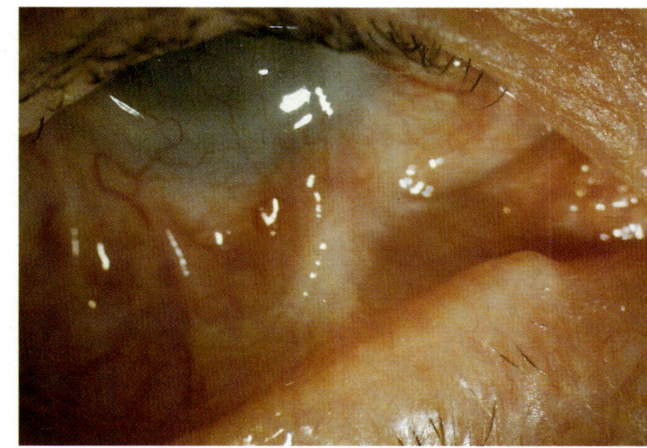

Figure 3.44 Ocular pemphigoid. The condition is thought to have an autoimmune basis. It is characterized by progressive scarring and shrinkage of the conjunctiva with severe sicca syndrome and may result in blindness. Systemic immunosuppressive therapy is necessary.

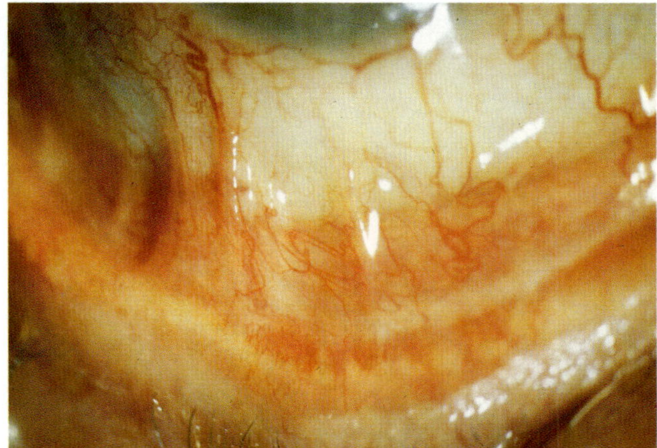

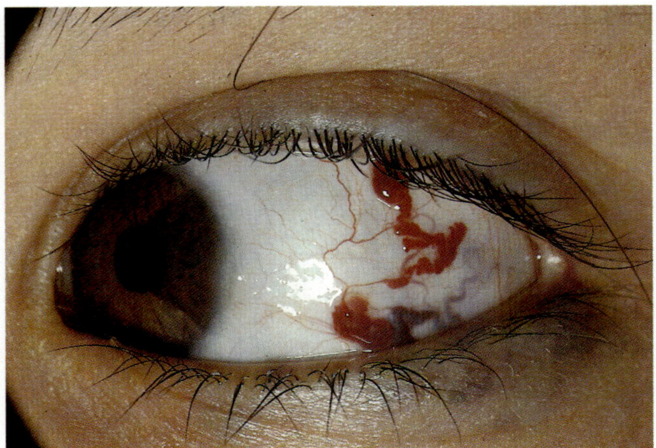

Figure 3.45 Congenital telangiectasia.

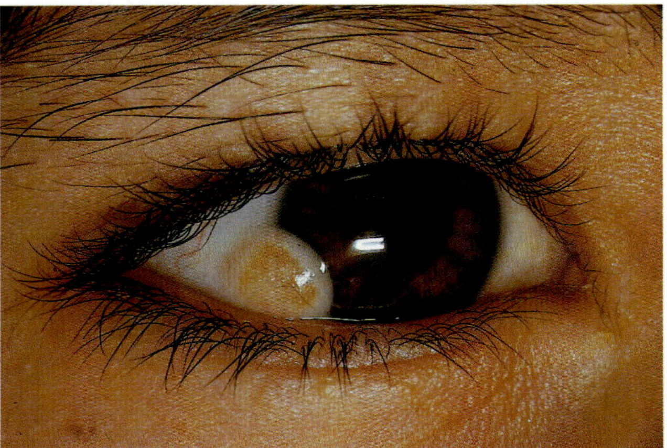

Figure 3.46 Epibulbar limbal dermoid cyst. Typically located temporally at the limbus. Congenital, benign tumor without growth, which may consist of different tissues.

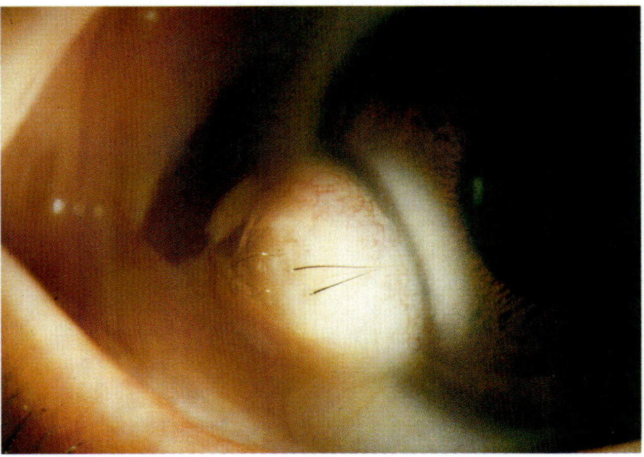

Figure 3.47 Dermoid cyst of the conjunctiva with fine hairs.

Figure 3.48 Conjunctival papilloma, caused by papilloma virus.

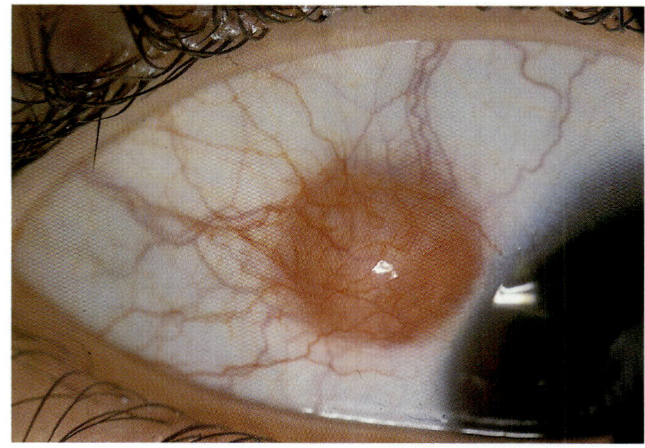

Figure 3.49 Conjunctival cyst. Etiology: superficial epithelium spread by trauma (e.g. surgery).

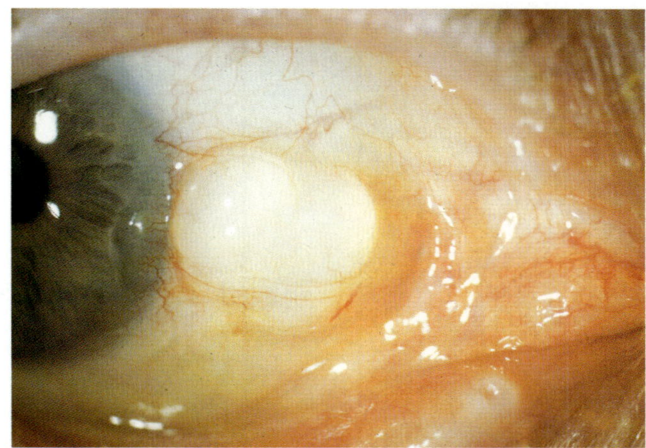

Figure 3.50 Conjunctival lipodermoid. Benign tumor, which consists of adipose tissue and extends into the orbit. Removal for cosmetic reasons.

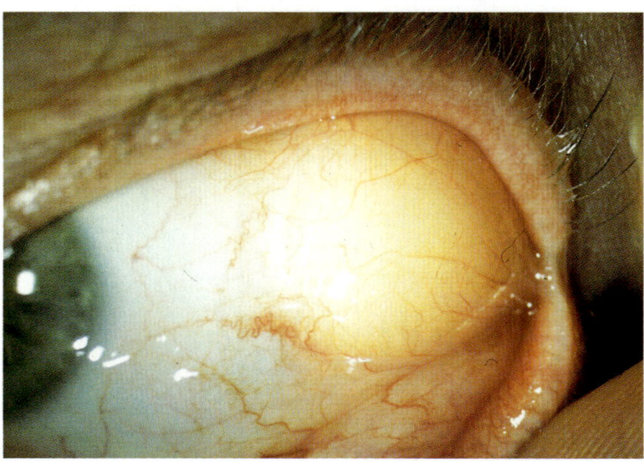

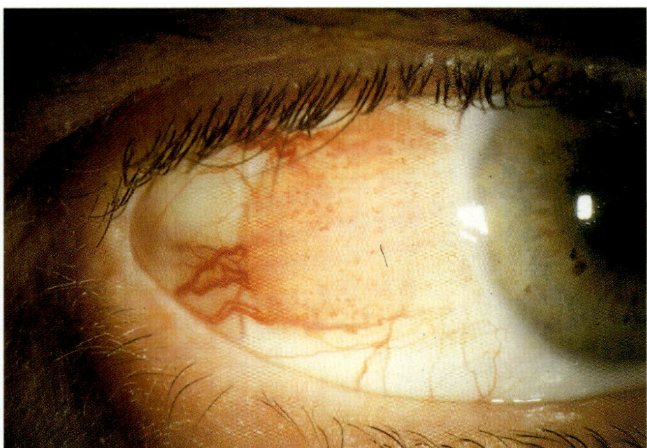

Figure 3.51 Conjunctival papilloma. Broad-based, flat tumor (sessile papilloma) consisting of fibrovascular tissue. The lesion is benign, malignant transformation is rare.

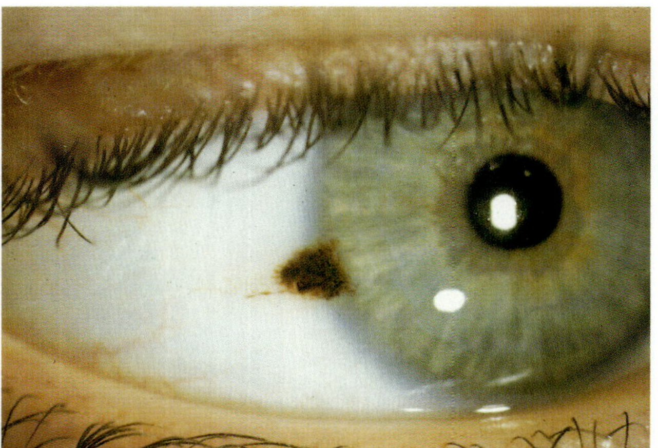

Figure 3.52 Perilimbal conjunctival nevus. Melanocytic nevi are benign lesions, which are stable, but may exhibit increasing pigmentation. Frequently located at the limbus or the plica semilunaris (see figure 3.53).

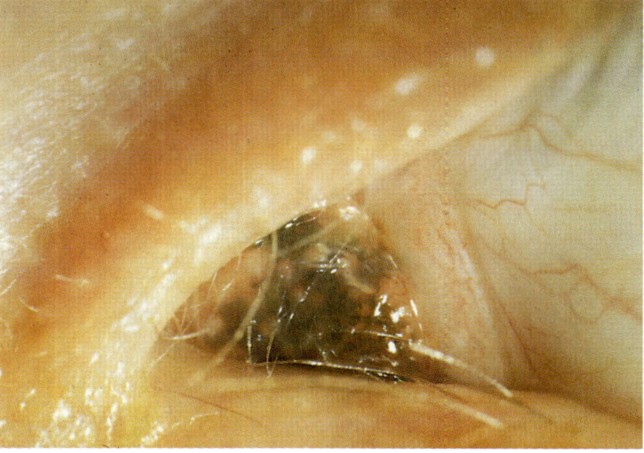

Figure 3.53 Nevus of the caruncle.

Figure 3.54 Congenital melanosis. Pigmentation of the episclera of grey-brownish color. The stable lesion is of variable extension and not elevated.

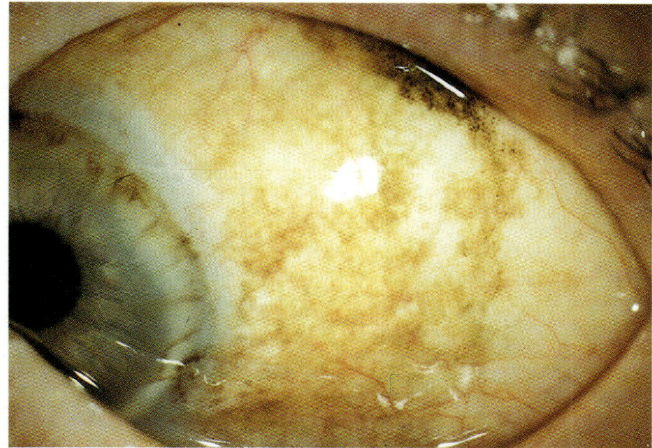

Figure 3.55 Pyogenic granuloma of the conjunctiva located at the lid margin. The condition may be caused by a perforated hordeolum or chalazion.

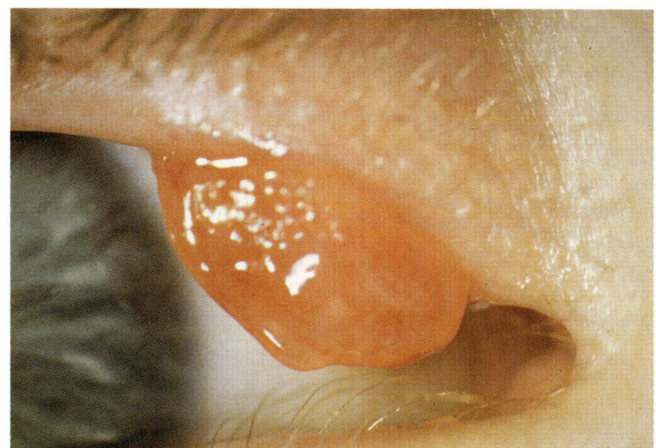

Figure 3.56 Benign lymphatic hyperplasia of the conjunctiva.

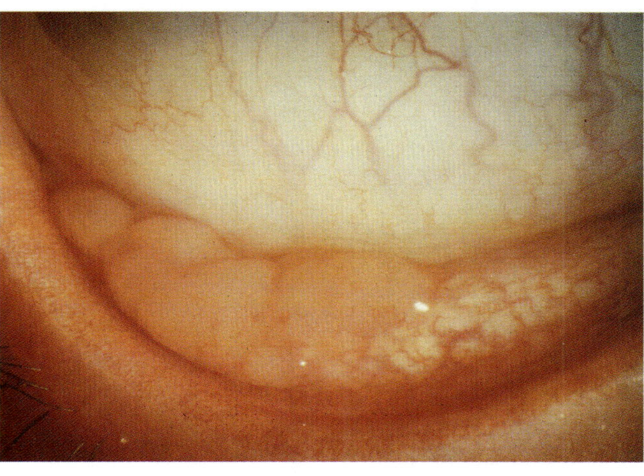

3.6 Malignant conjunctival tumors

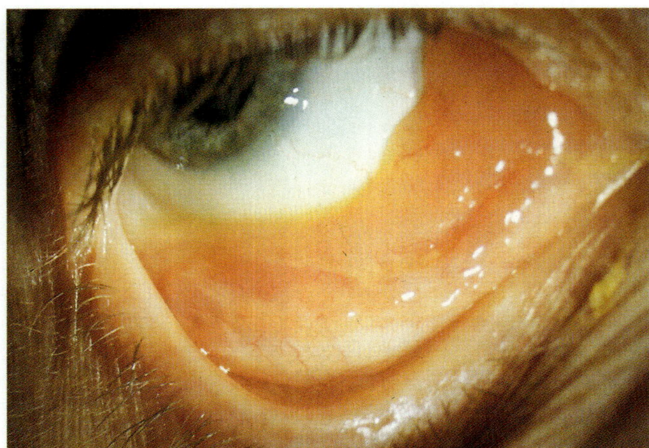

Figure 3.57 Malignant lymphoma of the conjunctiva. The tumor may be localized or represent a metastasis in systemic disease. Medical evaluation is required.

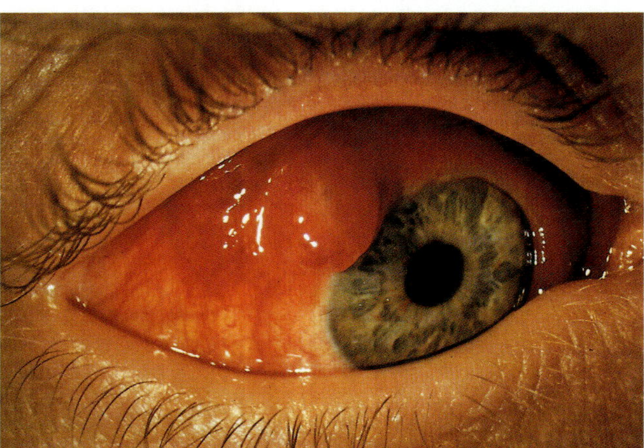

Figure 3.58 Kaposi sarcoma of the conjunctiva. Kaposi sarcoma mostly occurs in patients infected with HIV. Histologic evaluation shows endothelial cells and pericytes. Management: radiation therapy.

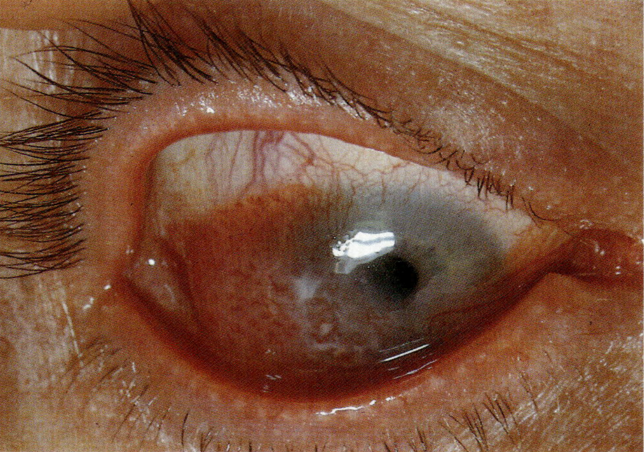

Figure 3.59 Conjunctival carcinoma. Frequently located at the limbus, growth towards the cornea. Intraocular involvement and metastases are rare. Fairly good prognosis after excision.

Figure 3.60 Perilimbal melanoma of the conjunctiva. Despite high malignancy preservation of globe intergrity can be achieved by local excision.

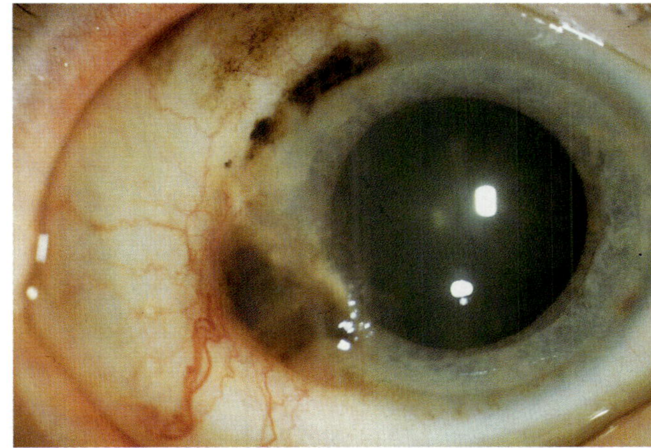

Figure 3.61 Status post surgical excision of the perilimbal melanoma shown in figure 3.60.

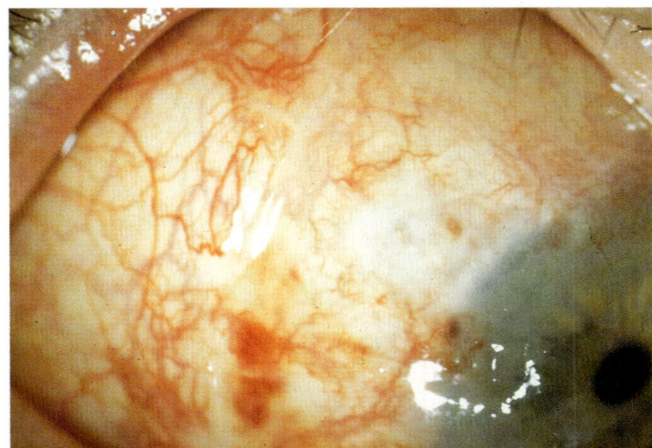

Figure 3.62 Perlimbal malignant melanoma of the conjunctiva.

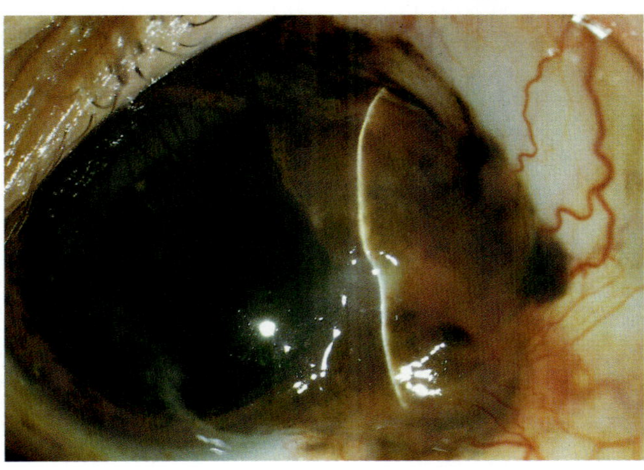

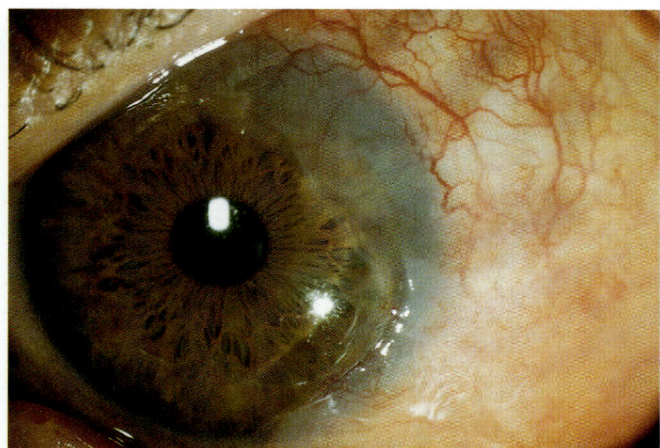

Figure 3.63 Status post surgical excision of the conjunctival melanoma shown in figure 3.62 with transplantation of buccal mucous membrane.

Cornea

4

4.1 Applied anatomy and examination techniques

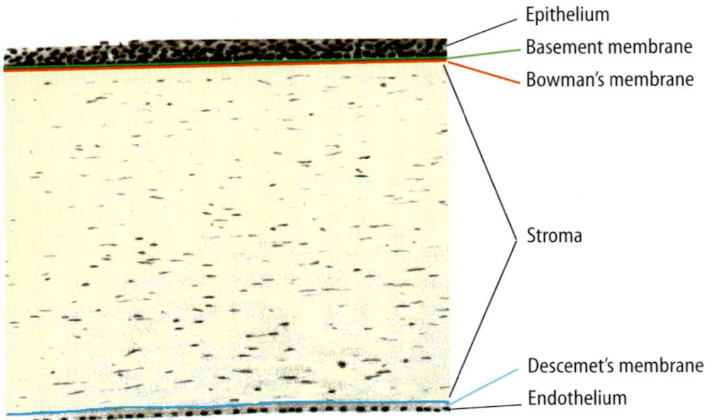

Figure 4.1 Schema of the corneal structure. The *epithelium* is multilayered and nonkeratinizing. It is divided by a basement membrane from Bowman´s layer. The intact epithelium forms a barrier, which prevents the tear film from entering the cornea and protects from pathogenic germs. Shed superficial cells are replaced by mitosis. Excellent ability to regenerate. *Bowman´s layer* is a part of the corneal stroma. It consists of collagen fibrils and is acellular. Scar formation when damaged. The corneal *stroma* consists of collagen fibrils, which are arranged in a lamellar pattern, fibroblasts (keratocytes) and ground substance, containing keratan sulfate, chondoitin sulfate and chondoitin. The regular arrangement of the collagen fibrils provides the transparency of the cornea. The stroma has the ability to regenerate, but the transparency is not maintained after regeneration. *Descemet´s membrane* is the basal lamina of the endothelium. It is relatively thick, of high elasticity and resistance. It is often unaffected after injury to superficial corneal layers. The endothelium is a single layer of hexagonal cells, which are responsible for the deturgescence of the stroma. In structural or functional defects of the corneal endothelium, transit of anterior chamber fluid into the stroma occurs, resulting in stromal edema. Reduction of cell number with age. There is no true ability to regenerate.

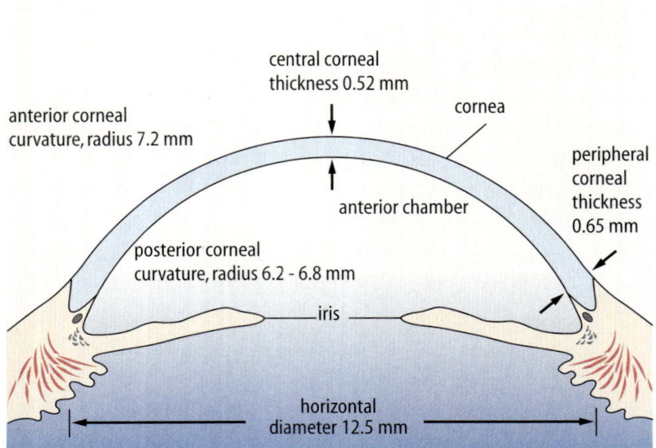

Figure 4.2 Schematic cross section through the cornea and the anterior chamber. The average horizontal diameter in the adult is 12,5 mm, in the infant up to age1 it is 10 mm (important data for the differentiation of congenital glaucoma). The corneal radius of curvature is smaller than the radius of curvaure of the eyeball. The cornea is wedge-shaped in the corneoscleral transition zone (limbus).

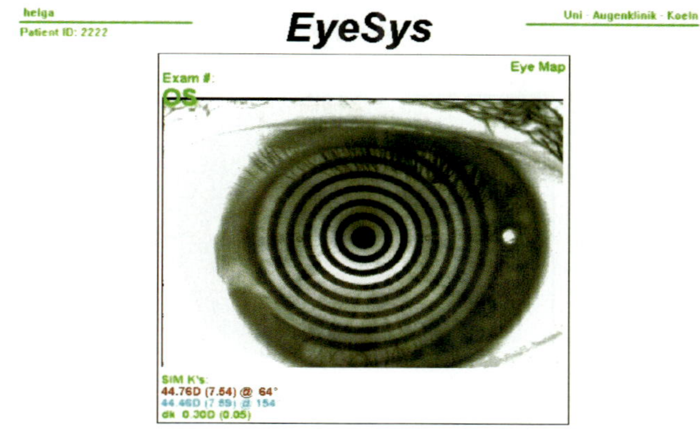

Figure 4.3 Keratoscope. With a keratoscope (photo keratoscope, video keratoscope) the corneal refractive power and astigmatism can be measured. The technique is based on the reflection of a circular target on the corneal surface. The distance of the single rings in various meridians provides information about the corneal surface. The figure shows a normal corneal surface depicted by computer aided keratoscopy. The concentric rings are regular and have the same distance from one another.

Figure 4.4 Normal keratoscope photograph, colored computer analysis. The refractive power can be color-coded. The figure (same patient as in figure 4.3) shows a normal corneal surface of almost uniform color.

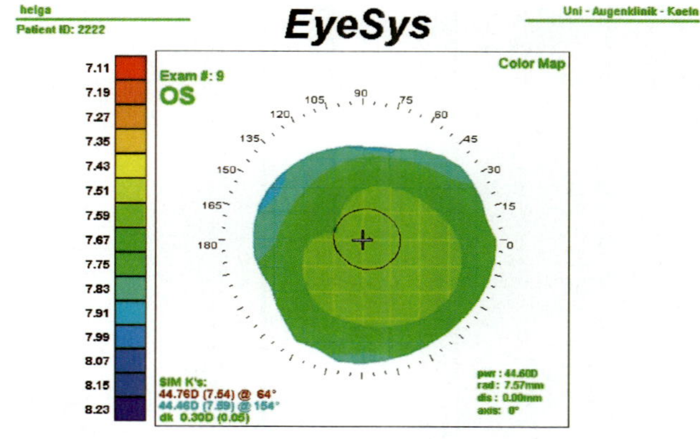

4.1 Applied anatomy and examination techniques

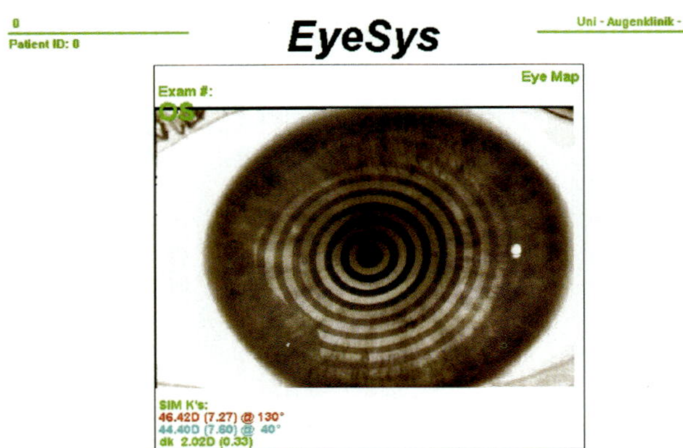

Figure 4.5 Keratoscope photograph. The image produced by reflection of a circular target reveals subtle changes (2 diopters of astigmatism). The concentric rings are more densly arranged in the axis corresponding to the steeper meridian.

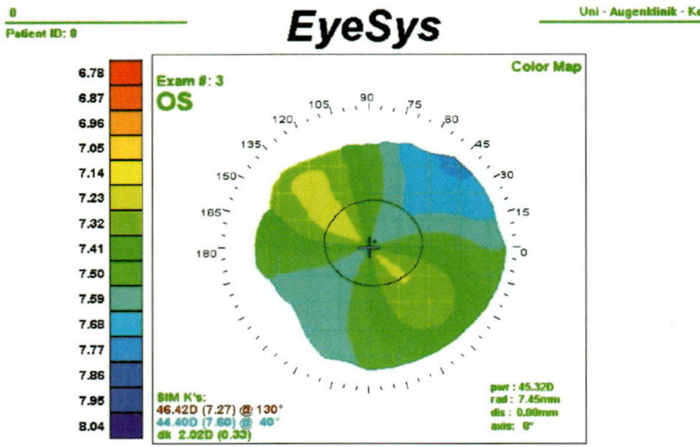

Figure 4.6 Keratoscope photograph, colored computer analysis, same patient as in figure 4.5. The color analysis clearly depicts the astigmatism. *Blue* color indicates the axis of flatter curvature, *yellow* the axis of steeper curvature.

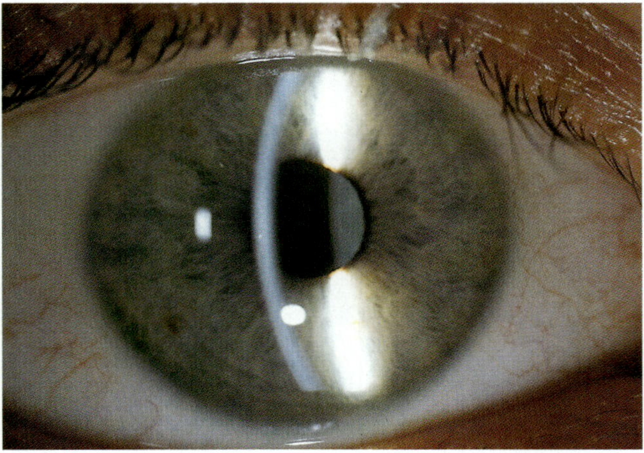

Figure 4.7 Cross section of the normal cornea viewed with a slit lamp.

Figure 4.8 Specular microscopy, normal endothelium. The polygonal, mostly hexagonal cells are of regular size and shape. The cell count varies between 3500 and 4000 cells per square millimeter. A sufficient number of functioning endothelial cells is crucial for the deturgescence of the cornea by means of the endothelial pump mechanism.

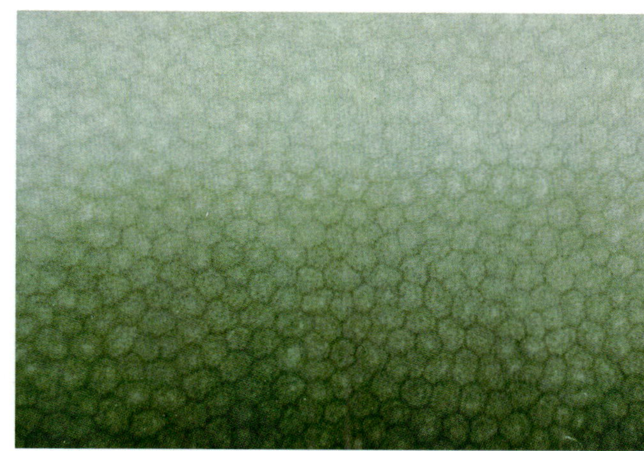

Figure 4.9 Specular microscopy, pathologic endothelium. The loss of endothelial cells with age or trauma is compensated by an enlargement of the cells. There is little or no ability for mitosis. The pathologic endothelium shows a variation in cell size with atypical shapes. Despite a highly reduced cell number, the deturgescence of the cornea can be maintained, provided the endothelial pump mechanism is intact.

Figure 4.10 Aesthesiometer of Cochet and Bonnet. The corneal nerve supply is derived from the trigeminal nerve. The sensitivity decreases from the center to the periphery. With the aesthesiometer a quantitative measurement of corneal sensitivity can be performed. Processes along the trigeminal nerve, infection with herpes simplex and herpes zoster virus lead to a reduction or loss of corneal sensitivity. In herpetic changes, the evaluation of corneal sensitivity is an important diagnosic tool.

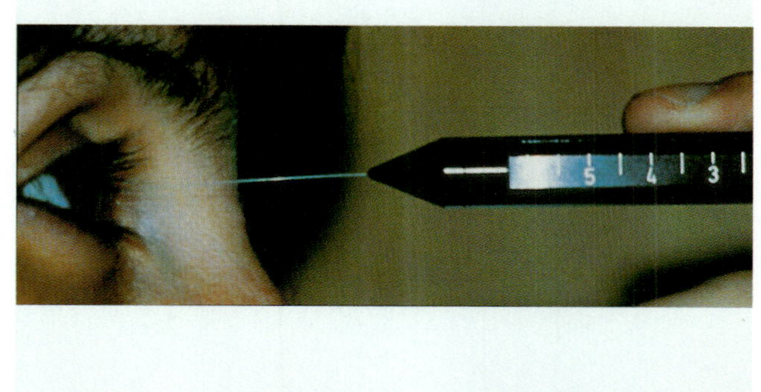

4.1 Applied anatomy and examination techniques

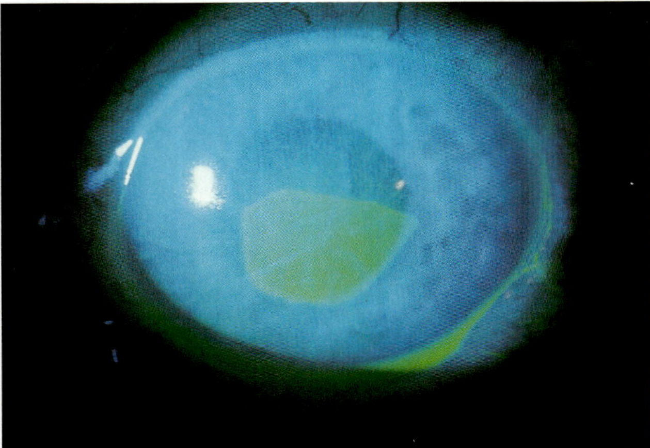

Figure 4.11 Fluorescein staining of the cornea. Fluorescein dye stains areas in which the corneal surface is not intact. Staining is an important diagnostic tool for the detection of epithelial defects. The figure shows a large epithelial defect (erosion). The area takes a *green* stain.

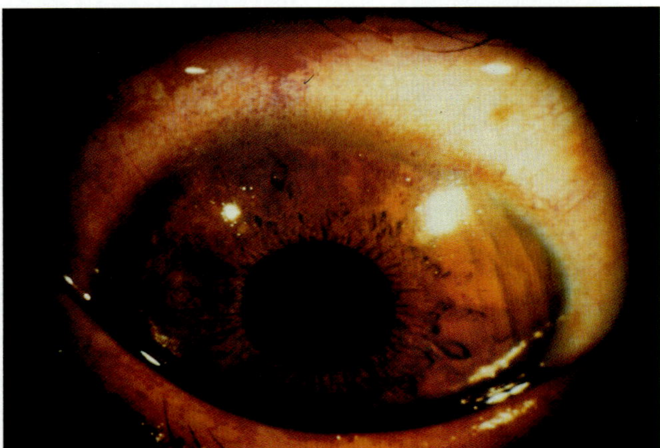

Figure 4.12 Rose bengal staining. Unlike fluorescein, rose bengal dye stains devitalized epithelial cells as well as intact epithelial cells with lacking mucoid layer. In the figure, the affected area at the superior limbus takes a blue-reddish stain.

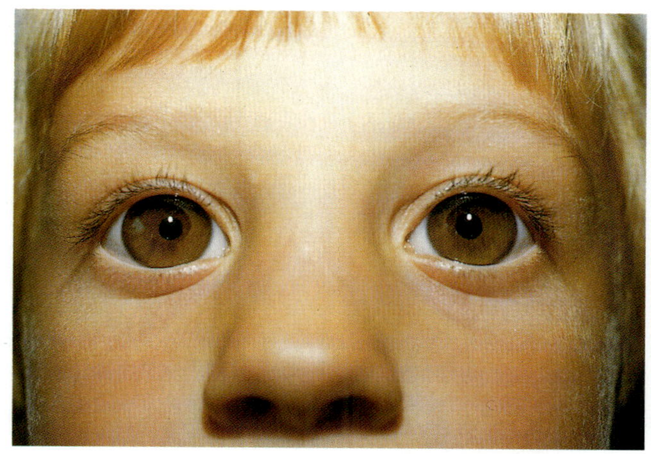

Figure 4.13   Megalocornea. Cornea with normal structure, but enlarged horizontal and vertical diameters (horizontal diameter is 16 mm). Megalocornea is determined an inherited condition which may be associated with other changes in the anterior segment. The corneal structure is normal, opacities are not found. Intraocular pressure is normal, although measurement may be difficult. The condition has to be differentiated from buphthalmos in congenital glaucoma. The simple megalocornea does not require treatment.

Figure 4.14   Megalocornea, lateral view.

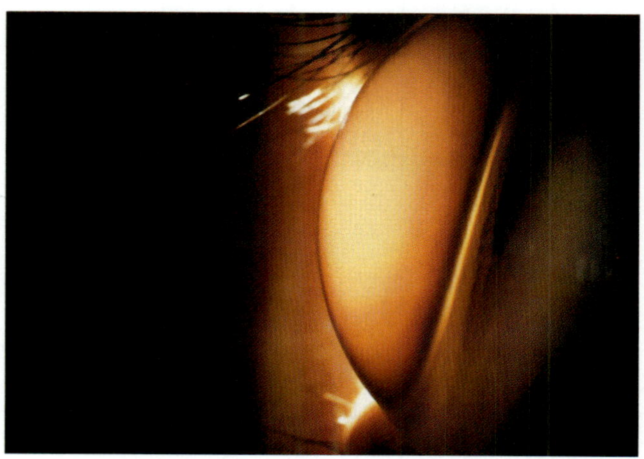

4.2 Developmental anomalies

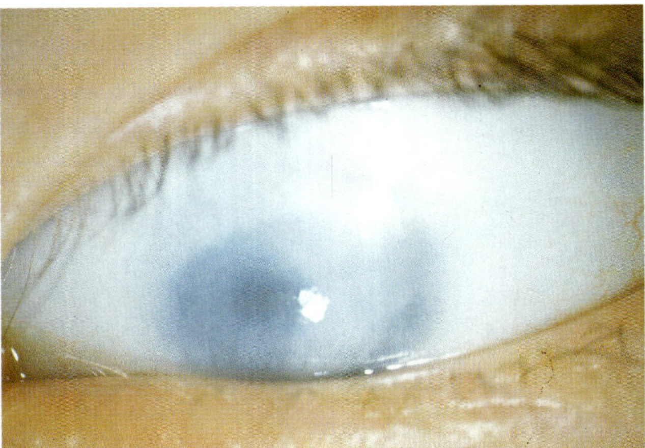

Figure 4.15 Sclerocornea. Sclerocornea is a nonprogressive hereditary corneal opacity, which may be associated with other abnormalities in the anterior segment. No possibilities of treatment.

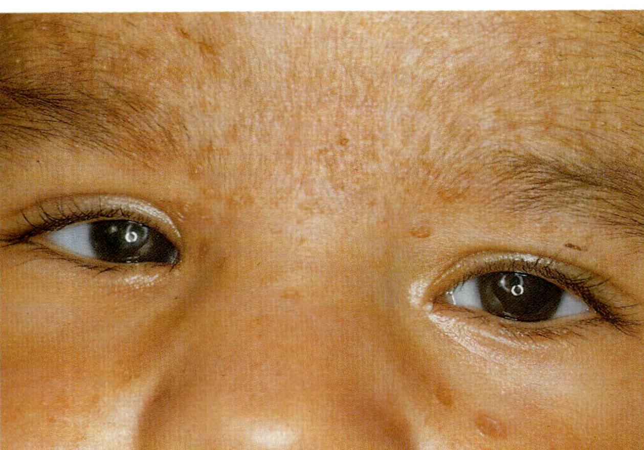

Figure 4.16 Microcornea. Reduced corneal diameter with otherwise normal corneal structure. Microcornea is an inherited condition. An association with other ocular abnormalities may be present. An elevation of intraocular pressure has to be ruled out (angle-closure). IOP measurement may be difficult.

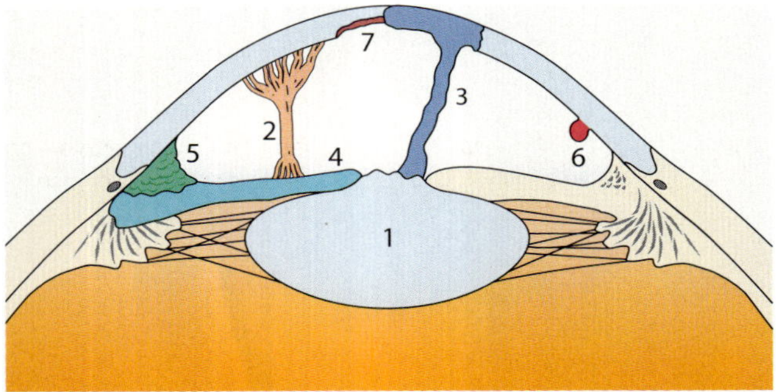

Figure 4.17 Schema of various congenital corneal opacities and anterior synechiae (anterior chamber cleavage syndrome). The opacities and anterior synechiae result from an impaired differentiation of the anterior chamber during embryologic development. Depending on their localization, the changes cause visual impairment. Severe glaucoma is frequent (see chapter 9). (1-3) Peters´ anomaly; (4-6) Rieger´s anomaly; (5,6) Axenfeld´s anomaly; (6) posterior embryotoxin; (7) posterior keratoconus.

Figure 4.18 Axenfeld´s anomaly. The ring of Schwalbe (transition of Descemet´s membrane to the trabecular meshwork, see figure 4.2) is prominent. It appears as a greywhite, concentric corneal opacity parallel to the limbus. Anterior synechiae can be found between the prominent ring of Schwalbe and the iris (compare with figure 4.17).

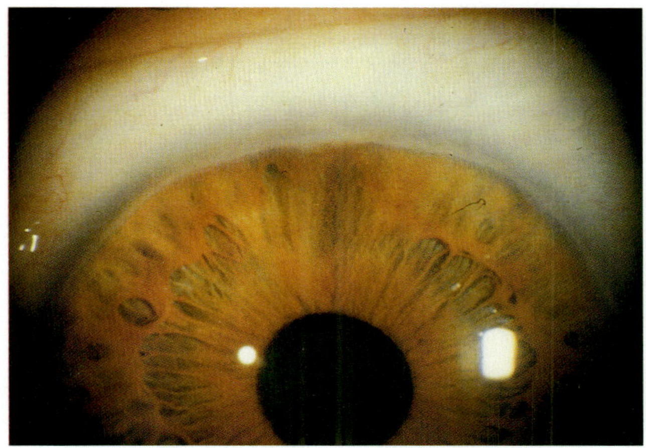

Figure 4.19 Peter´s anomaly. The condition presents with a central corneal opacity and synechiae of variable extent. In this case, a broad synechia between the opaque cornea and the anterior lens surface exists. The is no known therapy for functional improvement.

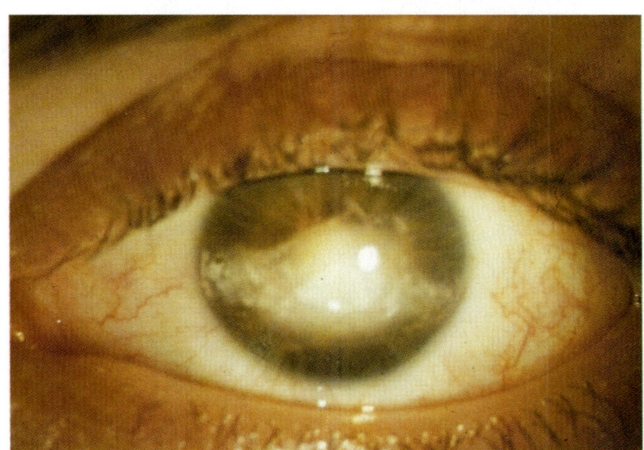

General: Degenerative changes of the cornea mostly occur with age or secondary to exogenous noxious agents. In contrast to the dystrophies, degenerative changes are often more pronounced in one eye.

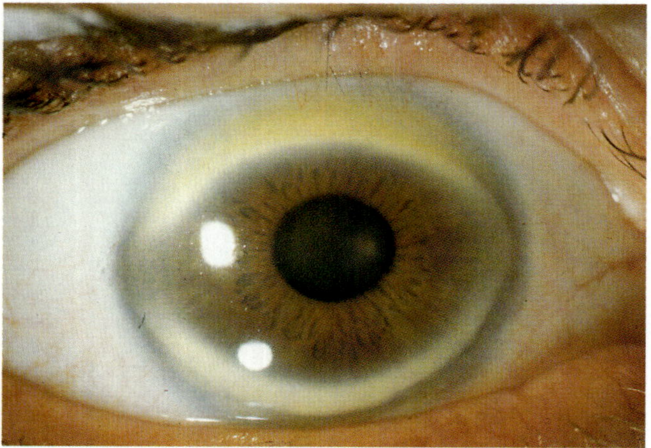

Figure 4.20   Arcus lipoides. The figure shows a yellow-white circular opacity in the peripheral cornea. The lesion consits of lipids, which are deposited in the corneal stroma. The opacity is separated from the limbus by a clear interval (more pronounced in the inferior circumference). Arcus lipoides has a high prevalence, particularly in elderly persons (arcus senilis). Arcus lipoides in a young person requires evaluation for hyperlipoproteinemia. Unilateral occurence may be associated with vascular changes on the unaffected side.

Figure 4.21   Limbal gyrdle of Vogt, yellow-white opacity in the limbal region, which unlike arcus lipoides is confined to the interpalpebral cornea. The condition can be found in up to 60% of the elderly population. There is no progression, no treatment is required.

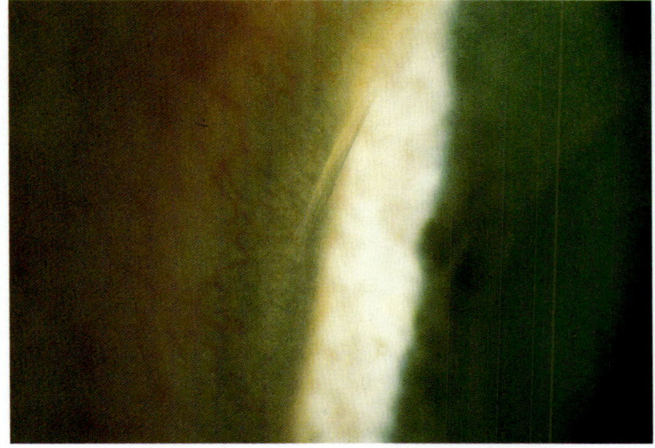

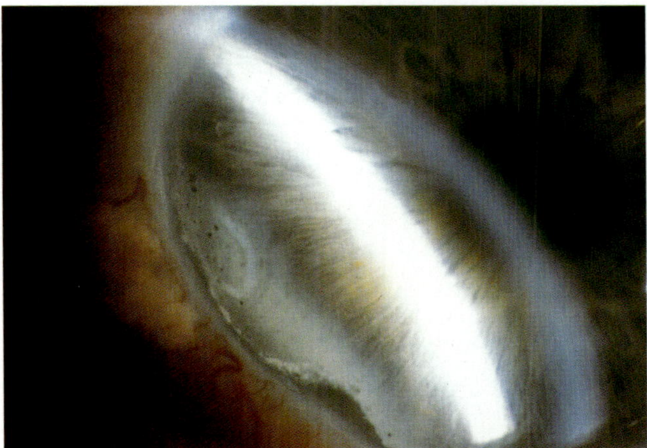

Figure 4.22   Band keratopathy, peripheral form. Grey-white calcium deposits underneath the epithelium, which are separated from the limbus by a clear interval. The dense opacity may be interrupted by small clear zones at several points. The calcium deposition may arise from localized ocular disorders (the figure shows a patient with glaucoma) or from systemic disorders involving the calcium-/phosphate metabolism. Systemic disorders, in children especially renal disorders, have to be ruled out, if the condition is not related to an ocular pathology.

4.3 Degenerative changes of the cornea

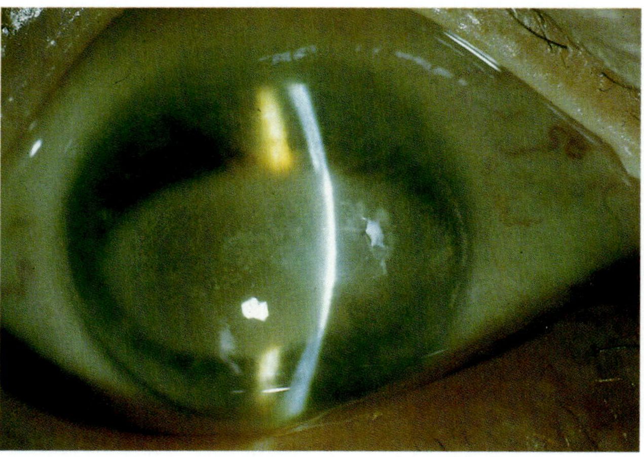

Figure 4.23 Band keratopathy involving the central cornea. In advanced stages, the band-shaped opacity extends over almost the entire cornea, sparing only a narrow interval at the limbus. The condition may arise from long-standing ocular diorders as well as from numerous systemic disorders (see figure 4.22). Disturbances of the calcium-/phosphate metabolism have to be ruled out. Vision can be severly impaired. The calcium deposits can be removed with hydrochloric acid or EDTA. Frequent recurrences.

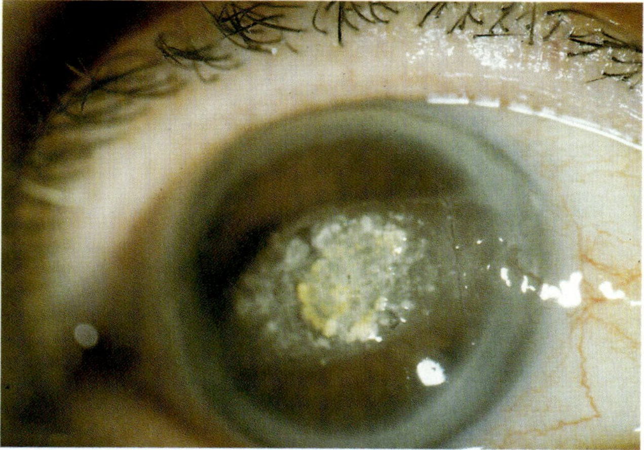

Figure 4.24 Spheroid degeneration. Yellow subepithelial and stromal deposits are found in spheroid degeneration. The resulting uneven corneal surface leads to visual impairment as well as severe photophobia and pain. The condition is thought to be causally related to climatic conditions, such as frequent exposure to sunlight. Lamellar keratoplasty may be beneficial in advanced stages.

Figure 4.25 Terrien´s marginal degeneration. The clinical picture is characterized by thinning of the peripheral cornea with an intact epithelium, superficial vascularization and a yellow border of lipid. The condition usually progresses slowly and induces corneal astigmatism. The cause remains unclear, conservative treatment is unable to improve the condition. Surgery is required in advanced stages.

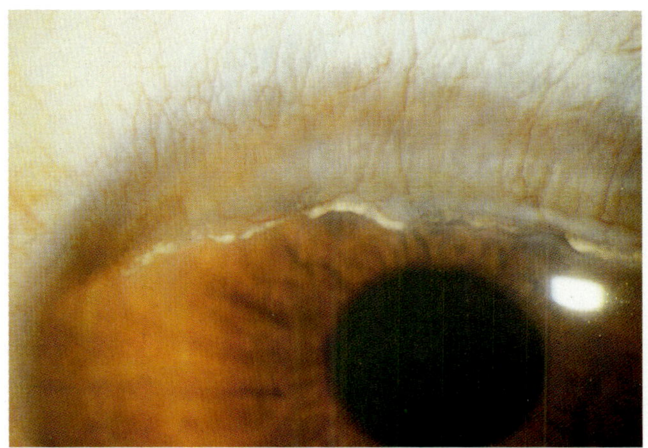

Figure 4.26 Terrien´s marginal degeneration with descemetocele. In some cases, the marginal thinning may progress to the extent that a descemetocele develops with risk of perforation. A partial lamellar keratoplasty may be considered.

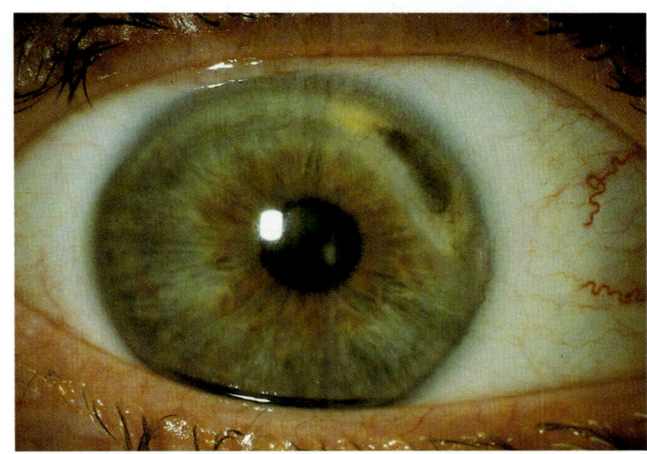

Figure 4.27 Salzmann´s nodular degeneration. The clinical picture is characterized by multiple bluish-white superficial nodules, mostly in the periphery and midperiphery. The degree of visual impairment depends on the localization of the lesions. The condition may be related to previous corneal inflammation and sometimes to trauma. In severly decreased vision, treatment may include sremoval of the nodules with excimer-laser or lamellar keratoplasty.

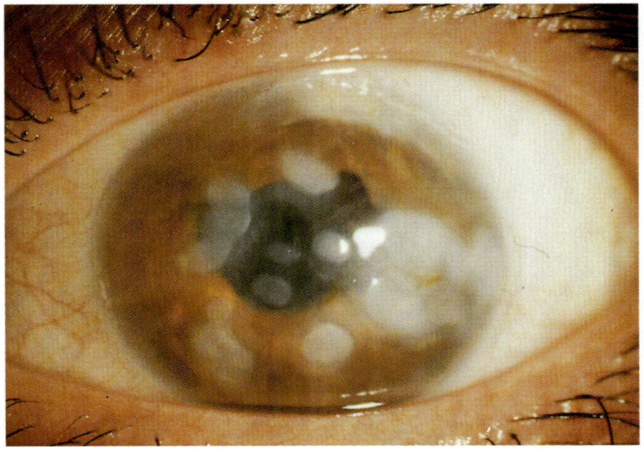

4.3 Degenerative changes of the cornea

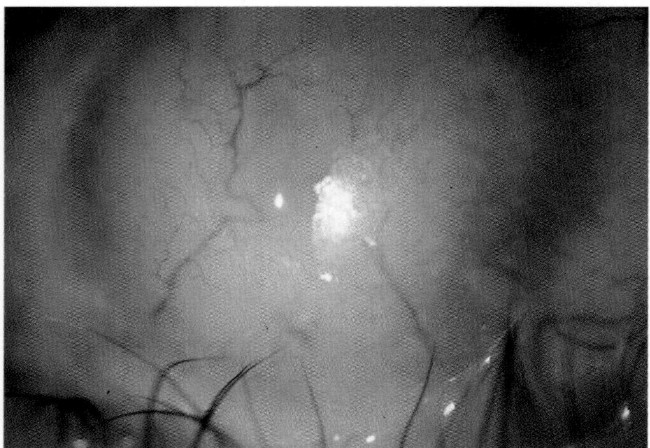

Figure 4.28 Corneal opacity and vascularization in ocular pemphigoid. Dense opacity of all corneal layers with superificial vessels arising from the conjunctiva (conjuntivalization). Findings like this often result from severe tear deficiency, for instance in ocular pemphigoid (see chapter 3).

General: Corneal dystrophies have to be differentiated from corneal degenerations. They are hereditary, bilateral with symmetric involvement and are mostly located centrally.

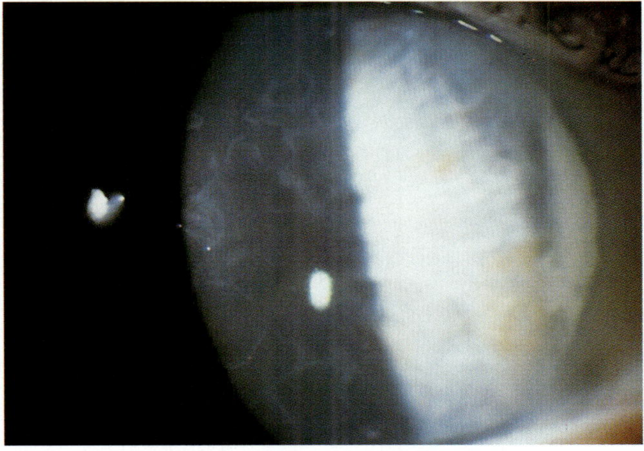

Figure 4.29   Epithelial dystrophy (map-dot-fingerprint). Anterior corneal dystrophy with typical formation of subepithelial ridges (fingerprints), intraepithelial microcysts (dots) and geographic opacities (maps). Histologic analysis reveals involvement of the basal epithelium and its basement membrane. The clinical picture is variable and the patients are often asymptomatic. The condition is complicated by the occurence of recurrent erosion. [The dense opacity at the limbus shown in the figure is not related to the described condition. It is a limbal gyrdle of Vogt (see figure 4.21)].

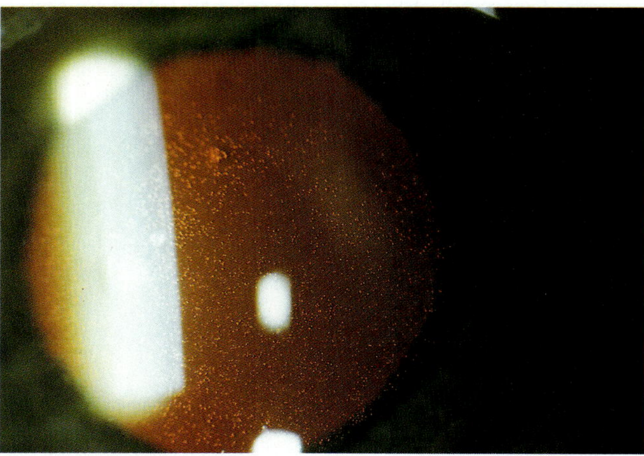

Figure 4.30 Meesmann´s dystrophy. Hereditary epithelial dystrophy, clinical picture with multiple intraepithelial cysts scattered across the entire cornea. Visual acuity is only mildly decreased, foreign body sensation and photophobia are the predominant symptoms. Complications are painful epithelial breaks. Usually no treatment is required. Recurrence after surgical treatment (excimer laser, lamellar keratoplasty) has been described.

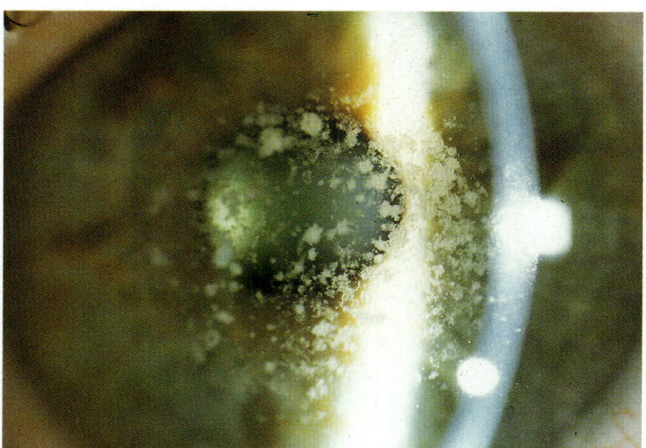

Figure 4.31 Granular dystrophy. Hereditary disorder, clinical picture with multiple grey-white, sharply demarcated opacities usually beginning in the epithelium, later found in the entire stroma. Visual acuity is mostly good for a long period of time, since the progression of the disorder is slow. When visual acuity is severly decreased, the treatment is penetrating keratoplasty. Recurrence in the graft may occur, since the disorder is thought to arise from the epithelium.

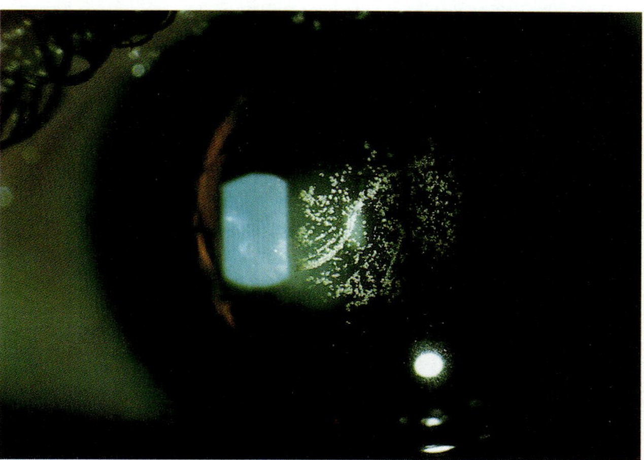

Figure 4.32 Granular dystrophy, status post penetrating keratoplasty, recurrence. The figure shows multiple opacities in the axial portion of the cornea, which are determined a recurrrence of the underlying disorder.

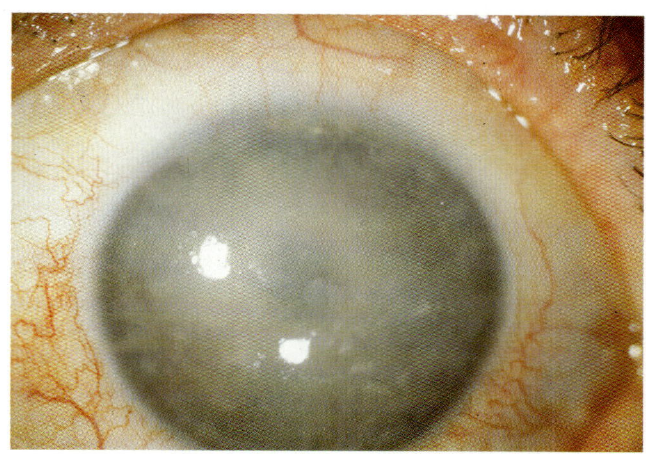

Figure 4.33   Macular dystrophy. Hereditary disorder, which begins in youth and leads to the development of confluent opacities throughout the entire stromal thickness. The progressive visual deterioration is often accomanied by recurrent epithelial breaks. The condition is thought to represent a systemic disorder of keratan sulfate metabolism. When visual acuity is severly decreased, the treatment is penetrating keratoplasty. Recurrence may occur, but has been decribed only after a long period of time.

Figure 4.34   Macular dystrophy, 20 years after penetrating keratoplasty (compare with figure 4.33). Clear graft, no signs of recurrence.

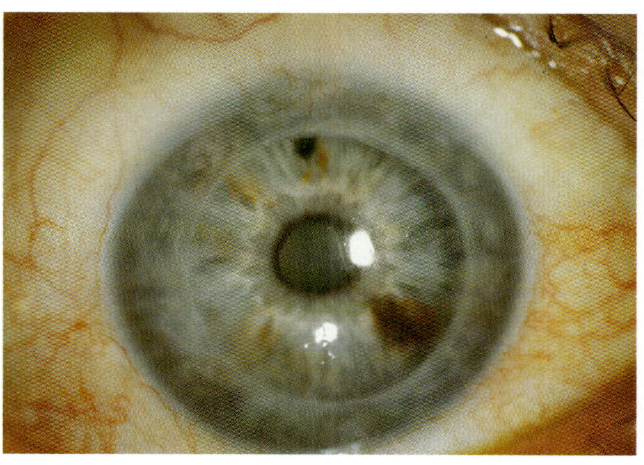

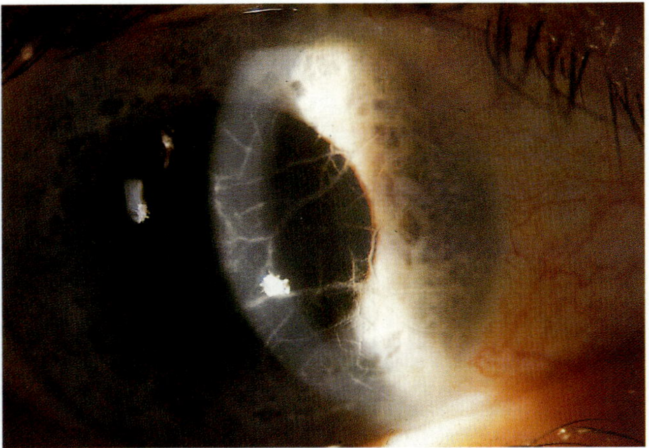

Figure 4.35 Lattice dystrophy. Hereditary disorder. The clinical picture is characterized by sub-epithelial and intrastromal branching lattice figures. The opacities are accumulations of amyloid material. The progredient opacities in the axial portion of the cornea leads to severe visual impairment. The condition is complicated by recurrent epithelial breaks with risk of infection. The treatment involves penetrating keratoplasty. Recurrence may occur.

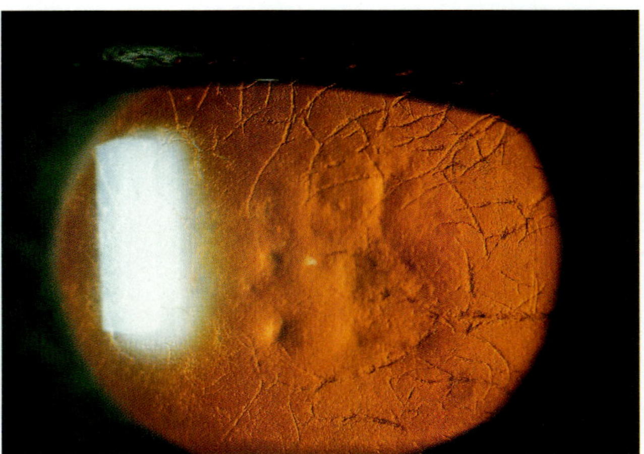

Figure 4.36 Lattice dystrophy (compare with figure 4.35), view with retroillumination. The pathognomonic branching lattice figures are best visible with retroillumination.

Figure 4.37 Crystalline dystrophy (Schnyder). Rare hereditary disorder, clinical picture with axial, ring-shaped corneal opacity consisting of fine crystal deposits. The condition slowly progresses, the peripheral cornea remains clear. The disorder may be associated with defects of systemic lipid metabolism. Visual acuity is usually good, therefore corneal grafting is not required.

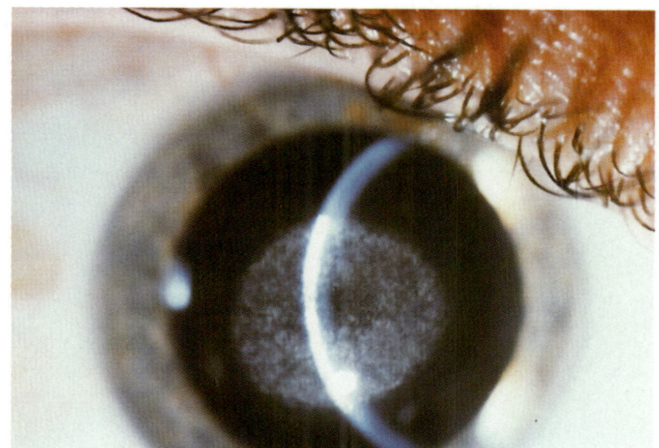

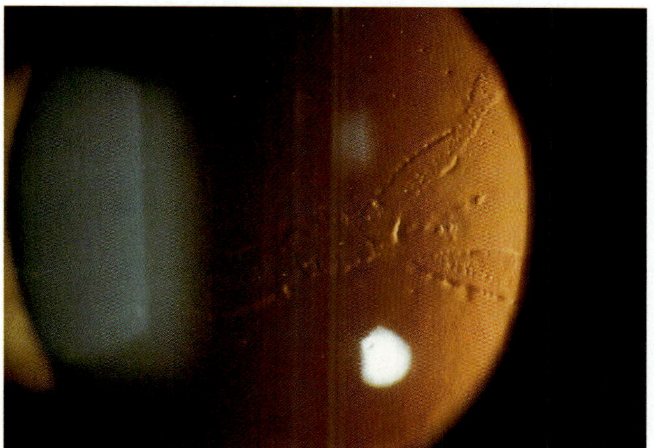

Figure 4.38 Posterior polymorphous dystrophy. Hererditary disorder, clinical picture with vesicular-appearing lesions on the posterior corneal surface and bandlike arrangement of lesions. Descemet´s membrane may show areas of glass-appearing thickening. The cornea remains clear only when limited regions are affected. The main symptom is photophobia. When the entire posterior corneal surface is involved, leading to persistent stromal edema, penetrating keratoplasty is required.

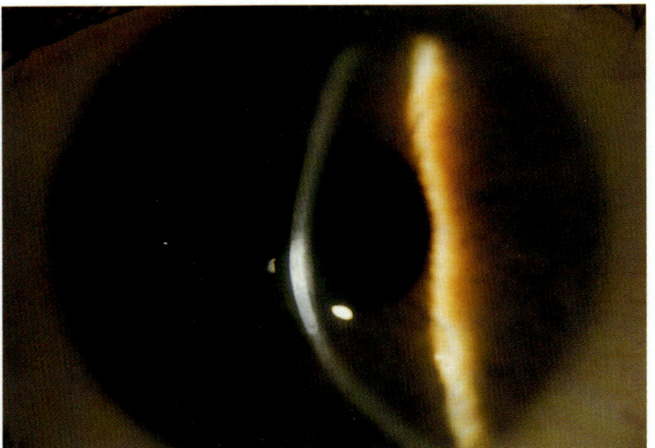

Figure 4.39 Keratoconus. Bilateral condition with cone-like ectasia of the cornea centrally or subcentrally. Progressive thinning, irregular astigmatism, slow or rapid progression. Manifestation at early age. The condition progresses rapidly between the age of 10 and 20, over the age of 30 it usually stabilizes or progression is relatively slow. Vertical lines in the deep stroma are seen (Vogt´s striae) next to the area of thinning. A ring-like deposition of hemosiderin pigment may be present at the base of the cone. The condition can occur in asssociation with various ocular and systemic disorders, including atopia and Down´s syndrome. The diagnosis in early stages is best made with a keratoscope. Initially, spectacle correction is possible. With more pronounced ectasia, rigid contact lenses are fitted in order to compensate for the irregular astigmatism. If lens fit is impossible, penetrating keratoplasty is required. The postoperative prognosis is good.

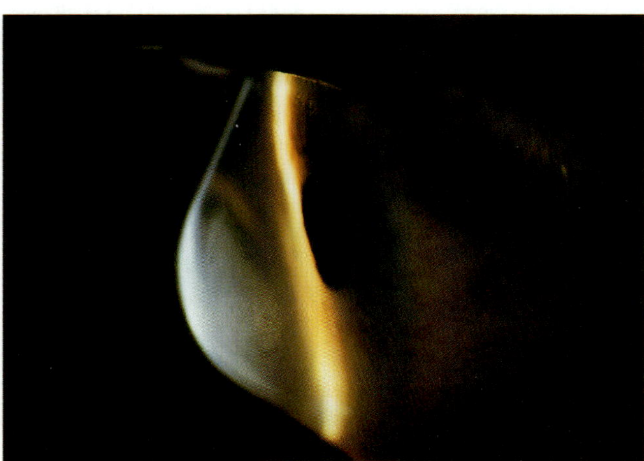

Figure 4.40 Acute hydrops. In advanced stages of keratoconus with extreme corneal thinning, a rupture of Descemet´s membrane can occur. The concomitant endothelial defect allows aqueous humor to transit into the stroma, leading to profound corneal edema. After healing of the rupture and bridging by endothelium, the marked corneal edema may slowly resolve. Penetrating keratoplasty is required, which can also be performed in the acute hydrops.

Figure 4.41 Acute hydrops. The circumscribed grey opacity of the cornea arises from a rupture of Descemet´s membrane and the endothelium. In the case shown here, the condition is relatively limited, spontaneous remission is possible. Penetrating keratoplasty should be performed due to residual scarring and distortion of the cornea.

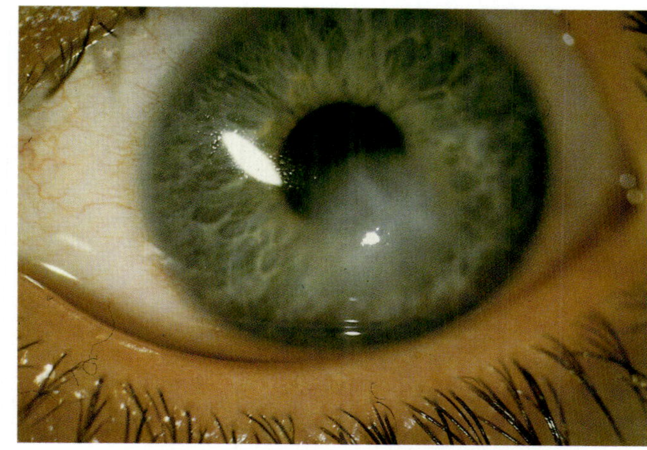

Figure 4.42 Acute hydrops. Patient with atopic dermatitis. The opacity caused by stromal edema extends to the limbus. Despite the severity of the condition, penetrating keratoplasty can be performed with a good prognosis.

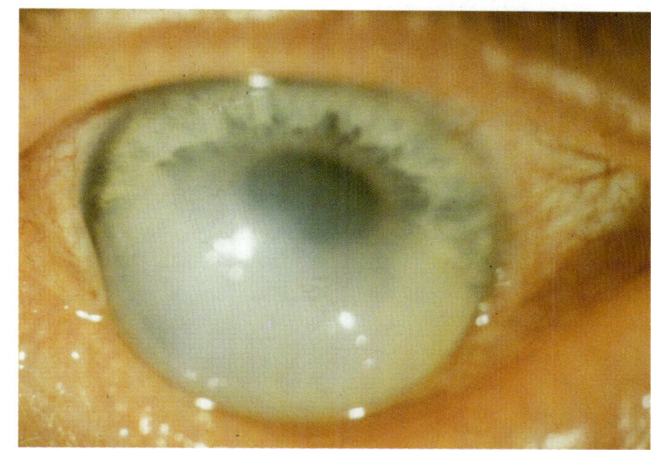

Figure 4.43 Status post penetrating keratoplasty (compare with figure 4.42. Clinical picture 1.5 years after surgery, clear graft, good visual acuity.

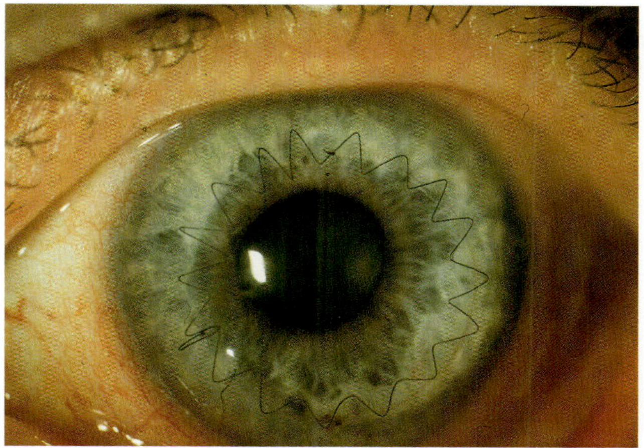

4.4 Corneal dystrophies

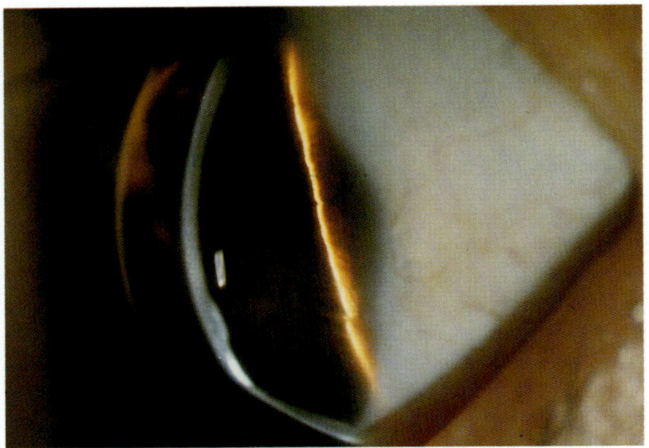

Figure 4.44 Pellucid marginal degeneration (cornea pellucida). The illustration shows marked thinning of the cornea at the inferior limbus. Despite the peripheral localization, the changes in pellucid marginal degeneration are similar to those found in keratoconus. Rarely rupture of Descemet´s memrane with edema occurs. The main problem is the progressive astigmatism. Correction with contact lenses is often impossible. Surgical treatment includes marginal lamellar keratoplasty, which is a technically demanding approach.

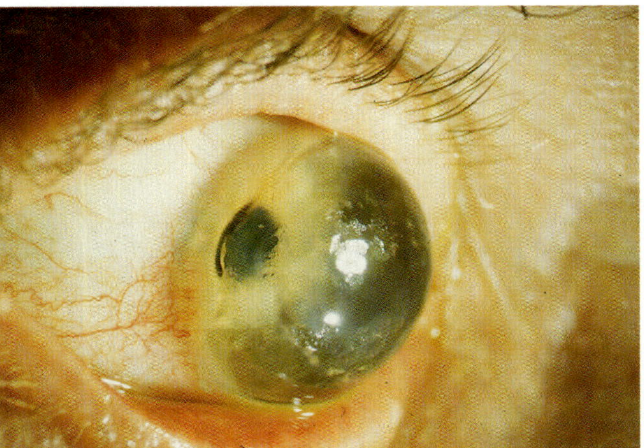

Figure 4.45 Keratoglobus. Extreme ectasia and thinning of the cornea, particularly peripherally. The cornea remains transparent. The protrusion of the cornea causes high myopia with uncorrectable irregular astigmatism. There is risk of perforation. Treatment may consist of lamellar keratoplasty.

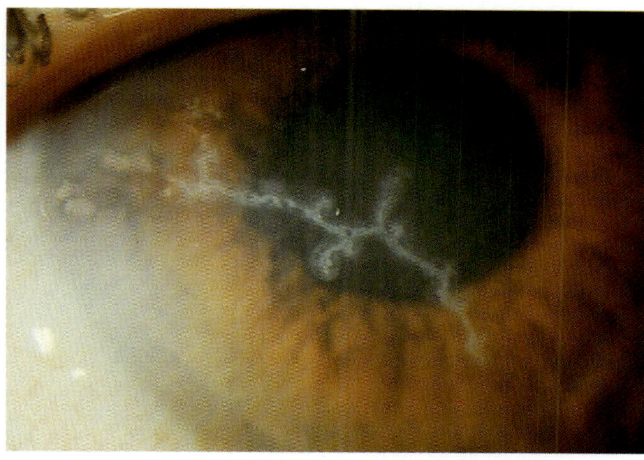

Figure 4.46 Dendritic keratitis. The epithelial infection of the cornea with herpes simplex virus has various clinical manifestations. The figure shows the characteristic picture of dendritic keratitis in the shape of a thin, irregular band with fine branching and terminal bulb formation. The epithelium is defective in these areas. Viruses can be found. The process is confined to the epithelium, the stroma is not involved. Corneal sensitivity measurement may be helpful for diagnosis (reduced sensation in herpes infection). The differential diagnosis includes trophic changes. Treatment consists of topical antiviral agents, in some cases in combination with epithelial abrasion. The condition quickly subsides, if the infection is restricted to the epithelium, but recurrence is possible.

Figure 4.47 Dendritic keratitis. The dendritic figure stains vividly with fluorescein dye. The finding is pathognomonic.

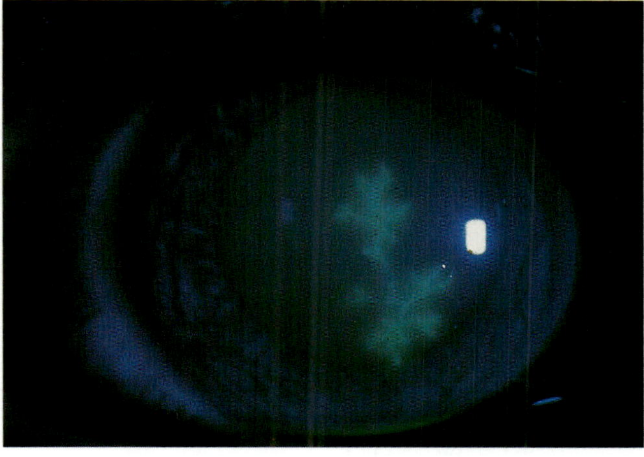

4.5 Corneal infections (viruses, bacteria, fungi, protozoa)

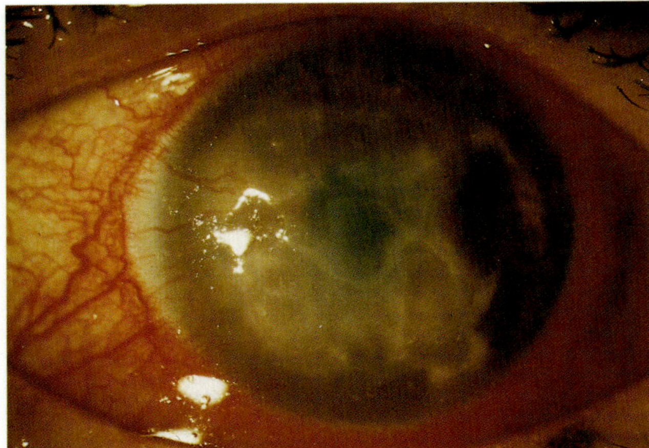

Figure 4.48 Metaherpetic keratitis. Status post long-term treatment of a herpes virus infection with trophic disturbances. The epithelial erosions extend to the anterior stroma. The condition is possibly causally related to trophic disturbances as well as toxicity of antiviral agents. Live virus is not found.

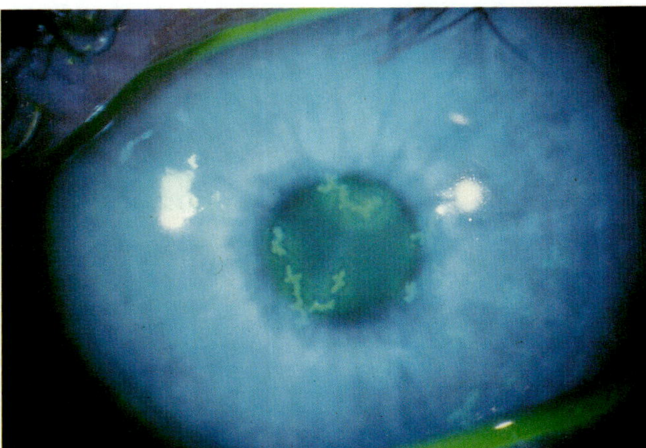

Figure 4.49 Dendritic keratitis in herpes zoster infection. Varizella-zoster virus can cause dendritic keratitis. In contrast to herpes simplex infection, the lesions (pseudodendrites) are smaller and do not have end-bulb formations (compare with figures 4.46 and 4.47). Treatment includes topical corticosteroids, a combination with antiviral agents is possible.

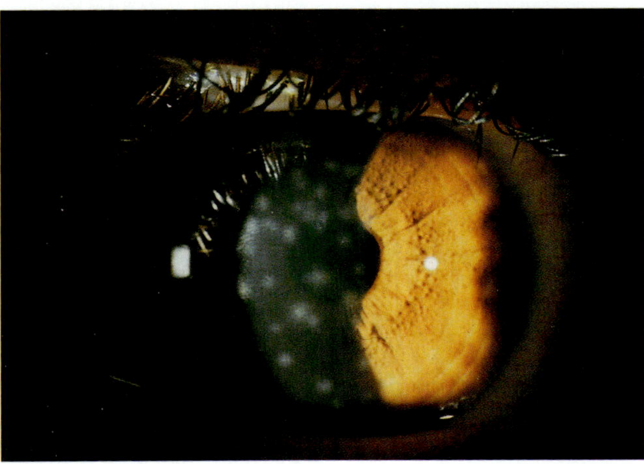

Figure 4.50 Epidemic keratoconjunctivitis (EKC). EKC is caused by adenovirus. The disorder is epidemic and the organism highly infectious. The clinical course is characterized by an initial acute conjunctivitis with hyperemia, chemosis and discharge (see chapter 3). After approximately 3 weeks subepithelial, nummular (coinlike) opacities may form. The opacities slowly diappear spontaneously. No proven therapy.

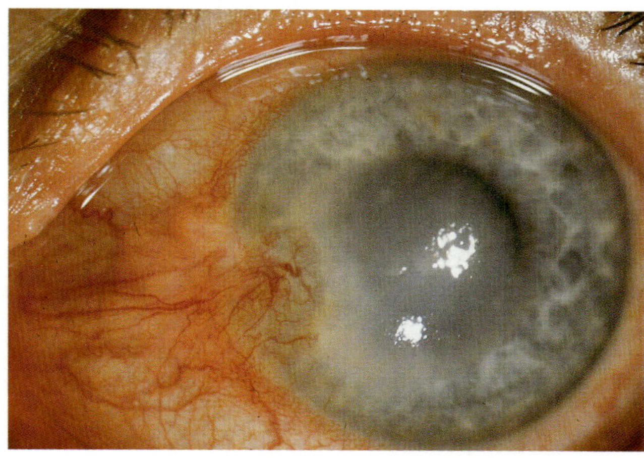

Figure 4.51 Disciform keratitis. Disciform keratitis is mostly a manifestation of herpes simplex virus infection, but may also be caused by other viruses. The typical clinical picture is that of a disc-shaped corneal opacity arising from stromal edema. A characteristic feature is the presence of keratic precipitates, which can be seen at the superior margin of the opacity in the figure. The condition is presumed to be a hypersensitivity reaction to viral infection; therefore, the treatment consits of topical corticosteroids in combination with antiviral agents. An elevation of intraocular pressure frequently occurs.

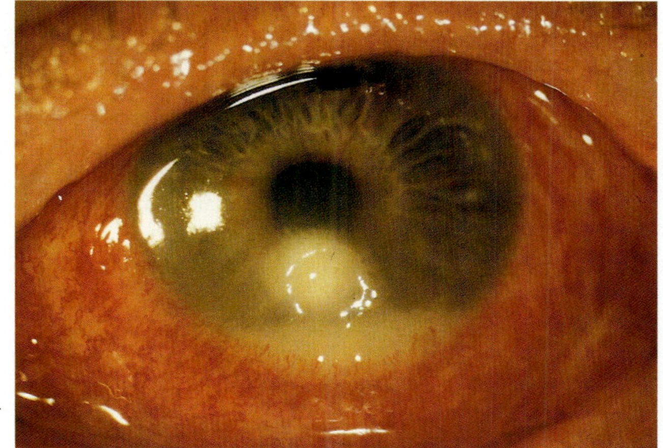

Figure 4.52 Infectious ulcerative keratitis caused by Staphylococcus in atopic dermatitis. The figure shows a round ulcer with deep stromal infiltration, which is well-demarcated towards the clear surrounding stroma, accompanied by hypopyon. The clinical picture is suspicious of Staphylococcus as causative organism, but a diagnosis can only be made by isolation of the organism from material obtained by corneal scraping. Treatment with broad-spectrum antibiotics is initiated beforehand. Patients suffering from atopic dermatitis are predisposed for infections, due to changes in the tear film, corneal surface and depressed cellular immunity.

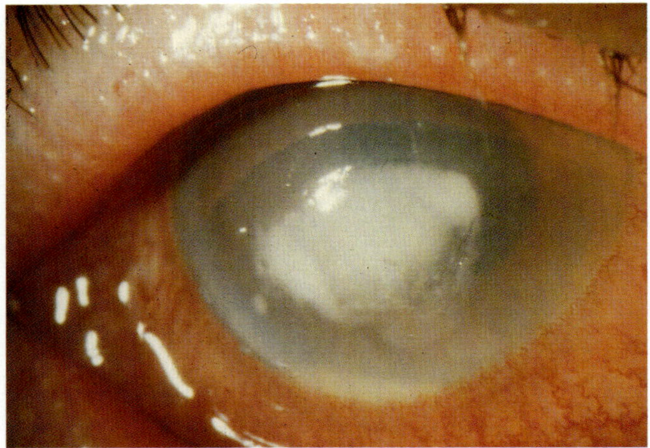

Figure 4.53 Infectious ulcerative keratitis in a patient with alcoholism. Dense, ill-defined area of infiltration, small hypopyon. The clinical picture may be suspicious of a mixed infection. Staphylococcus was isolated. Treatment with broad-spectrum antibiotics has to be initiated before identification of the infectious agent. Alcoholics have an increased incidence of corneal infections.

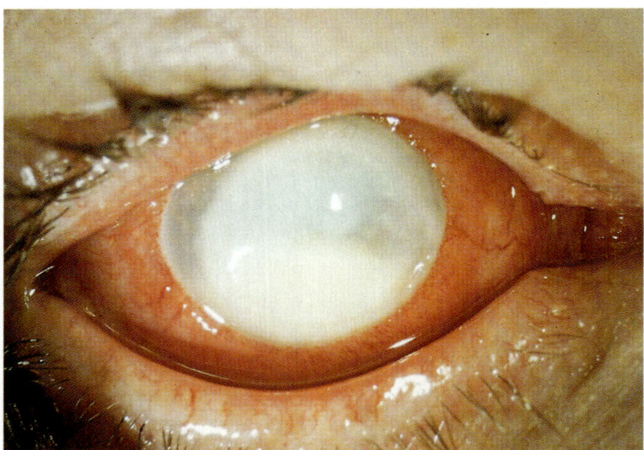

Figure 4.54 Infectious ulcerative keratitis, infection with Pseudomonas. Characteristic feature of bacterial infection with Pseudomonas aeruginosa is a rapidly spreading infiltrate with destruction of large areas of the cornea. Associated hypopyon. The high grade virulence of the germ is caused by lipases, proteases and toxins. Proteolytic enzymes lead to fast corneal destruction. The gram-negative rod Pseudomonas aeruginosa is ubiquitary. Corneal infections frequently occur after trauma or with specific predisposition (atopic dermatitis, diabetes mellitus, alcoholism, contact lens wear). In the present case (figure) keratitis developed after foreign body removal without susbsequent antibiotic treatment.

Figure 4.55 Infectious ulcerative keratitis in diabetes mellitus, status post ocular surgery. Isolation of Enterococci. As in Pseudomonas infection, the corneal infiltrate evolves rapidly and may lead to necrotic corneal destruction with perforation. A green hue is characteristic in this kind of infection. Immediate treatment with high-dose systemic and topical antibiotics is required.

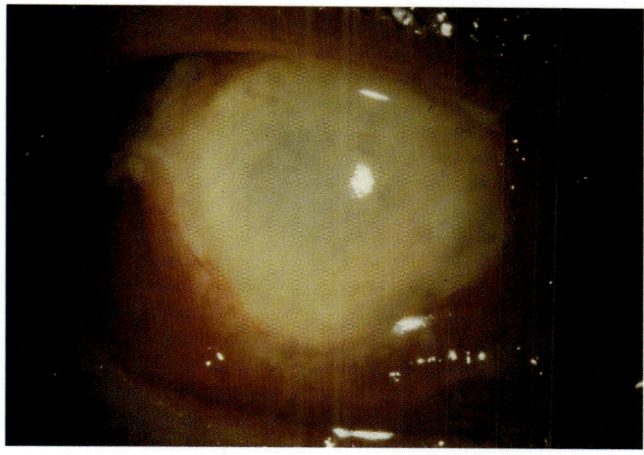

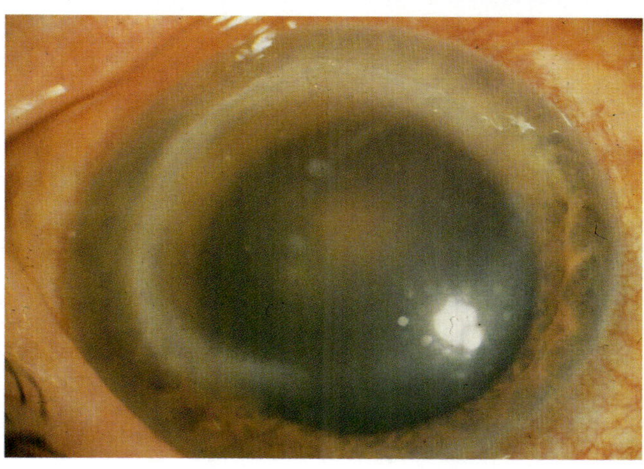

Figure 4.56 Acanthamoeba keratitis in a contact lens wearer. In the rare entity of Acanthamoeba keratitis, various corneal epithelial changes have been described. The clinical picture is nonspecific and may be difficult to differentiate from other infections , especially infections with herpes virus.

Annular infiltrates often form. A characteristic feature is severe ocular pain (radial neuritis). The infection mostly occurs in contact lens wearers with additional predisposing conditions (such as diabetes mellitus). The detection of the protozoa is difficult. Corneal biopsy may be required.

Trophozoites and cysts are found in infected corneas. Treatment is difficult. Diamidine and imidazole derivatives are currently recommended. Penetrating keratoplasty following medical treatment may be performed successfully.

4.5 Corneal infections (viruses, bacteria, fungi, protozoa)

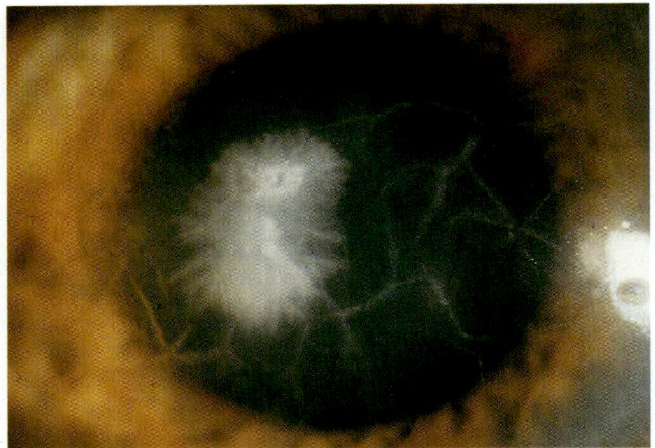

Figure 4.57 Infectious crystalline keratopathy in association with lattice dystrophy. The clinical picture is characterized by crystalline deposits, which show fine fan-shaped branches. There are no signs of ocular irritation! The epithelium is intact! The deposits are located in between the stromal lamellae. For that reason, the detection of the infectious agent is difficult. Chronic course. Long-term antibiotic treatment is required, sometimes keratoplasty. The condition arises from epithelial defects (compare with lattice dystrophy) or following penetrating keratoplasty.

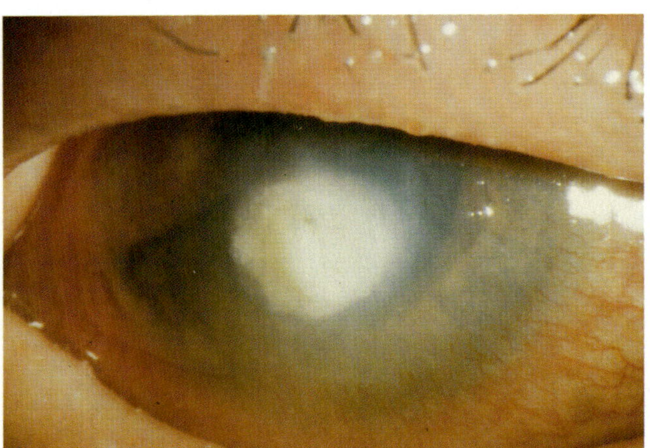

Figure 4.58 Fungal keratitis in a patient with atopic dermatitis. The infiltration caused by infection with yeasts is dense, sharply-demarcated and slightly prominent. Concomitant hypopyon may occur. Mycotic infections of the cornea occur with predisposition (such as atopic dermatitis) or following trauma. Immediate initiation of topical and sometimes systemic treatment with antifungal agents is mandatory. Early penetrating keratoplasty carries a fair prognosis.

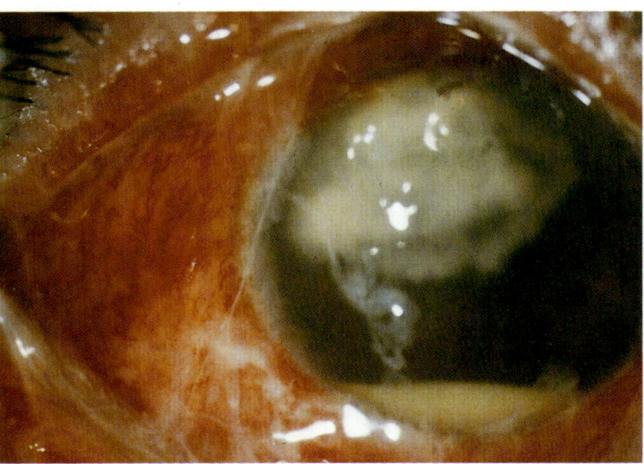

Figure 4.59 Fungal keratitis following anterior segment surgery (phaco, corneal incision). A dense, sharply-demarcated infiltration extends from the incision site to the upper third of the cornea. Concomitant hypopyon. Very rarely fungal infection follows surgical interventions. Immediate topical and systemic antifungal therapy is required.

Figure 4.60 Identification of fungal infection in excised cornea (compare with figure 4.59).

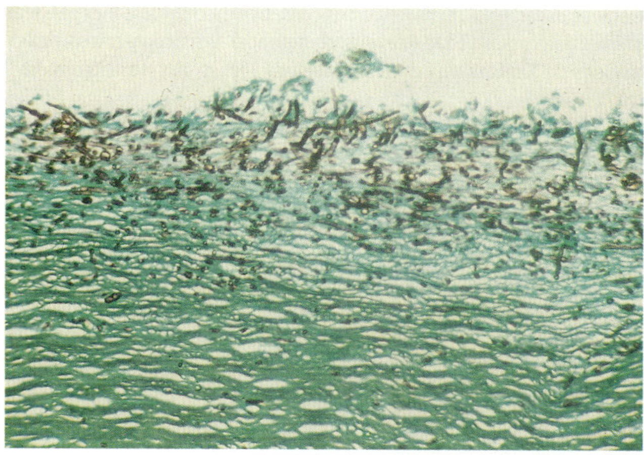

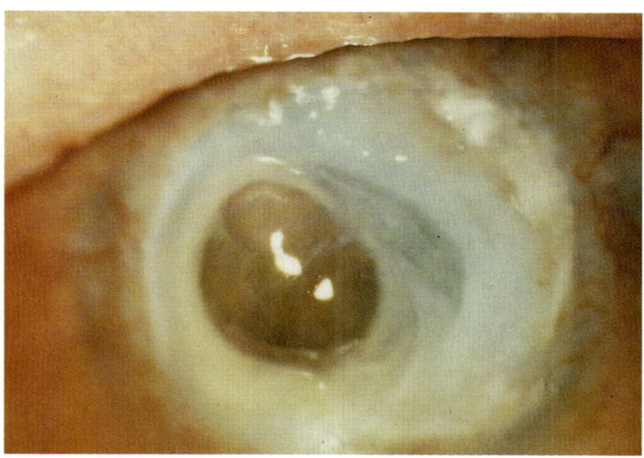

Figure 4.61 Descemetocele-perforation. Status post corneal infection with gramnegative bacteria. The superficial layers of the central cornea have melted away leaving a thin membrane (descemetocele), through which the iris is visible. In the nasal upper aspect, the descemetocele lies anterior to the iris tissue, inferior temporally a perforation has occured with prolapsed iris tissue. The remaining cornea is densely infiltrated. Conditions like this develop in patients with predisposition for corneal infections, highly virulent organisms and insufficient treatment.

4.6 Noninfectious keratitis

General: Keratitis can have various causative mechanisms independent of infectious agents (due to exposure, neuroparalysis, contact lens wear, inadequate lubrication, exogenous noxious agents, drug toxicity, irradiation).

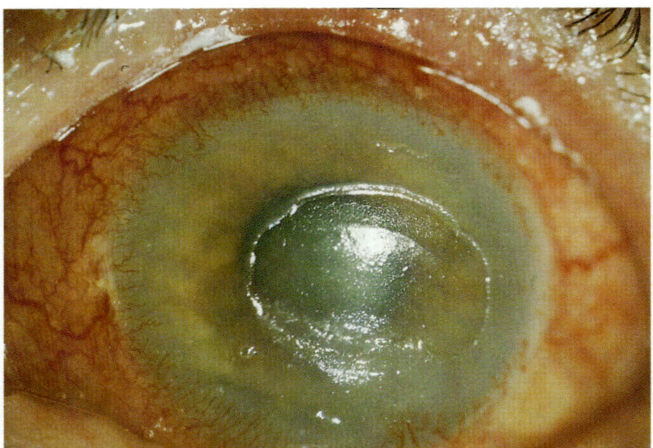

Figure 4.62   Exposure keratitis in lagophthalmos. In incomplete eyelid closure (in this case due to facial nerve palsy), the corneal surface dries out, resulting in a large erosion within the interpalpebral fissure. The resulting epithelial defect is sharply demarcated (see figure). Treatment includes surgery for improvement of eyelid position and corneal protection with lubricants and patching.

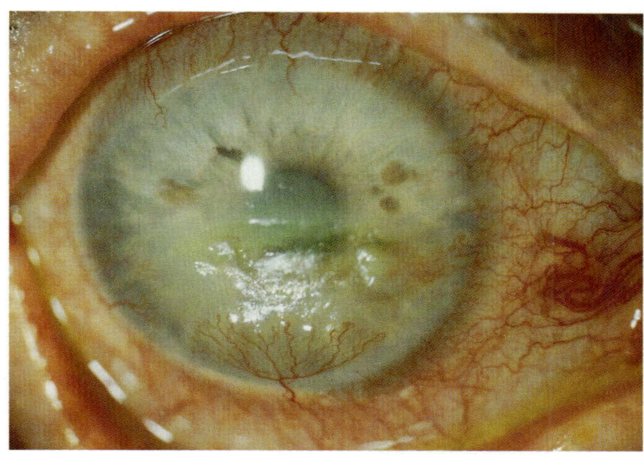

Figure 4.63 Neurotrophic keratitis following trauma of trigeminal nerve. A horizontal defect within the interpalpebral fissure with elevated, grey edges is characteristic. The defect involves the epithelium and the superficial stroma (long standing superficial defect). Sensitivity testing is important for the diagnosis. Neurotrophic keratitis can also develop after viral infection. An involvement of deeper ocular structures with iritis has been described. Treatment consists of ocular lubricants as well as topical antibiotics to protect against bacterial superinfection. Tarsorrhaphy can be considered for severe cases.

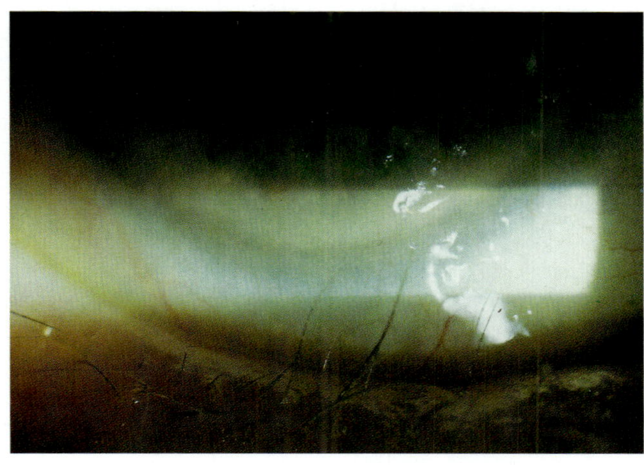

Figure 4.64 Misdirection of eyelashes, trichiasis. Misdirected eyelashes are a frequent cause of superficial defects of the cornea. There is an increased risk of bacterial infection. Treatment consists of removal of eyelashes with cryotherapy, sometimes eyelid surgery is required.

4.6 Noninfectious keratitis

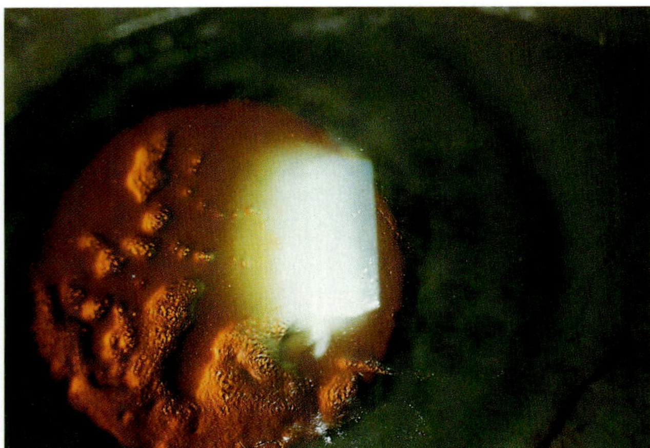

Figure 4.65 Corneal epithelial defects due to trichiasis, same patient as in figure 4.64. Retro-illumination reveals an uneven corneal surface with epithelial defects. The changes are caused by misdirected eyelashes.

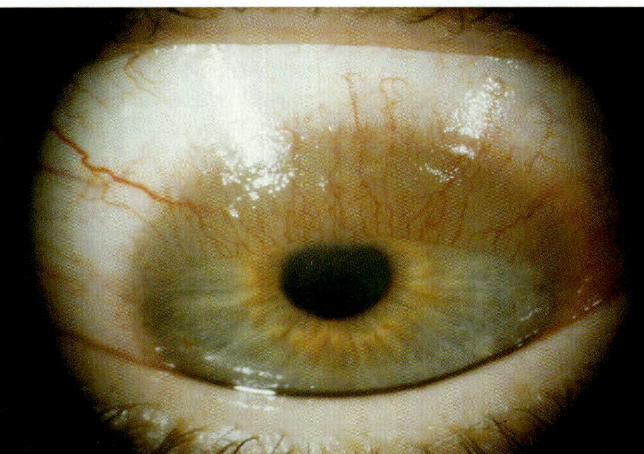

Figure 4.66 Pannus. Normally, the cornea is free of vessels. The formation of vascularized connective tissue in between the epithelium and Bowman´s layer is determined pannus. The condition may have various causes.

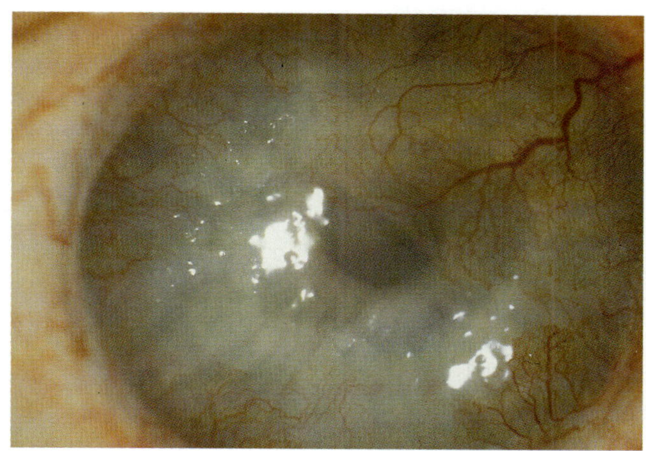

Figure 4.67 Conjunctivalization. An ingrowth of the conjunctiva to the cornea can be observed in various conditions. The conjunctiva can invade large areas of the cornea, leading to severe visual impairment. The condition is thought to be causally related to changes in the basal cells of the corneal limbus. These limbal cells can be damaged by trauma, chemical burns, surgery, hypersensitivity and contact lenses. The transplantation of intact limbal tissue is one possible therapeutic concept. Long-term results have not yet been provided.

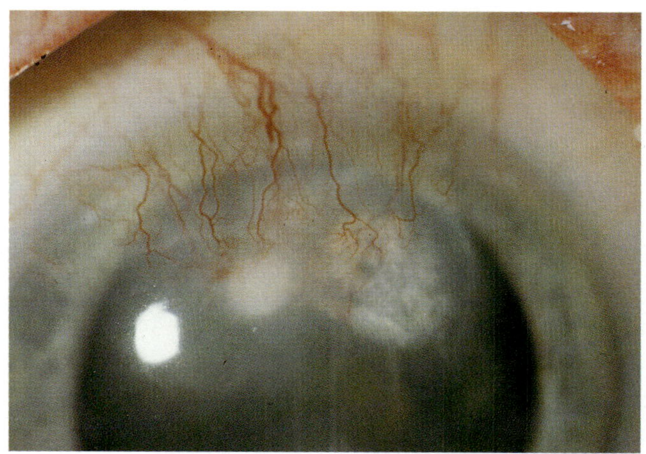

Figure 4.68 Superficial vascularization, status post herpes keratitis. In infectious processes of the peripheral cornea, subsiding of the inflammation is often accompanied with corneal vascularization starting from the limbus. The finding is usually stationary. Treatment consists of ocular lubricants. Depending on the caustive mechanism, treatment with topical corticosteroids can be considered.

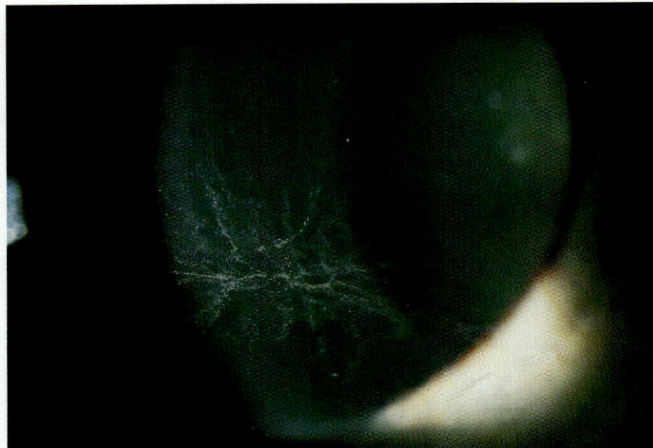

Figure 4.69 Cornea verticillata following amiodarone therapy. After treatment with certain drugs or in connection with systemic diseases, a whirl-like opacification of the corneal epithelium develops. The figure shows fine, grey-brown, whirl-like condensations in the interpalpebral cornea following long-term treatment with amiodarone. The abnormality does usually not result in vision loss.

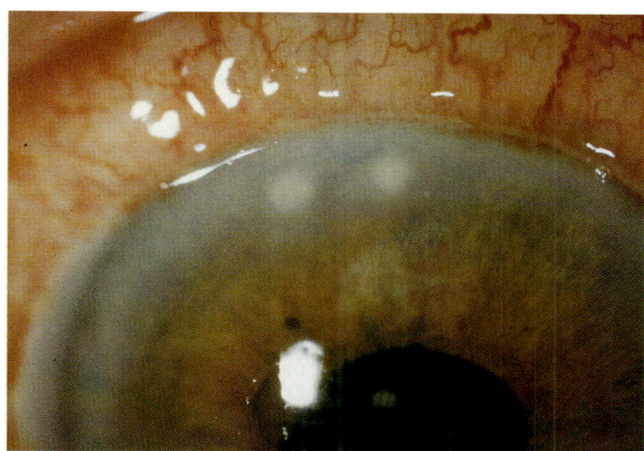

Figure 4.70 Staphylococcal marginal keratitis. The condition is characterized by infiltrates in the peripheral cornea, which are separated from the limbus by a lucid interval. Superficial ulceration may develop with rupture of the epithelium overlying the infiltrates. The condition is interpreted as a hypersensitivity reaction to staphylococcal toxins. Treatment consits of topical steroids following short-term application of topical antibiotics. The infiltrates usually resolve quickly under treatment.

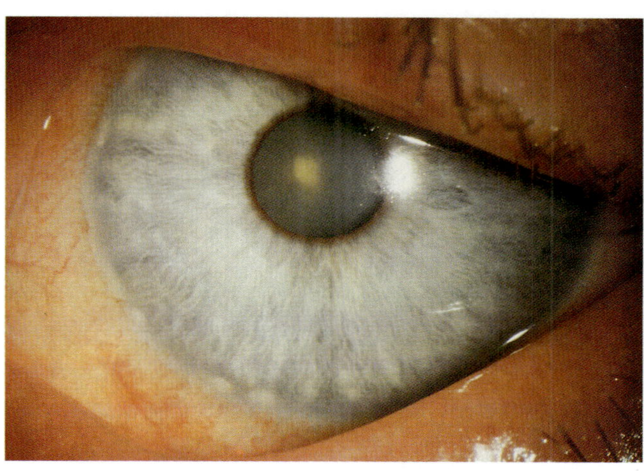

Figure 4.71 Multiple marginal infiltrates. Cause, therapy and course see figure 4.70.

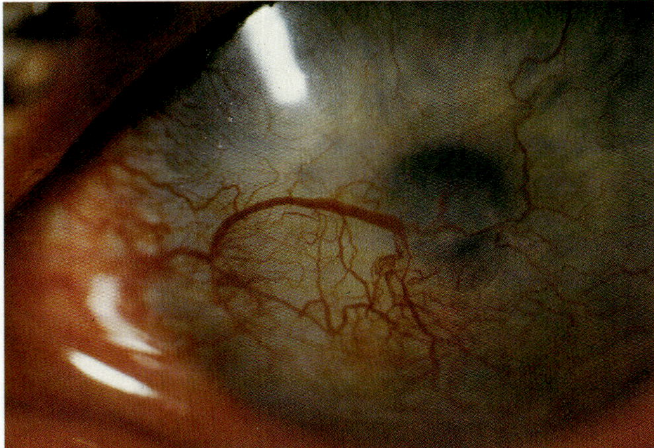

Figure 4.72 Conjunctivalization. Following long-term hypersensitivity reaction with conjunctivitis and superficial keratitis, the conjunctiva has invaded the corneal surface. The condition is thought to be related to damage of the limbal stem cells.

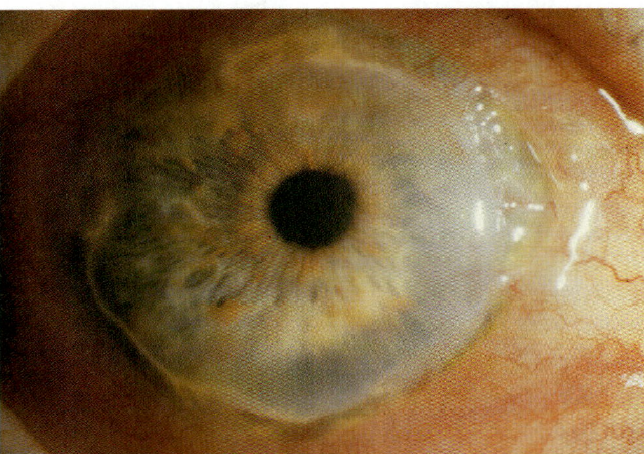

Figure 4.73 Marginal corneal melting in Wegener granulomatosis. The typical corneal manifestation of Wegener granulomatosis includes peripheral infiltrations associated with melting, which may result in centrally progressive circular ulceration with rolled-under edges. The systemic vasculitis has various ocular manifestations. The corneal changes are characteristic and sometimes lead to the diagnosis. Systemic immunosuppressive treatment with corticosteroids and cytostatic agents can relieve the condition. Topical treatment shows no effect.

Figure 4.74 Marginal corneal melting suggestive of systemic connective tissue disease, such as Wegener granulomatosis or collagenosis.

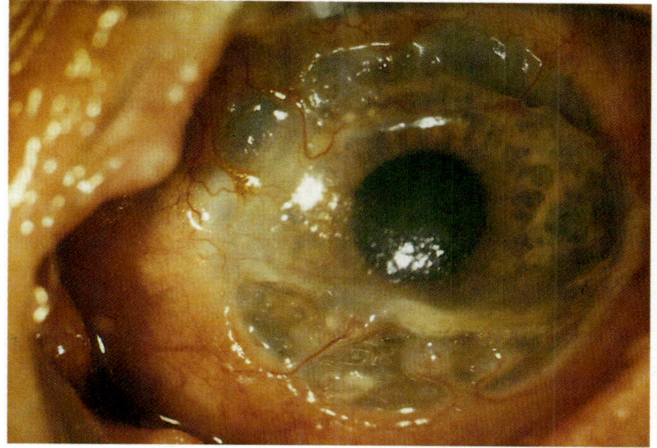

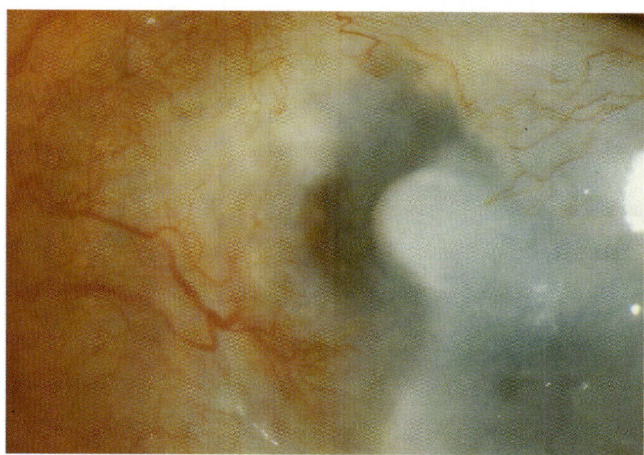

Figure 4.75 Mooren´s ulcer. Peripheral progressive melting of corneal epithelium and superficial stroma. Characteristic features are the undermined central edges of the ulcerative process and the associated severe pain. The deeper corneal layers are preserved with progressive scarring. Perforation does usually not occur. The condition is a localized autoimmune inflammatory process. Systemic connective tissue disease must be exluded. No effective treatment is available. Systemic immunosuppression is not indicated. Conjunctival resection adjacent to the ulcer is recommended.

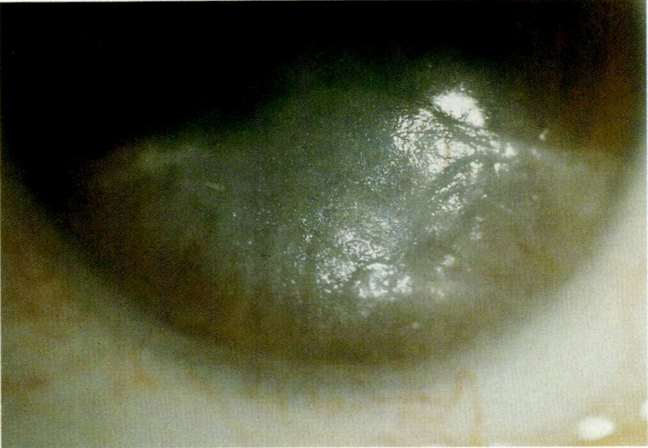

Figure 4.76 Systemic amyloidosis, corneal deposits. The grey-white, slightly elevated lesions consist of deposited immunoglobulins. No inflammation is present. Central localization results in severe visual impairment. Corneal deposits are a rare manifestation of this entity. Other ocular changes, such as ophthalmoplegia resulting from polyneuropathy may occur more often. An amyloidosis restricted to the cornea is found secondarily to degenerations or dystrophies (compare with 4.4).

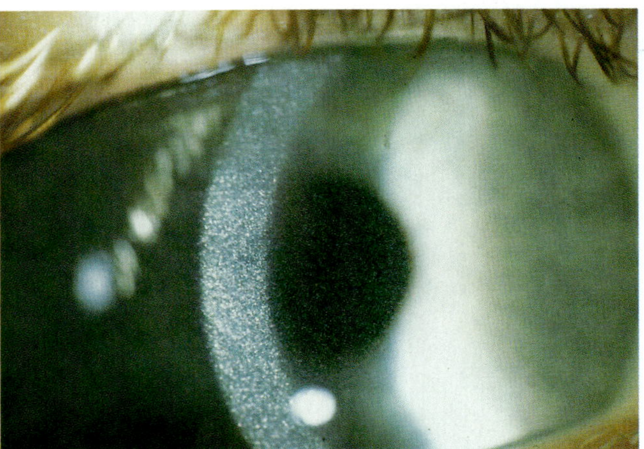

Figure 4.77 Cystinosis. Crystalline corneal deposits. In cystinosis, crystalline deposits are found in various ocular tissues. The figure shows fine crystals throughout the entire cornea. The deposition begins peripherally in the superficial corneal layers and advances to the entire corneal thickness. Corneal and retinal changes representing ocular involvement in infantile cystinosis develop in the first months of life. The ocular findings are pathognomonic. In cases without retinopathy, visual acuity is fairly good. The patients complain of severe photophobia. Treatment with cysteamine eyedrops can be considered.

Figure 4.78 Cystinosis. Corneal findings, enlarged view. The crystalline deposits are located in the keratocytes.

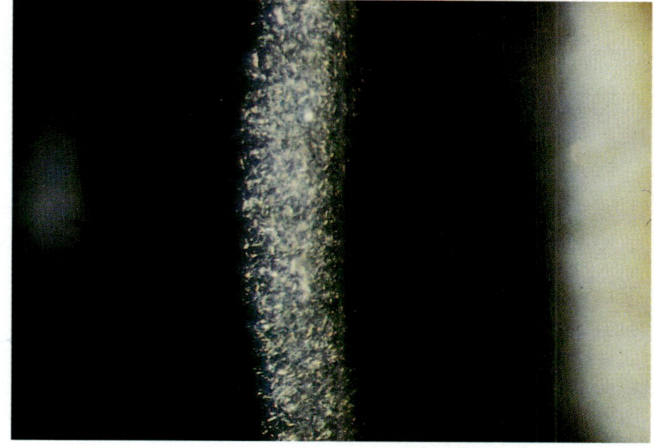

Figure 4.79 Diffuse corneal opacity resulting from fine, granular deposits. This finding is suggestive of paraproteinemia. Systemic evaluation should be performed.

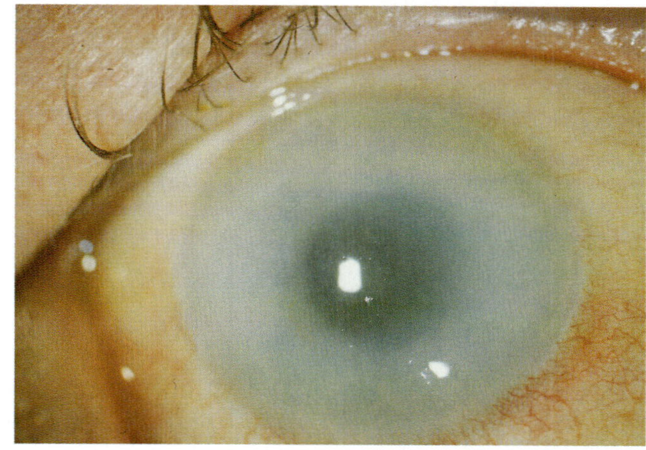

Figure 4.80 Kayser-Fleischer ring, Wilson´s disease. The cornea shows a band of red-brown color at the limbus. The pigmentation starts in the superior and inferior aspects of the corneal periphery and then spreads towards the horizontal plane. It consits of copper deposits in the deep corneal layers (Descemet, endothelium). In advanced stages, the finding is macroscopically visible. The Kayser-Fleischer ring is pathognomonic and may lead to an early diagnosis. The corneal changes can disappear with D-penicillamine treatment.

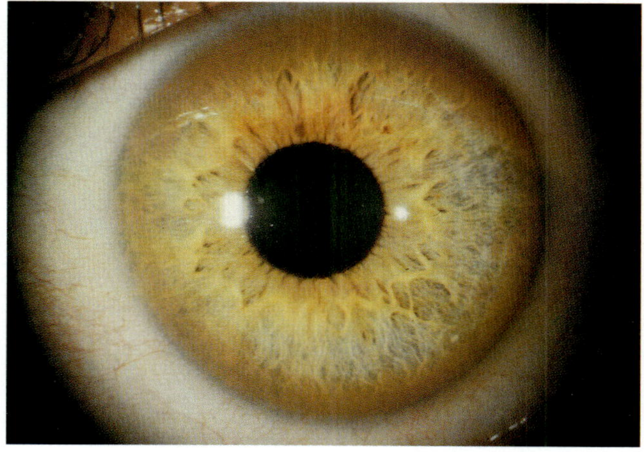

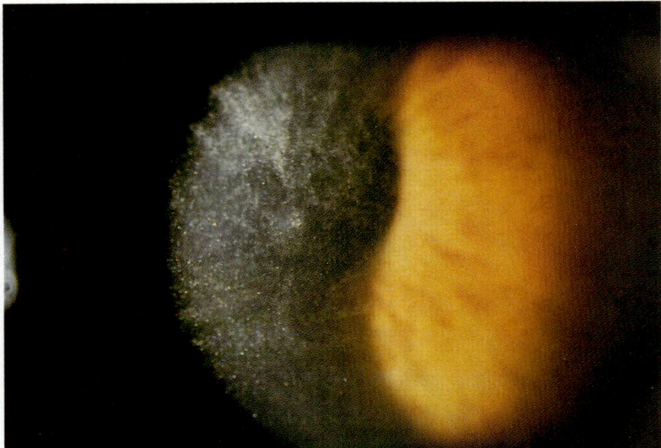

Figure 4.81 Cornea verticillata, Fabry´s disease. The characteristic corneal finding consits of fine, grey- white, whirl-like opacities in the subepithelial layers. The opacities result from deposition of glycoshingolipids. Visual impairment is rare. The ocular findings occur early, they are pathognomonic.

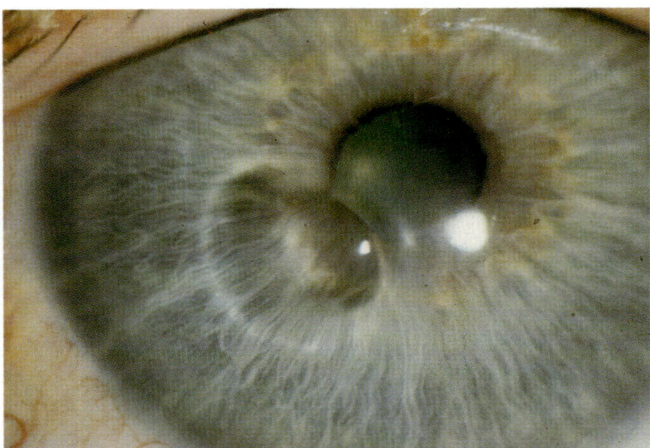

Figure 4.82 Descemetocele in rheumatic disease. In rheumatic disease, peripheral and paracentral keratolysis occurs. The figure shows a paracentral desecemetocele without signs of inflammation. Corneal melting in rheumatic diseases is characteristically symptom-free. The cause remains unclear, there is no effective treatment. Recurrences of keratolyses after keratoplasty are frequent.

General: Tumors consisting of corneal tissue are rare, neoplastic changes usually occur at the limbus.

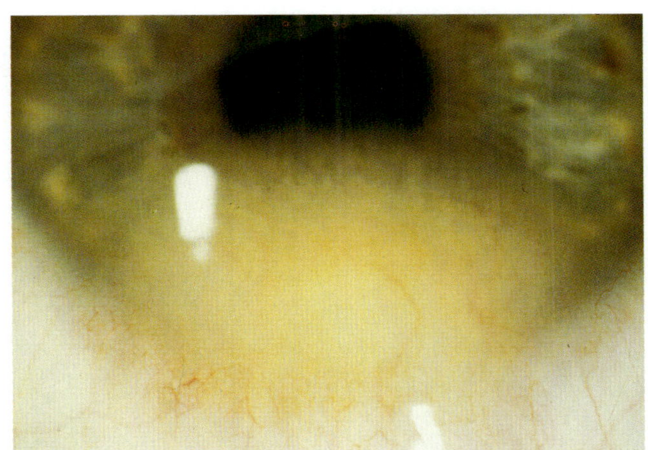

Figure 4.83   Fibrous histiocytoma. The tumor consists of fibroblasts and histiocytes. It arises from the limbus and infiltrates the cornea. The tumor is benign and does not metastasize. Treatment consists of surgical excision.

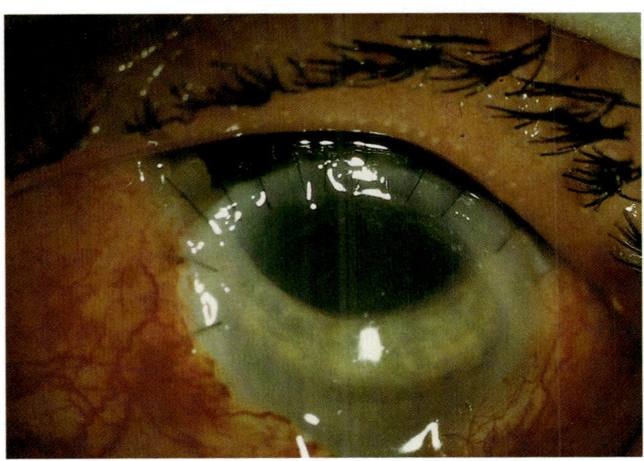

Figure 4.84   Fibrous histiocytoma, status post surgical excision and keratoplasty. The tumor, which had spread into the deeper corneal layers and the sclera was completely excised.

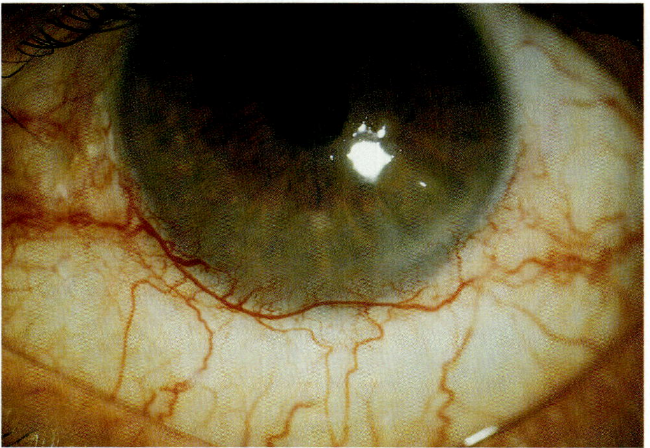

Figure 4.85 Carcinoma in situ. The intraepithelial neoplasia is located at the limbus, growth is slow. The clinical diagnosis is difficult. Increased filling of the conjunctival vessels at the limbus is a conspicuous feature. Corneal superficial changes occur as a result of limbal destruction. The condition is painful, irrespective of the low degree of corneal changes. In this case (figure), the diagnosis was made by corneal biopsy. Therapy consits of surgical excision followed by lamellar keratoplasty.

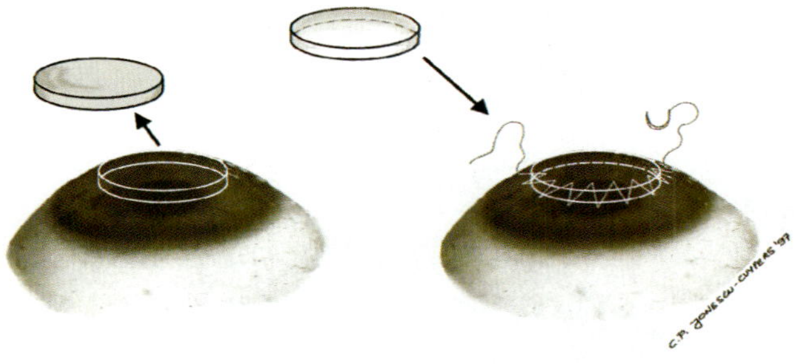

Figure 4.86 Penetrating keratoplasty, surgical technique. In penetrating keratoplasty, a central corneal button is trephined and a graft button is sutured in place.

The prognosis depends on the underlying diagnosis. Postoperative problems arise from immunologic reactions and superficial changes. In lamellar keratoplasty, only the superficial layers of the cornea are replaced. Immunologic reactions are less important, since the endothelium is preserved.

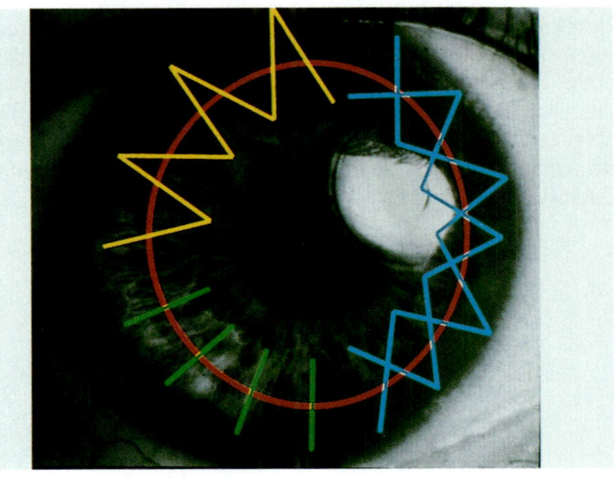

Figure 4.87 Schema of different suturing techniques in penetrating keratoplasty. *Yellow* single running suture; *blue* double running suture; *green* interrupted sutures. Interrupted sutures are indicated if loosening is expected in the post-operative course.

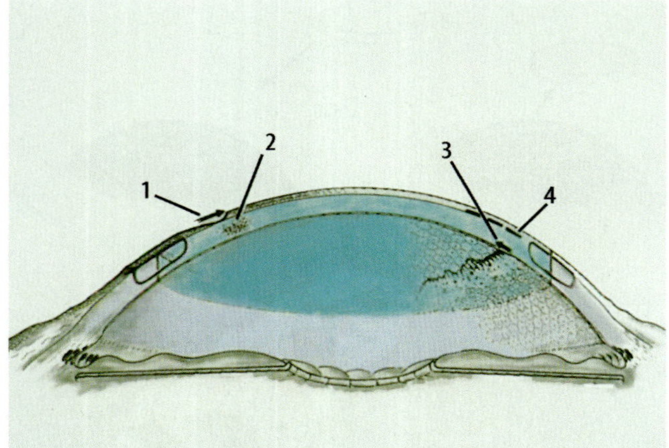

Figure 4.88   Main types of corneal allograft immune reaction. Schema of the various localizations of immune reactions in the graft tissue. Immune reactions can occur separately in the individual corneal layers and offer a distinct clinical picture, (1) epithelial, (2) stromal, (3) endothelial, (4) subepithelial.

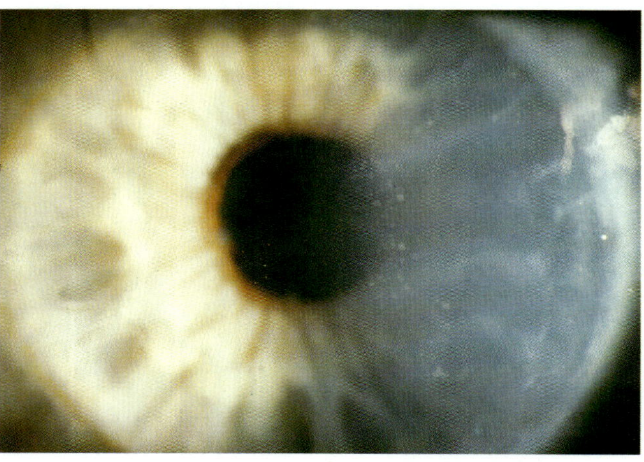

Figure 4.89   Endothelial immune reaction. Opacification of one third of the corneal graft. Fine keratic precipitates form an irregular line at the central margin of the opacity. In this immunologic process, cytotoxic lymphocytes transited from the host cornea to the graft. The endothelium has been destroyed and corneal edema has ensued in the affected area. The linear keratic precipitates mark the border of the corneal area affected by the immunologic process. The line is termed Khodadoust-line. Intensive immunosuppressive treatment is indicated. Clearing of the cornea can thereby be achieved, although the endothelium remains partially damaged.

Figure 4.90 Status post penetrating keratoplasty. Immune reaction with few precipitates. Precipitates, which are restricted to the graft cornea, are a sign of immunologic reaction. In this case (figure), the endothelium has not been completely destroyed. The graft cornea is still clear. A clear graft cornea can be preserved with immunosuppressive treatment.

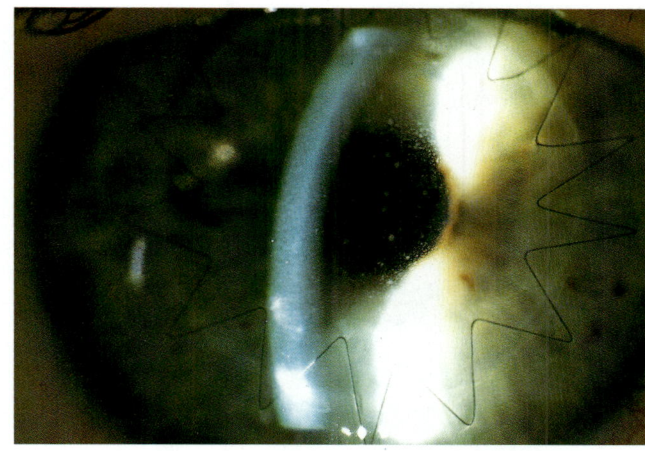

Figure 4.91 Status post penetrating keratoplasty. Subepithelial immune reaction. Characteristic picture: small, round, grey opacities in the superficial corneal layers, restricted to the graft tissue. The opacities are a sign of immunologic reaction. The reaction can be controlled with immunosuppressive treatment (topical corticosteroids). There is no permanent damage, since the endothelium is not involved.

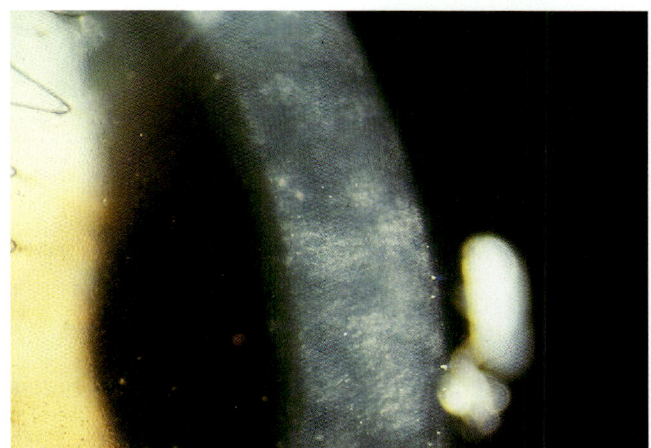

Figure 4.92 Radial keratotomy. In radial keratotomy, the cornea is radially incised to alter the corneal curvature in such a manner, that myopia is corrected. RK is used to correct low to moderate myopia. Disadvantages of the procedure: fluctuation of refraction causing fluctuation of vision, glare, occasionally increased risk of infection, reduced corneal stability towards trauma.

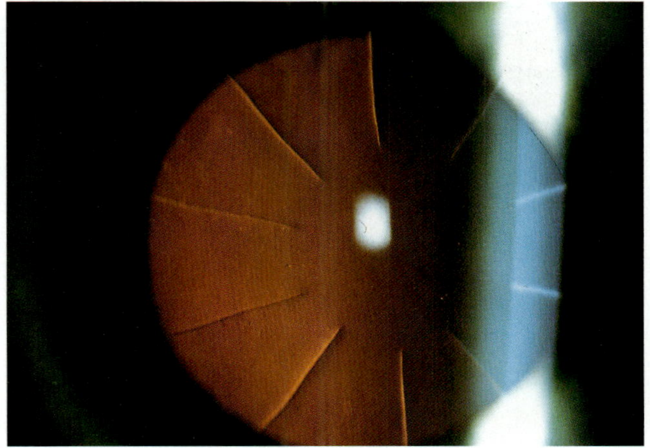

4.10 Keratoplasty and refractive corneal surgery

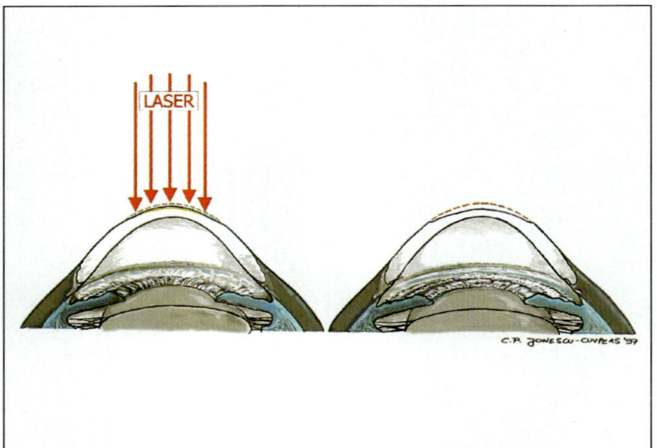

Figure 4.93 Photorefractive keratectomy (PRK, Excimer laser), schema. A flattening of the cornea can be achieved by laser ablation of the superficial layers in order to correct initial myopia. The technique is used to correct low to moderate myopia. The results in low myopia are very good.

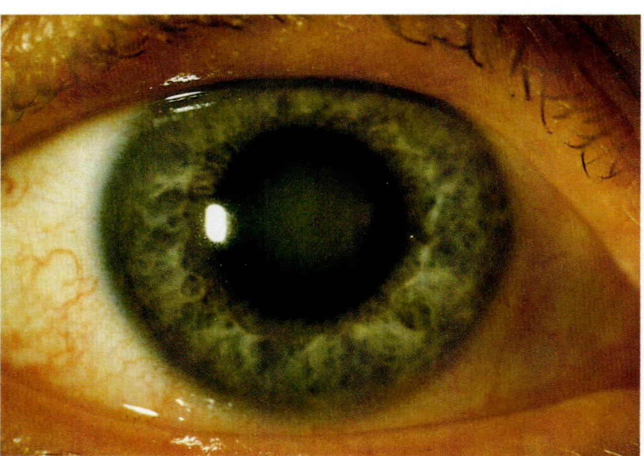

Figure 4.94 Status post photorefractive keratectomy (PRK, Excimer laser). A fine reticular haze in the area of corneal ablation is a frequent complication following PRK. The opacity usually resolves under treatment with topical corticosteroids.

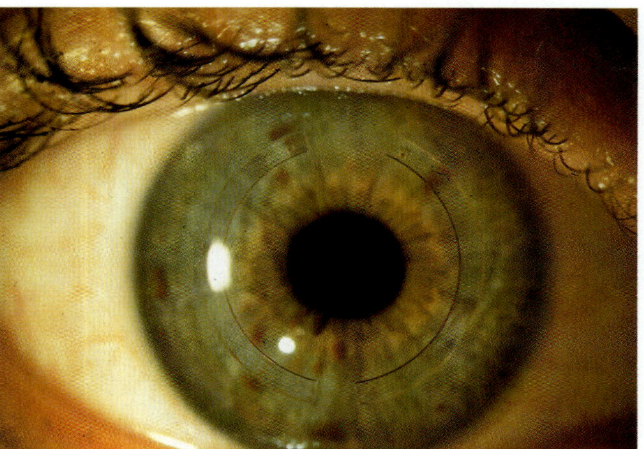

Figure 4.95 Intracorneal ring. An intracorneal ring has recently been applied in the correction of myopia. The polymethylmethacrylate (PMMA) ring is implanted into the corneal stroma in the mid-periphery. The obtained refraction can be controlled by variation of the thickness of the ring. Increasing clinical experience is being gained.

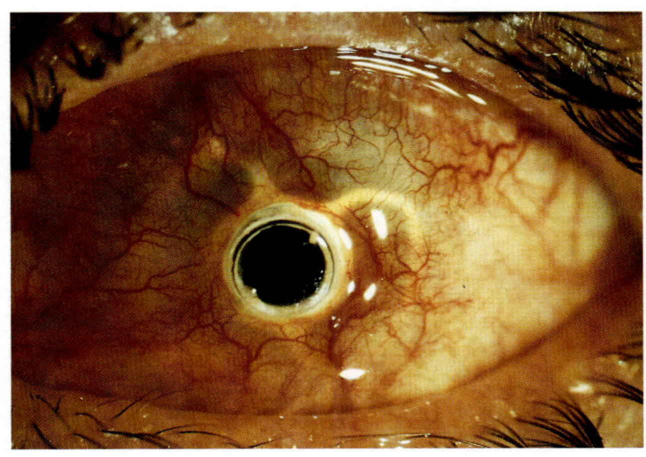

Figure 4.96 Keratoprosthesis. Severly damaged eyes with contraindications for penetrating keratoplasty are considered for permanent implantation of an artificial cornea, provided that the deeper ocular segments are intact.

Sclera

5

5.1 Applied anatomy and examination techniques

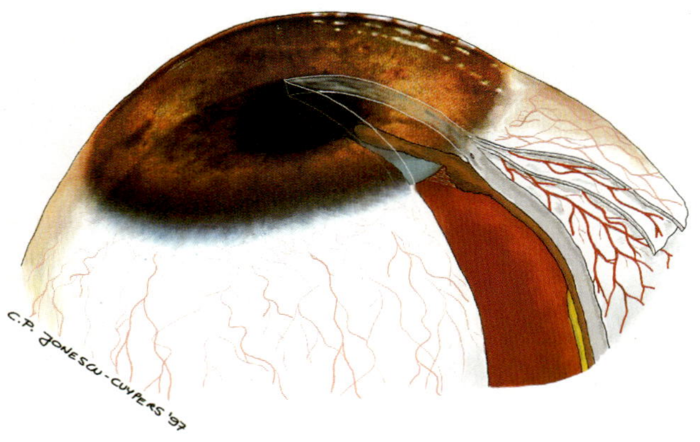

Figure 5.1 Anatomy of the sclera with adjacent cornea (schematic drawing). The sclera is a rigid, opaque tissue, which extends from the limbus to the optic nerve and covers 90% of the globe. The sclera varies in thickness with 0.3 mm immediately behind the rectus muscle tendinous insertions, 0.5 mm at the equator and 1.0 mm at the posterior pole. The anterior portion forms the scleral spur at the corneoscleral junction (compare with chapter 4). The sclera itself is relatively avascular, it is supplied by the overlying dense episcleral vasculature. The irregular arrangement of collagen fibrils of variable size accounts for the opaqueness of intact scleral tissue. Inflammations can lead to a rearrangement of the collagen fibrils, resulting in a change of color, which may resemble thinning of the tissue.

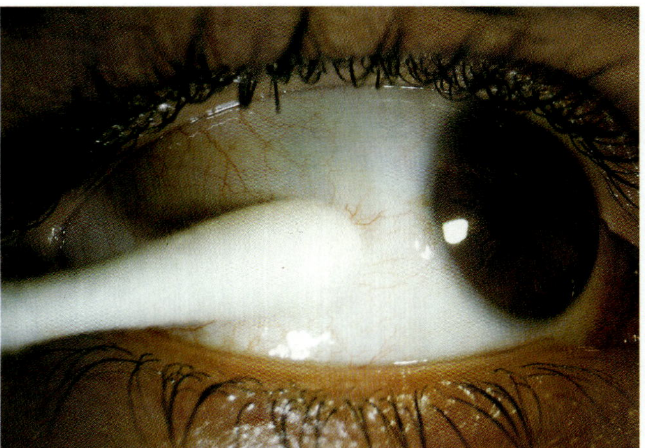

Figure 5.2 Scleral examination, pressure sensitivity testing. This test provides important diagnostic information in the red eye. It can easily be performed with a Q-tip. In episceritis, there is no or mild pain, whereas in scleritis, the patient complains of severe pain. Besides pressure sensitivity testing, the evaluation of vascular injection (compare with figures 5.7 and 5.8) and scleral thickness (compare with figure 5.15) are important for the diagnosis.

Figure 5.3 Senile scleral plaque. The figure shows an oval, grey, well-circumscribed area located anterior to the medial rectus muscle. The condition is considered an aging change. The scleral structure is altered in the affected area, there is no thinning.

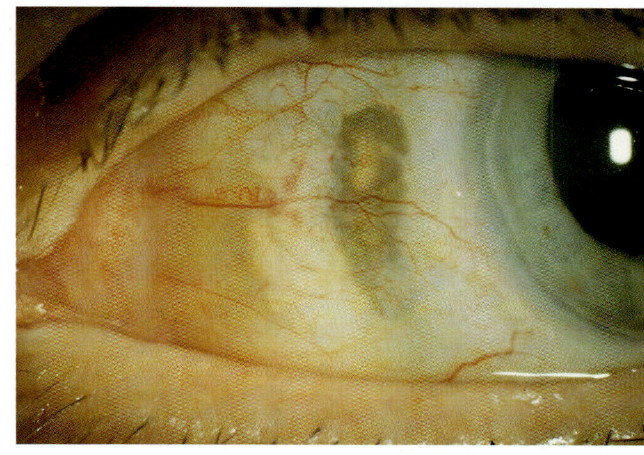

Figure 5.4 Melanosis. A localized, non-progressive dark-grey pigmentation of the sclera mostly is a harmless finding caused by migration of melanocytes. Extensive dark pigmentation can occur in systemic disorders (ochronosis, osteogenesis imperfecta, Ehlers-Danlos syndrome). The blue sclera found in osteogenesis imperfecta results from scleral thinning. Systemic evaluation is important.

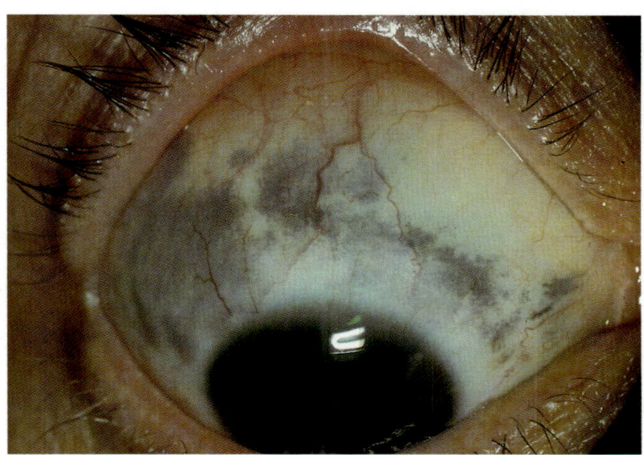

Figure 5.5 Scleral icterus, jaundice. The yellow hue of the sclera can be so intense, that the ophthalmologic finding may lead to the diagnosis of a hepatic / biliary disorder. Systemic evaluation is important. Reversible changes that resemble scleral icterus may occur after i.v. injection of fluorescein dye (compare with retinal examination).

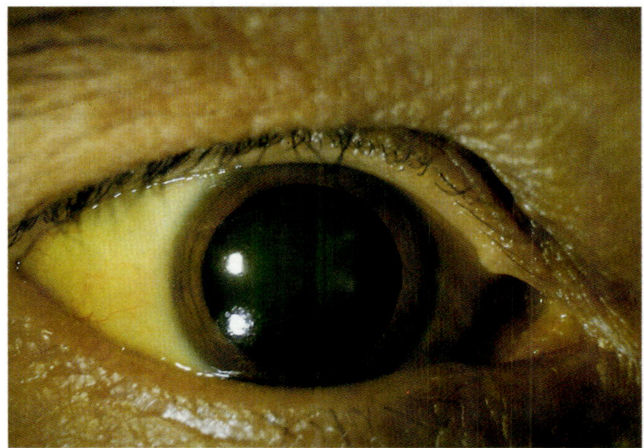

5.3 Inflammations

General: Inflammations of the sclera can occur as episcleritis and scleritis. A differentiation of the two distinct entities is important because of their different prognosis. Both may appear diffuse or nodular, their appearance upon slitlamp examination is similar.
Compare with figure 5.2 for examination techniques.

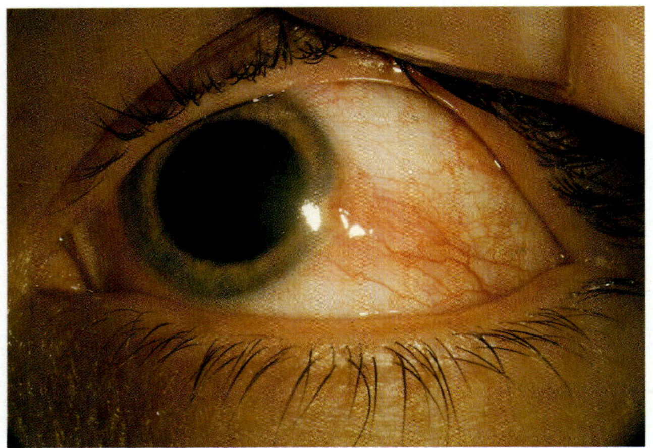

Figure 5.6 Episcleritis, sectorial, circumscribed. The figure shows congested vessels of linear arrangement within the interpalpebral fissure and minor corneal involvement. This is the characteristic picture of episcleritis. Important diagnostic features are the linear, radial arrangement of vessels and their non-adherence to the sclera. Watery discharge is ususally present. Episcleritis and the concomitant corneal changes usually resolve spontaneously without complications. Locally applied nonsteroidal anti-inflammatory drugs (NSAIDs) or corticosteroids may be used. In recurrent disease medical evaluation should be conducted in order to rule out rheumatic disease.

Figure 5.7   Diffuse episcleritis. Episcleritis can affect large areas of the ocular surface. Diagnosis compare with figure 5.6. The differentiation from scleritis may be difficult. Medical evaluation in recurrent disease.

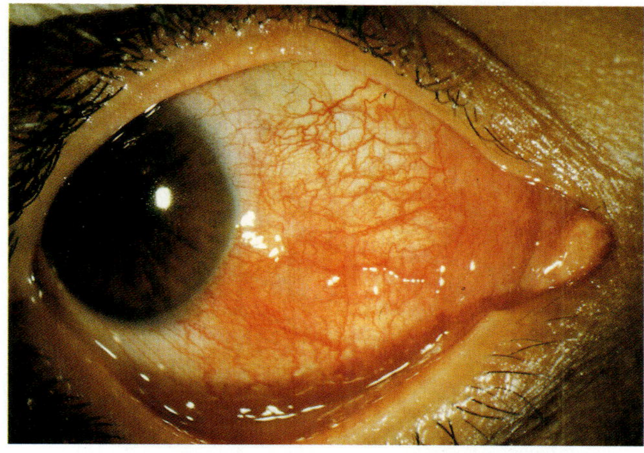

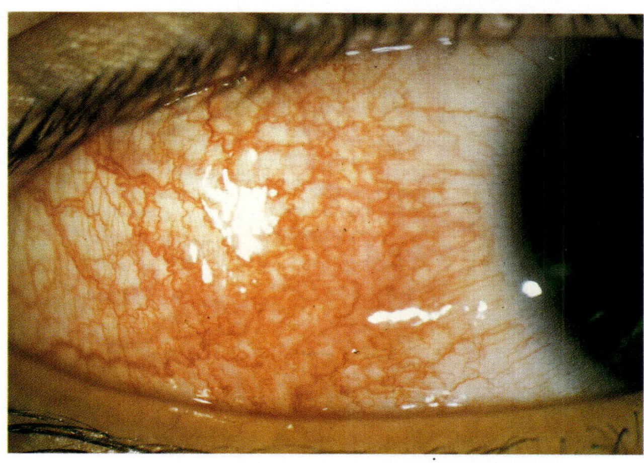

Figure 5.8   Scleritis. Unlike episcleritis, scleritis has a poor prognosis. The differentiation from episcleritis may be very difficult, for scleritis is always accompanied by episcleritis. The arrangement of the congested vessels is irregular, there may be a bluish tinge. Marked pressure sensitivity is the most important diagnostic feature. In scleritis, the involvement of the cornea and the deeper ocular tissues is more frequent. Scleritis may be the manifestation of immunologic disorders, e.g. collagenosis and vasculitis. Medical evaluation is therefore mandatory. Treatment is to be directed towards the underlying condition. Topical treatment is purely symptomatic.

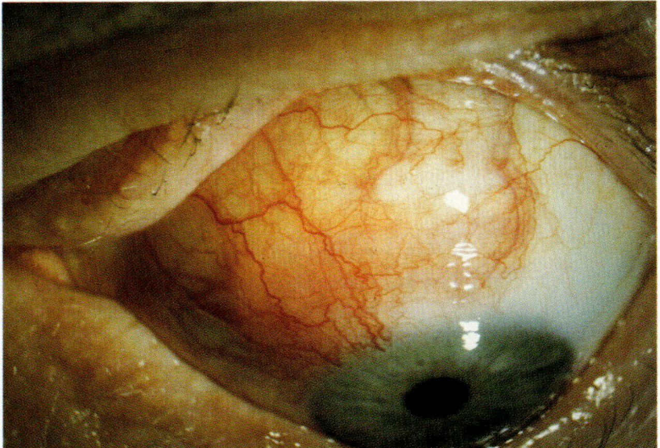

Figure 5.9   Nodular scleritis. The figure shows an elevated area of light color at the 12 o´clock position, which is surrounded by congested vessels. Local vaso-obliteration may have occured in this case. Systemic disease, such as generalized collagenosis or vasculitis has to be ruled out. In the later course, severe thinning of the sclera may occur. Treatment is to be directed towards the underlying disorder.

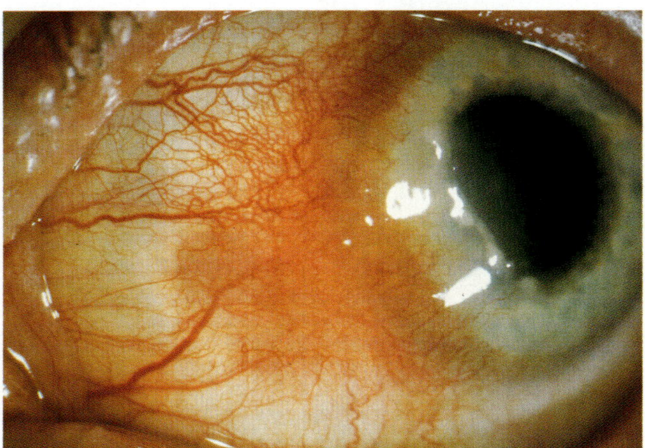

Figure 5.10   Scleritis with corneal involvement. The figure shows marked vascular injection at the limbus from the 7 to 10 o´clock position with grey-white opacities at the borders. Every scleritis localized at the limbus can lead to corneal involvement with melting of corneal tissue. The process cannot be influenced by topical treatment. Underlying systemic disease has to be ruled out (compare with figure 5.8 and 5.9). In this particular case, no systemic disease was found. Nevertheless, systemic evaluation should be conducted on a regular basis.

Figure 5.11 Status post limbal keratitis with progressive corneal opacity. A dense infiltration of the cornea can occur following scleritis. Vascularization and opacification can progress towards the central cornea. In this particular case, penetrating keratoplasty had to be conducted. Histologic examination showed inflammatory cells. Systemic evaluation did not reveal any underlying disease. Nevertheless, further medical follow-up is needed.

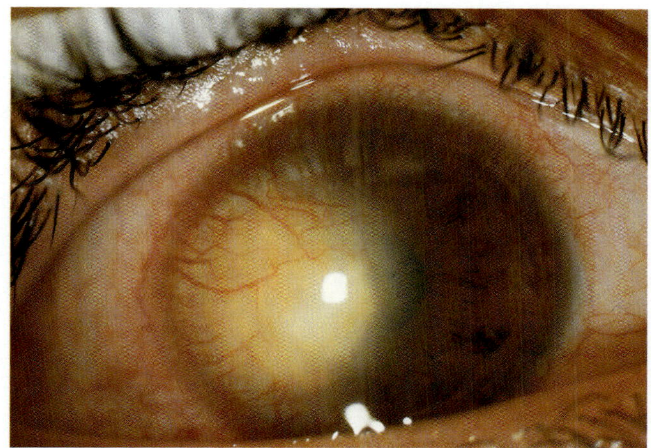

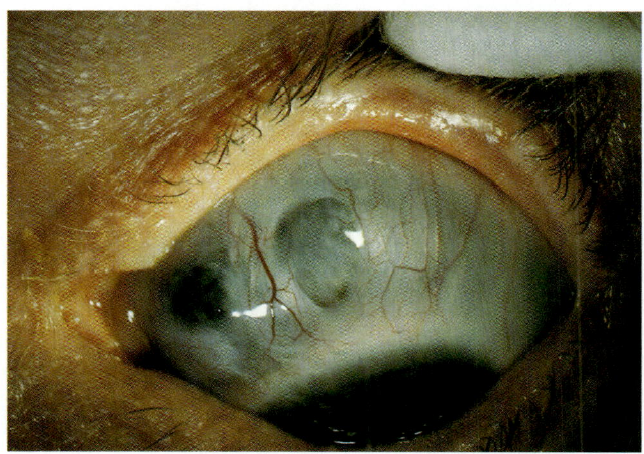

Figure 5.12 Necrotizing anterior scleritis in the absence of inflammation (scleromalacia perfomans). The figure shows massive thinning of the sclera in the superior half of the circumference, at some points nasally, the underlying choroid is covered only by a thin membrane. The striking features of this condition are the insidious onset and the absence of inflammation and pain. Vasoobliteration in the episclera is considered a cause. Regarding underlying disease compare with scleritis. No topical treatment has proven effective. Systemic treatment is to be directed towards the underlying systemic disorder, if present.

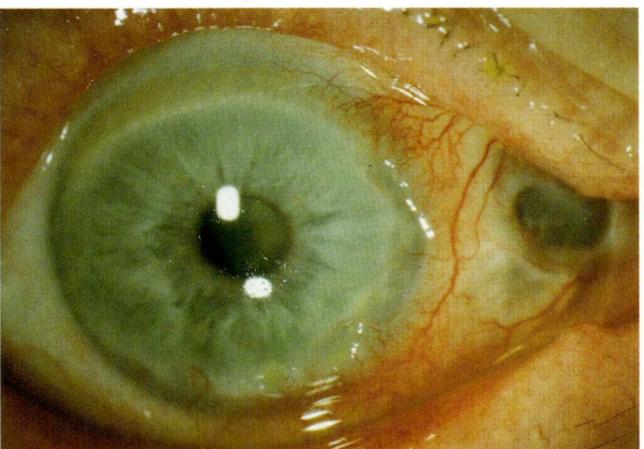

Figure 5.13 Wegener´s granulomatosis, scleromalacia with corneal melting. The figure shows a circumscribed area of extreme scleral thinning in the nasal aspect of the interpalpebral fissure. The choroid, which is covered only by a thin membrane, has a bluish tinge. Between the 2 and 3 o´clock position at the limbus keratolysis has caused a groove. Findings like this are frequent in Wegener´s granulomatosis. The ocular findings may represent the first organ manifestation. No topical treatment has proven effective. Usually fast resolution under systemic treatment.

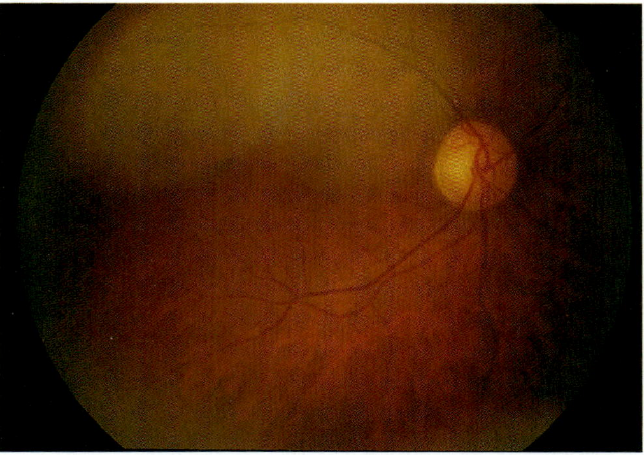

Figure 5.14 Posterior scleritis. The figure shows a grey, elevated area superior to the disc, which represents retinal edema caused by involvement of the retina and choroid in scleritis. The diagnosis is difficult, because the sclera is not visible in this region. Visual impairment, pain and sometimes signs of orbital involvement with diplopia and ophthalmoplegia indicate the presence of posterior scleritis. The diagnosis is made with ultrasonography (compare with figure 5.15).

Figure 5.15 Measurement of scleral thickness in posterior scleritis. Same patient as in figure 5.14. The ultrasonographic B-scan shows marked thickening of the sclera in the affected area. *Top* thickened sclera in the affected area, *bottom* nomal sclera.

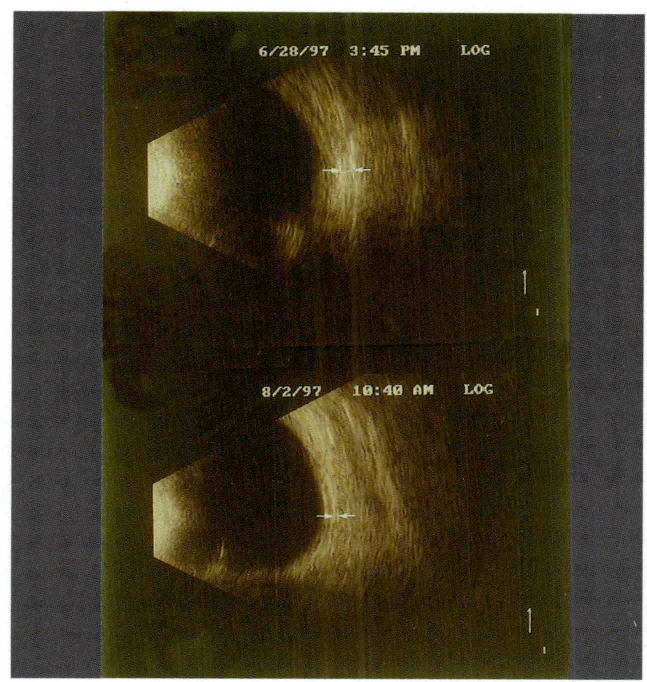

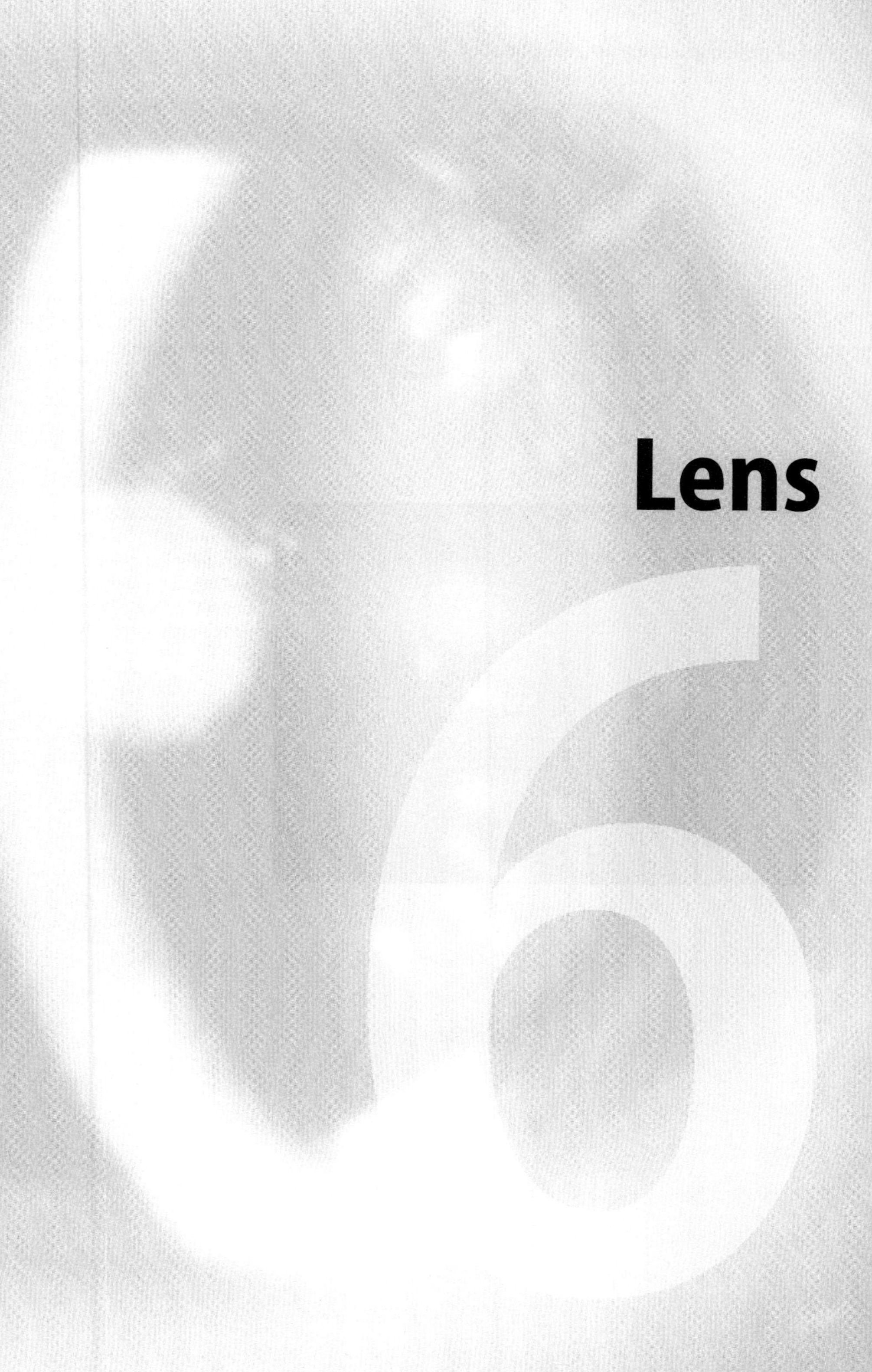

6

Lens

6.1 Applied anatomy and examination techniques

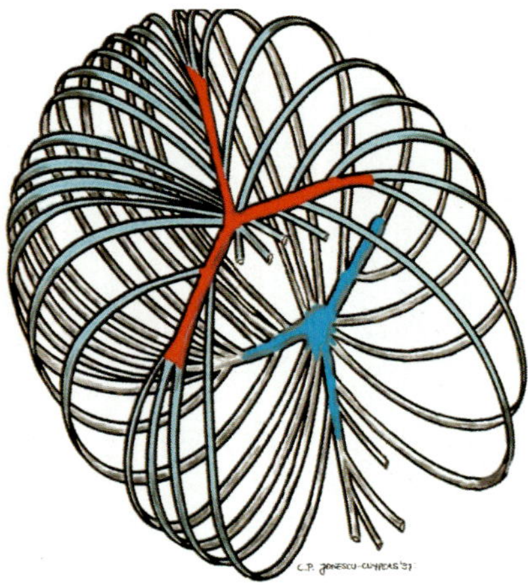

Figure 6.1 Arrangement of the lens fibrils in the fetal nucleus, which is still visble in the adult eye, schematic drawing. The nuclear fibrils forms an upright „Y" at the anterior pole and an inverse „Y" at the posterior pole. A congenital opacity following this arrangement is called „suture cataract", *red* anterior Y-suture, *blue* posterior Y-suture.

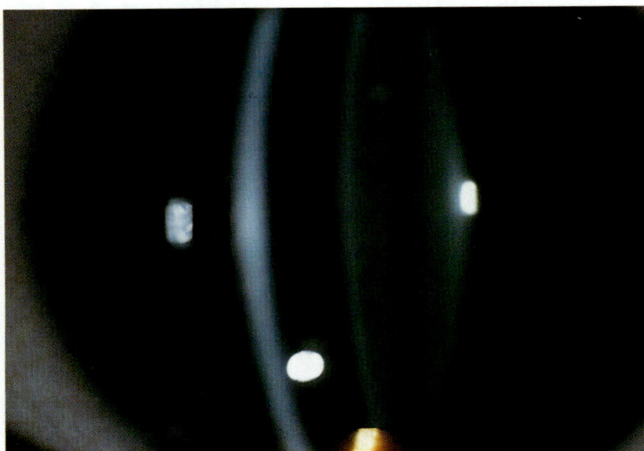

Figure 6.2 Optical section through the lens of a child. The narrow slit lamp beam reveals a relatively flat, highly transparent lens with only a thin cortex, the lens consists mainly of nucleus.

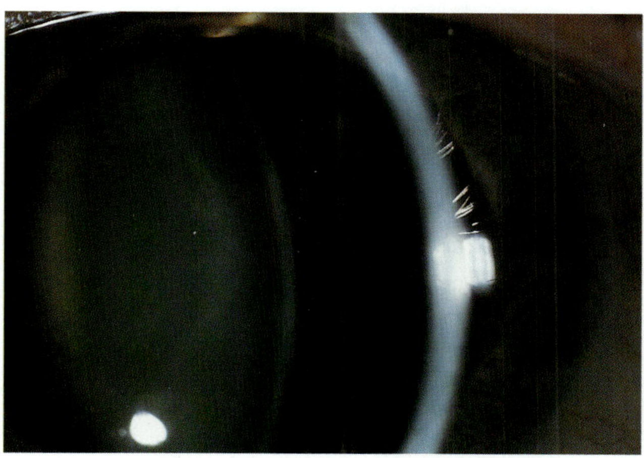

Figure 6.3 Optical section through the lens of an elderly person. Note that the axial diameter of the lens is larger – due to an enlargement of the nucleus and a lifelong increase of lens-thickness by appositional growth of lens fibers, arising from the eqatorial, subcapsular lens epithelium. The lens is less transparent than the lens of a child, the distinct zones of optical discontinuity are well visible. The curvatures of the lens are variable, the convexity of the anterior and posterior lens surfaces have increased with age. An increase in density of the nucleus leads to myopia, so-called "refractive myopia".

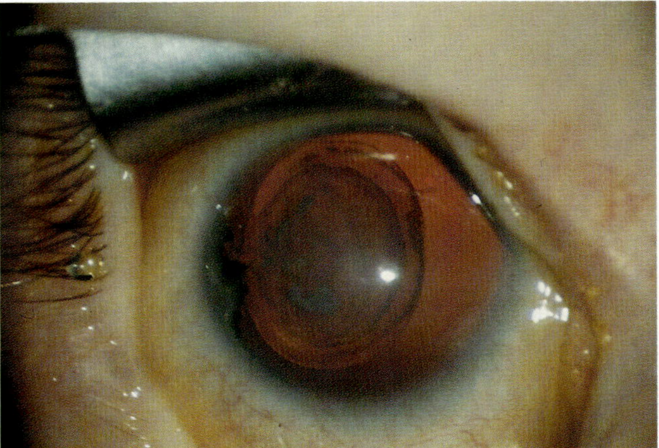

Figure 6.4 Lens with pathologically small diameter (microphakia) and increased curvature (spherophakia) as well as marked congenital opacification of the embryonic lens nucleus. In this case, the congenital microspherophakia is associated with aniridia, rendering this condition a combined dysplasia of lens and iris.

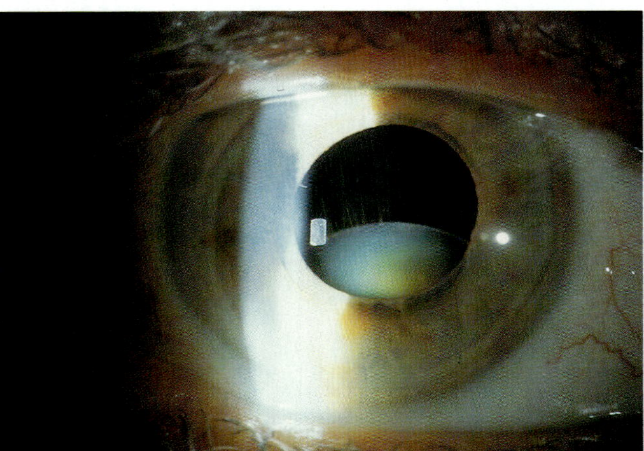

Figure 6.5 Lens subluxated inferiorly with incipient nuclear cataract. The metabolism of the subluxated lens is disturbed, a cataract develops. At the lens equator, fine, disinserted zonular fibers are visible. The subluxated lens subdivides the pupil, the optical axis lies superior to the lens equator. The patient sees as in uncorrected aphakia.

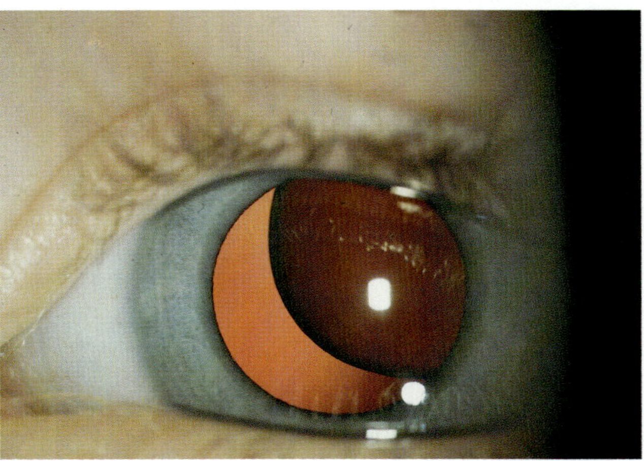

Figure 6.6 Subluxated lens in Marfan syndrome viewed with retroillumination. The lens, which is subluxated supero-temporally, lies outside the optical axis. It does no longer form part of the dioptrics of the eye. Unlike the subluxated lens in figure 6.5, this lens is clear (note red fundus reflex).

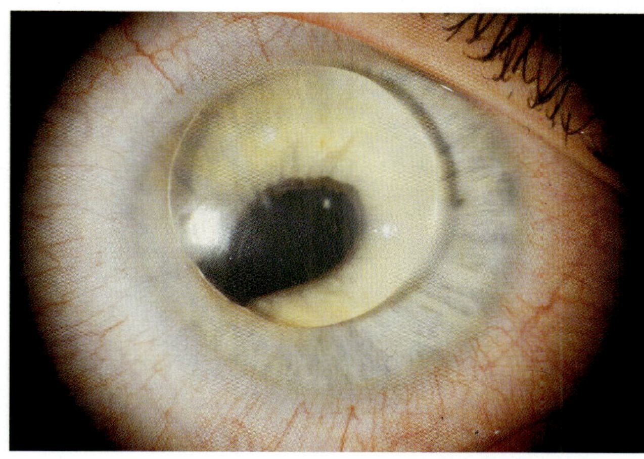

Figure 6.7   Clear lens luxated into the anterior chamber in a 18 year-old patient with Marfan syndrome. The small lens with increased anterior and posterior curvatures (microspherophakia) is luxated into the anterior chamber. The zonular fibers of the lens remain attached only in a small area from the 8 to 9 o´clock position, causing a notch in the pupillary margin. An extraction of the luxated lens from the anterior chamber has to be peformed immediately in order to avoid a pupillary block with a dramatic rise of IOP.

Figure 6.8   Markedly long fingers of the patient with luxated lens (figure 6.7), so called "arachno-dactyly", characteristic feature of Marfan syndrome with hyper-extensible joints.

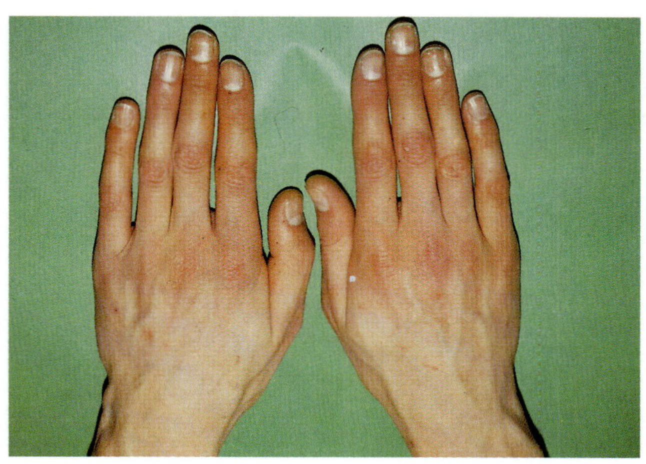

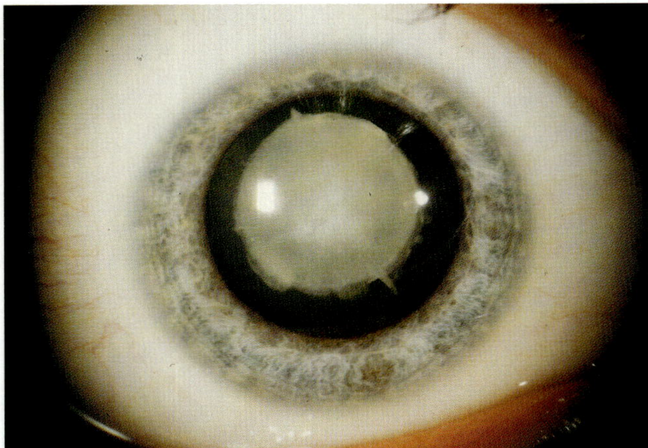

Figure 6.9 Congenital nuclear cataract. The embryonic lens nucleus is milky, opaque. Discrete wedge-shaped cortical opacities are present at the equator.

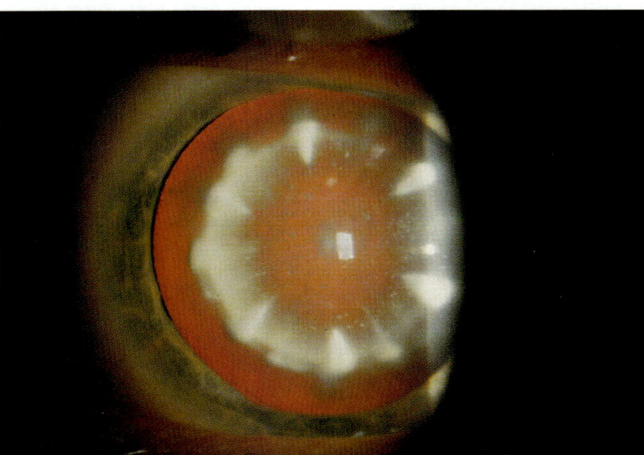

Figure 6.10 Congenital nuclear cataract in a 3 year-old child, viewed with retroillumination. The epinucleus surrounding the embryonic nucleus shows wedge-shaped opacities, so called "cuneifom" cataract.

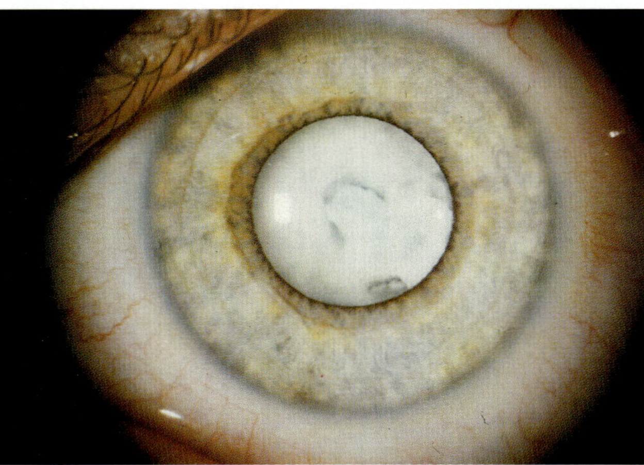

Figure 6.11 Mature, congenital cataract in an infant. The pupil is completely opaque, causing total visual deprivation. Lens extraction has to be performed as soon as possible in order to prevent amblyopia.

Figure 6.12 Congenital posterior polar cataract, viewed with retroillumination. Confined to the axial area is a cone-shaped opacity, of which the top is directed to the center of the lens. In retroillumination, the polar cataract can be well distinguished from the surrounding transparent lens tissue. If visual deprivation occurs, surgical extraction is needed.

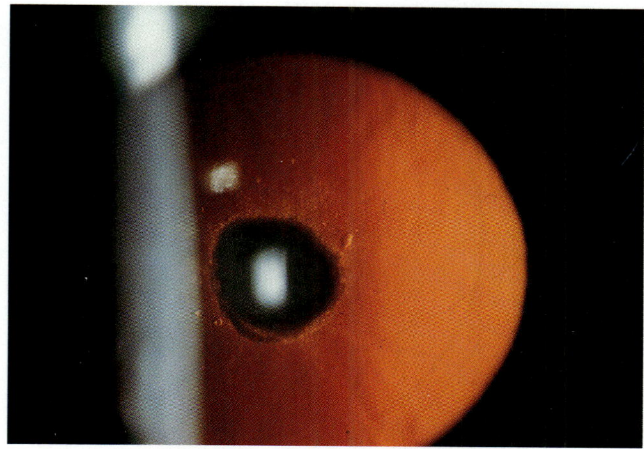

6.4 Cataract: acquired/involutional/age-related

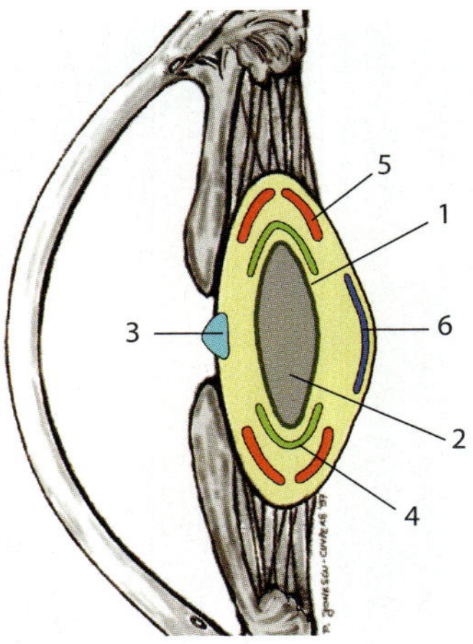

Figure 6.13 Various kinds of opacities in the human lens, schematic drawing. Age-related, acquired cataracts can affect the cortex, the nucleus or both. (1) lamellar cataract, (2) nuclear cataract, (3) capsular cataract, (4) cortical cataract (coronary), (5) cortical cataract (cuneiform), (6) posterior subcapsular cataract.

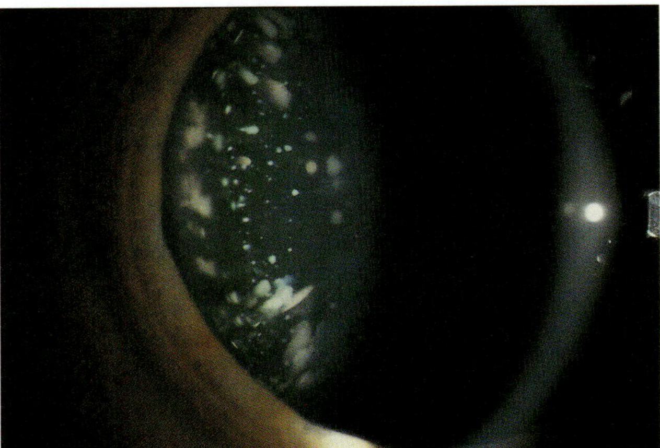

Figure 6.14 Cerulean cataract. This cataract consist of small, wedge-shaped opacities that have a bluish hue, similar to copper vitreole – therefore described as cerulean *(latin* copper) cataract. The droplet-shaped, bluish opacities in the cortex mostly occur at a young age and are non-progressive.

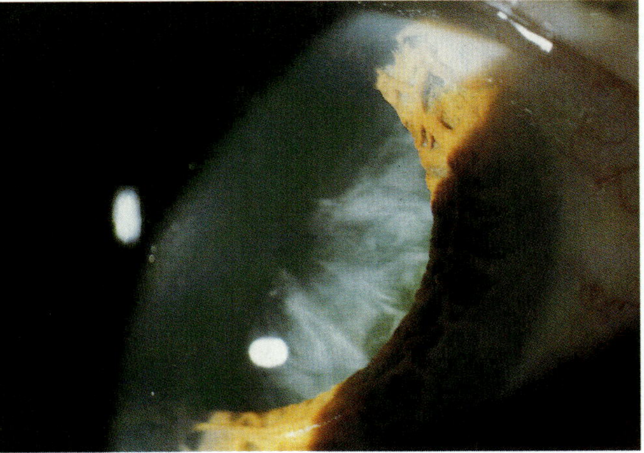

Figure 6.15 Spoke-shaped cortical opacities, cuneiform cataract.

Figure 6.16 Nuclear cataract in high myopia. The optical section viewed with the slit lamp reveals a greenish, dense opacity of the lens nucleus. This kind of cataract frequently occurs in highly myopic eyes in advanced age.

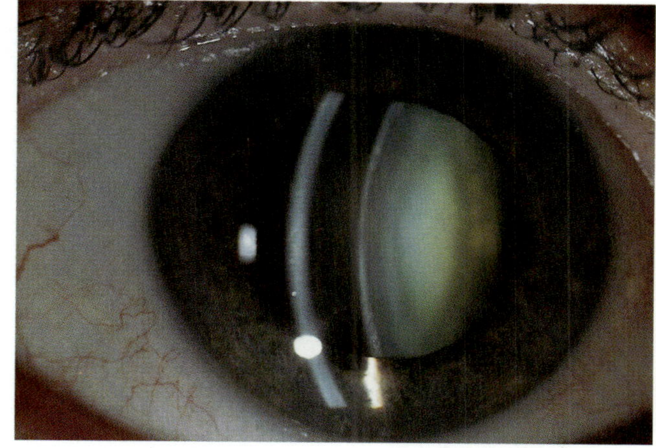

Figure 6.17 Waterclefts in the anterior lens cortex. Separation of tissue layers within the lens cortex leads to an accumulation of fluid and formation of so-called "waterclefts". Due to the different refractive indices of the lens tissue and water, this condition may produce monocular diplopia.

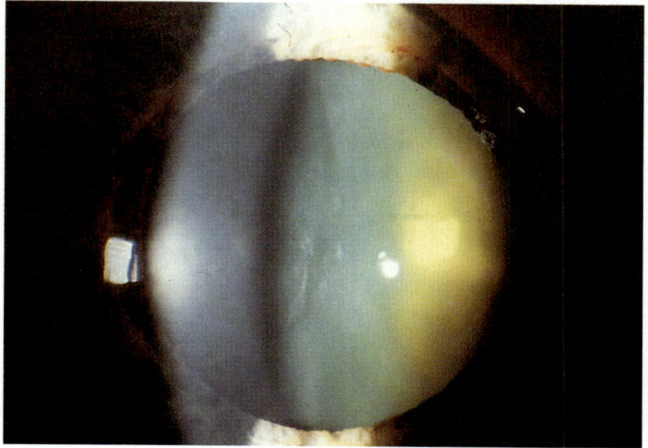

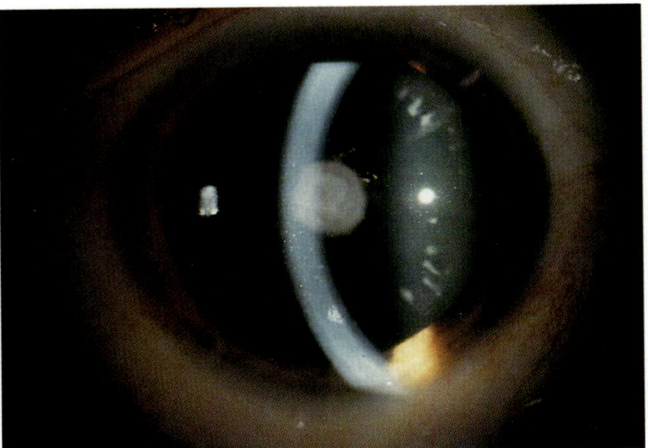

Figure 6.18 Anterior polar cataract. A cone-shaped white opacity is found on the anterior lens surface. In this case, discrete, wedge-shaped cortical opacities are an additional finding. Lens opacities are the more visually significant, the closer they lie to the nodal point of the eye´s compound optical system. The nodal point of the eye´s dioptric system lies posterior to the lens in the anterior vitreous. For that reason, a posterior polar cataract impairs vision significantly more than an anterior polar cataract.

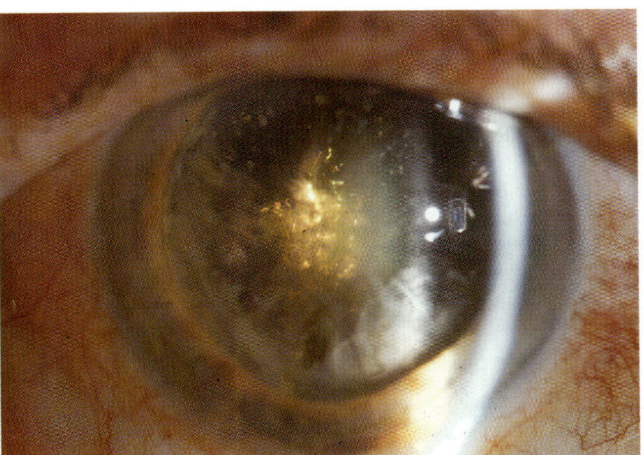

Figure 6.19 Crystalline inclusions in the anterior lens cortex and the nucleus, so-called "christmas tree cataract". The narrow beam of the slit lamp is reflected by the crystalline lipid inclusions. The condition bears a resemblance to a lit up christmas tree. The high refractiveness of this cataract induces glare.

Figure 6.20 Morgagnian cataract. The brownish, opaque lens nucleus has sunk within the lens. In this advanced form of age-related cataract, the cortex becomes liquefied and the hard, dark colored nucleus sinks to the bottom of the capsular bag, it appears in a semicircle behind the pupil. This hypermature cataract can cause phacolytic uveitis or phacogenic glaucoma.

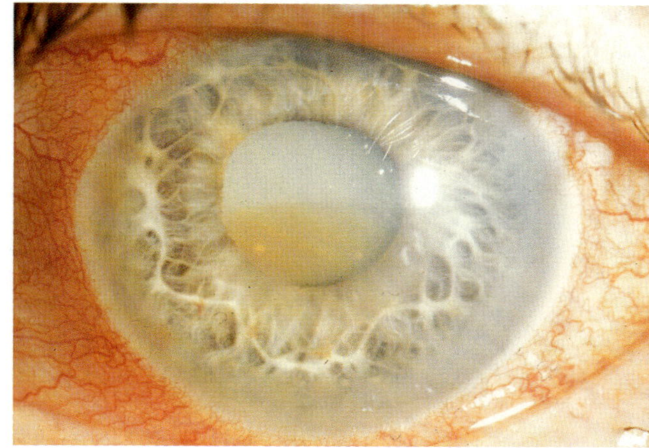

Figure 6.21 Cataracts extracted from human eyes. *Left* cataracta nigra, dark coloration of the lens nucleus in long-standing cataract. *Right* milky-white opaque lens following intracapsular lens extraction.

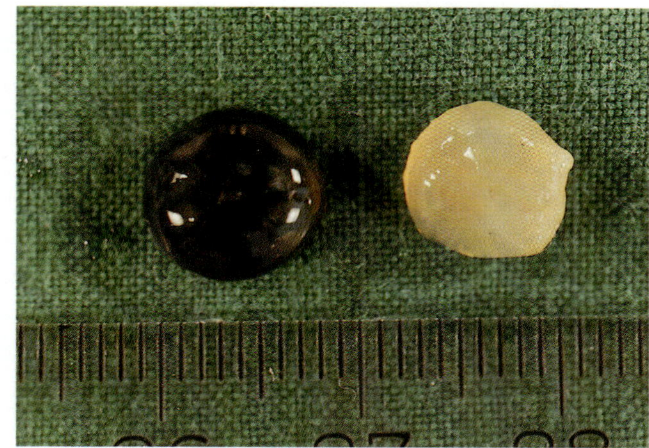

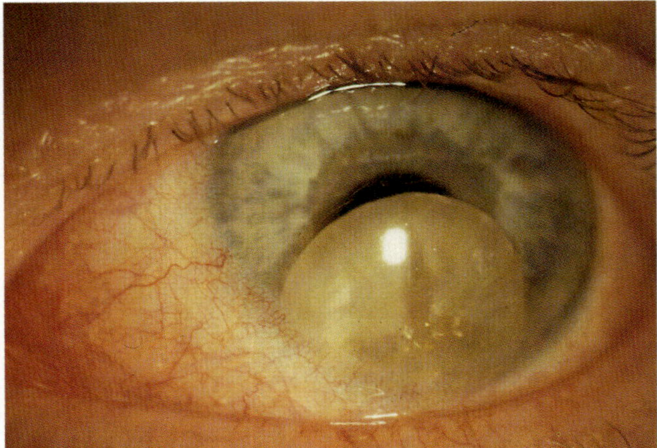

Figure 6.22 Cataract luxated into the anterior chamber following blunt trauma. The shock wave exerted on the globe has ruptured the fragile zonular fibers and luxated the opaque lens through the pupil into the anterior chamber. An immediate extraction of the lens is mandatory in order to prevent damage to the corneal endothelium.

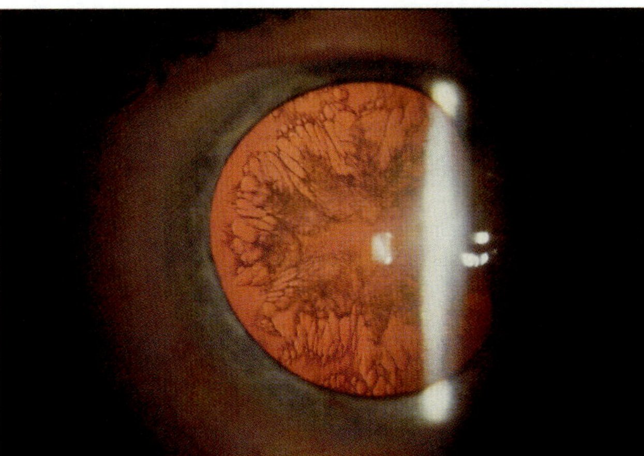

Figure 6.23 Contusion cataract. In blunt trauma, micro-perforation of the lens capsule often occurs. With water entering the posterior subcapsular lens cortex, a so-called "contusion rosette" develops.

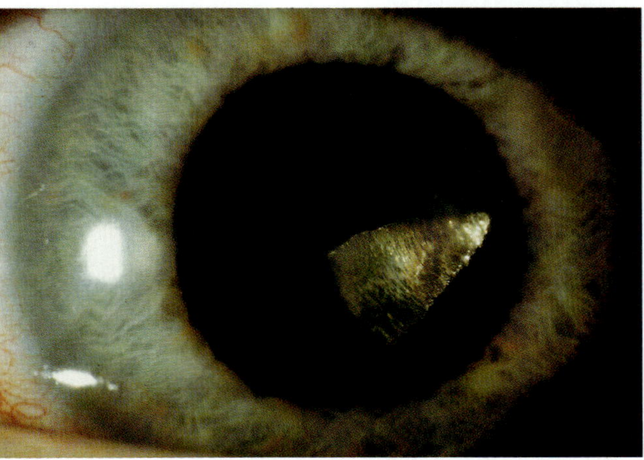

Figure 6.24 Metallic foreign body in the lens. A metallic, triangular foreign body is stuck in the lens, it entered the globe through a conjunctival and scleral perforation. The photograph was taken soon after the trauma, no cataract has yet developed.

Figure 6.25 Complicated cataract in siderosis bulbi. The patient retains an iron-bearing intraocular foreign body. The release of ionized iron causes an intoxication of the retina, resulting in blindness. A cataract develops with apposition of brownish material.

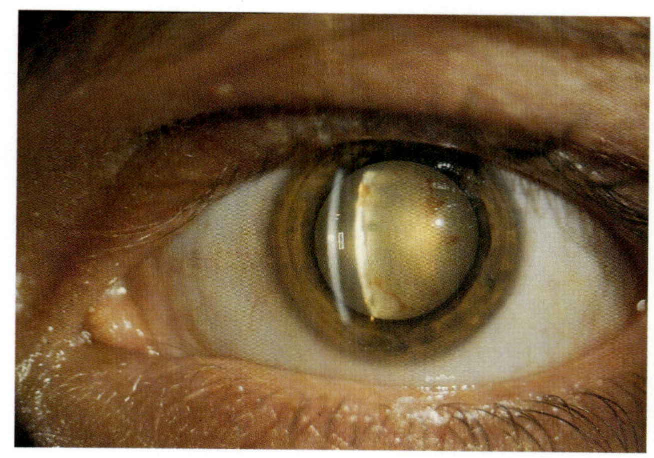

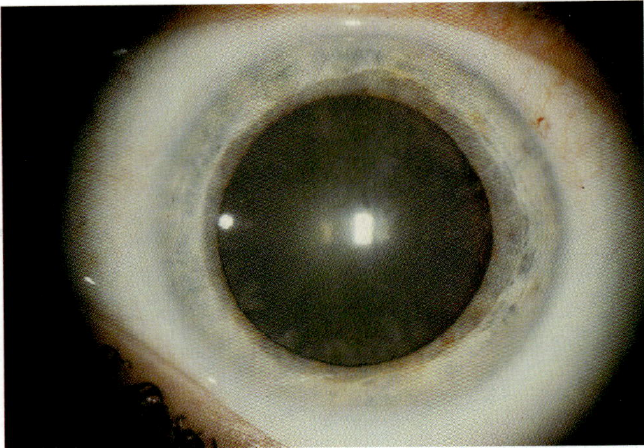

Figure 6.26 Myotonic cataract. The cataract associated with myotonia is most pronounced in the posterior lens cortex. If the lens metabolism is impaired in the presence of an underlying systemic defect, the posterior portion of the lens cortex is affected at first. Due to the attachment of the vitreous body, the posterior lens is not supplied by the aqueous humor as is the anterior lens. A discrete, powdery opacity in the posterior sucapsular lens cortex develops.

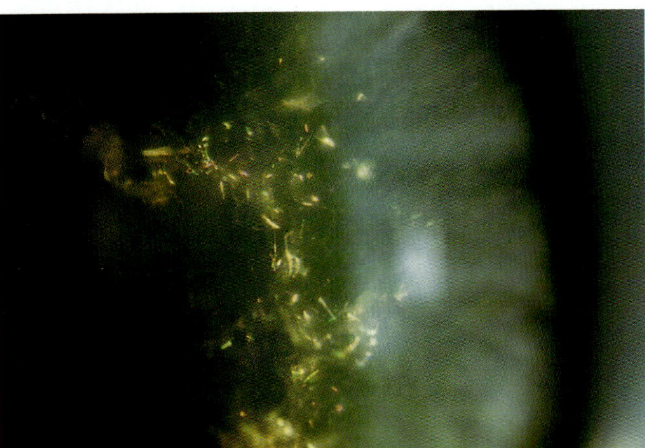

Figure 6.27 Crystalline cortical cataract associated with tetany. The epinuclear portion of the cortex shows light-refracting opacities induced by an altered calcium metabolism.

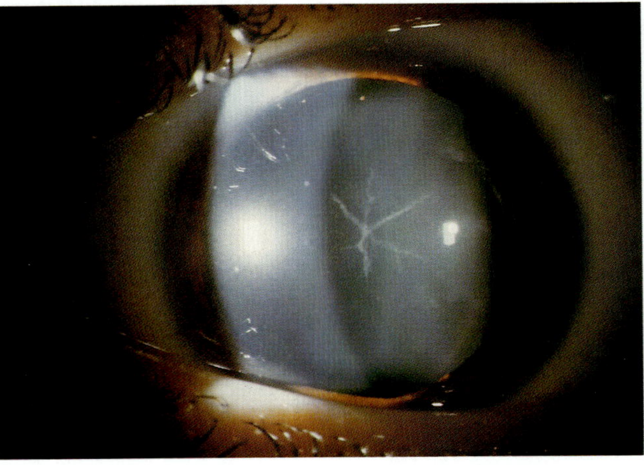

Figure 6.28 Suture cataract associated with galactosemia. The cataract associated with galactosemia is the only reversible cataract. A reversal of the opacities occurs, if galactose is removed from the diet.

Figure 6.29   Posterior subcapsular cataract following longstanding corticosteroid treatment. Subcapsular lens opacities develop in patients receiving chronic systemic corticosteroid treatment, depending on the duration of treatment and the cumulative dosis.

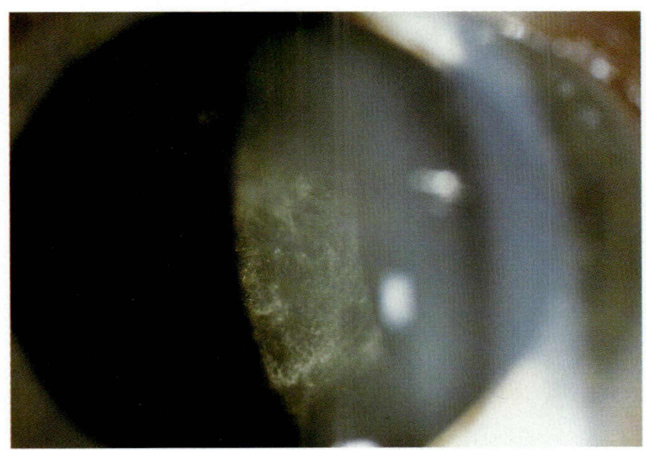

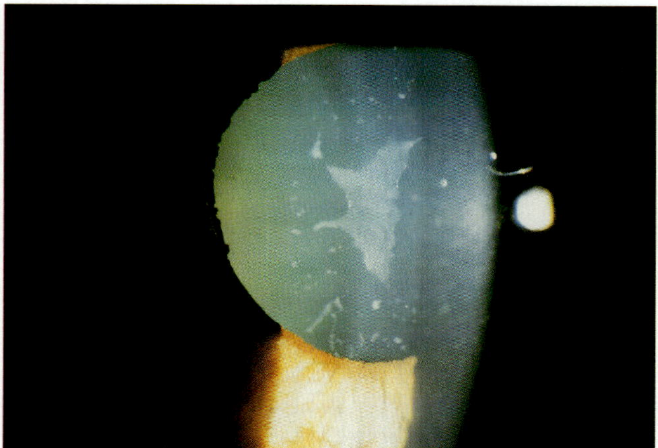

Figure 6.30   Subcapsular, anterior lens epithelial necrosis following acute glaucoma, so-called "glaukomflecken". With very high levels of intraocular pressure, localized necroses of the lens epithelium under the lens capsule develop. Biomicroscopically, they appear as discrete white opacities underneath the lens capsule.

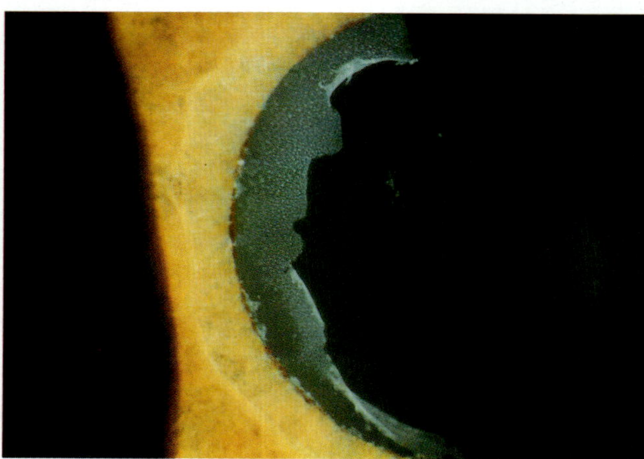

Figure 6.31   Pseudoexfoliation syndrome (PXS). Deposition of so-called "pseudoexfoliative material" an amyloid-like protein, on the midperipheral anterior lens surface is seen in pseudoexfoliation syndrome. The pseudoexfoliative material originates from a defective biosynthesis of intracellular matrix and is not only present on the anterior lens surface, but also in the outflow pathways, the pupillary border, the posterior chamber, the zonular fibers and the ciliary processes.

Figure 6.32 Fibrotic posterior capsular opacification following extracapsular cataract extraction. The remaining posterior lens capsule is wrinkled and opacified. The opacified posterior capsule can be opened with a photodisruptive laser (Nd:YAG) in order to obtain clear media in the optical axis.

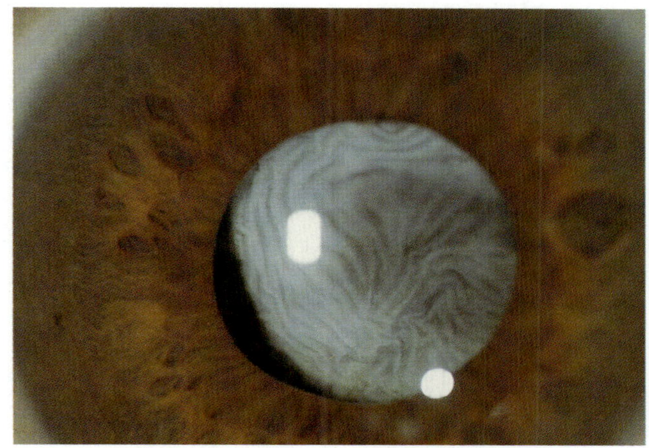

Figure 6.33 Proliferation of lens cells following extracapsular lens extraction and penetrating keratoplasty. Note the translucent spheres in the inferior pupillary space, so-called "Elschnig´s pearls". They represent proliferations of residual lens epithelial cells.

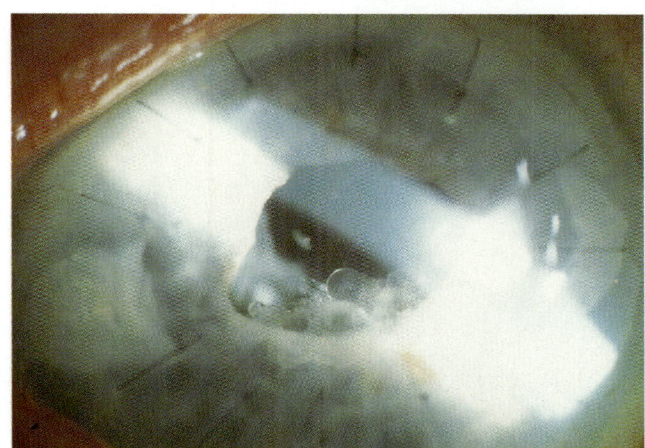

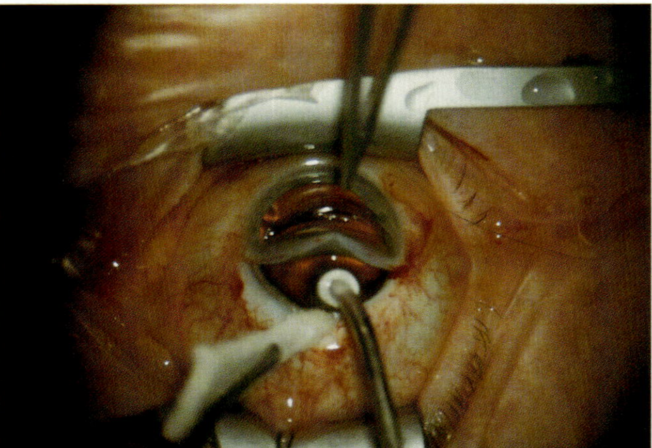

Figure 6.34 Removal of the entire lens with its capsule. The intracapsular cryo extraction is perfomed rarely. The technique is indicated in subluxation of the lens, when the zonular apparatus is not suitable for extracapsular surgery and implantation of an artificial lens.

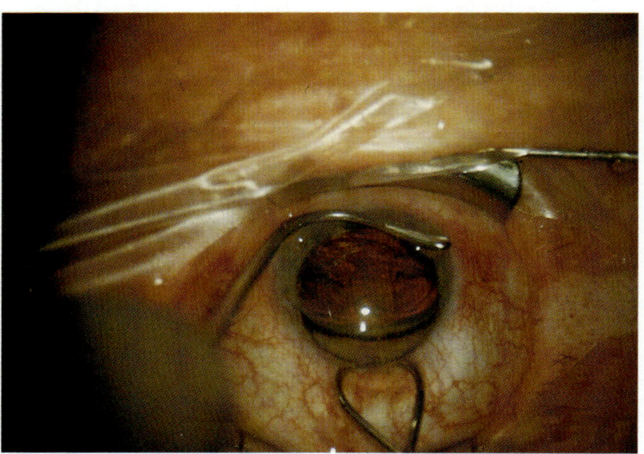

Figure 6.35 Removal of the lens nucleus by expression via a corneal wound during extracapsular cataract surgery. A 10 mm incision was made in the peripheral cornea with a diamond knife. The anterior lens capsule has been opened under viscoelastic material in the anterior chamber. The lens nucleus is loosened from cortical material and delivered by providing external pressure towards the lens equator at the 6 o´clock position and towards the scleral lip of the wound at 12 o´clock position.

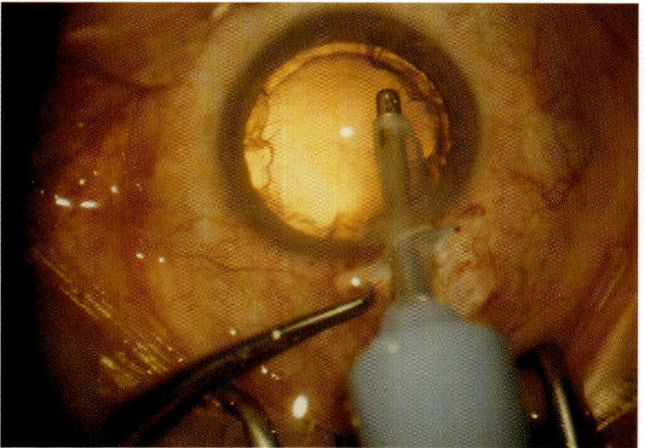

Figure 6.36 Removal of remaining cortical material in the capsular bag with an irrigation/aspiration device during extracapsular surgery. Remaining lens epithelium and cortical material are removed from the capsular bag, inside which an artificial lens is being placed during cataract surgery.

Figure 6.37 Phacoemulsification of a cataract. In phacoemulsification, the hard lens nucleus is emulsified and aspirated with an ultrasonic probe. The advantage of this technique over extracapsular surgery with expression of the lens nucleus is the smaller incision of the globe and the stability of the anterior chamber during the procedure.

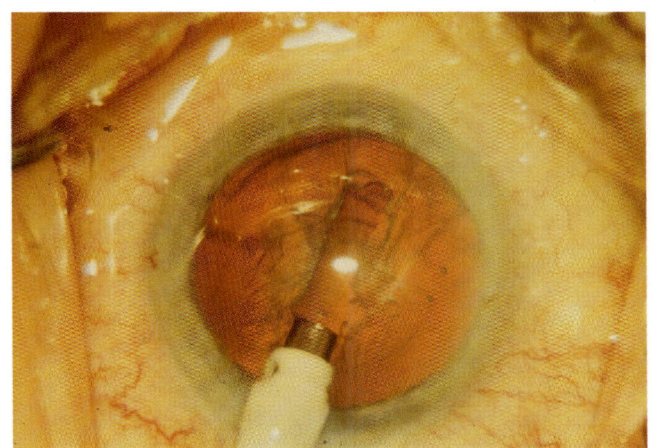

Figure 6.38 Implantation of an artificial foldable lens in the capsular bag following removal of the lens nucleus by phacoemulsification and aspiration of remaining cortical material and lens epithelium. The folded artificial lens is inserted into the capsular bag via a 3 mm corneoscleral incision. The artificial lens is stabilized in the capsular bag by two semicircular haptics.

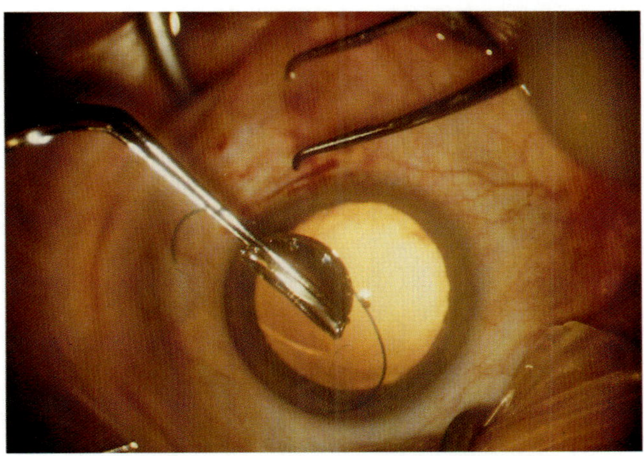

Figure 6.39 Artificial lens fixated in the capsular bag in the posterior chamber. The oval anterior capsular opening can be viewed with retroillumination. The remaining portions of the anterior lens capsule enclose the rim of the lens and fixate it in the capsular bag.

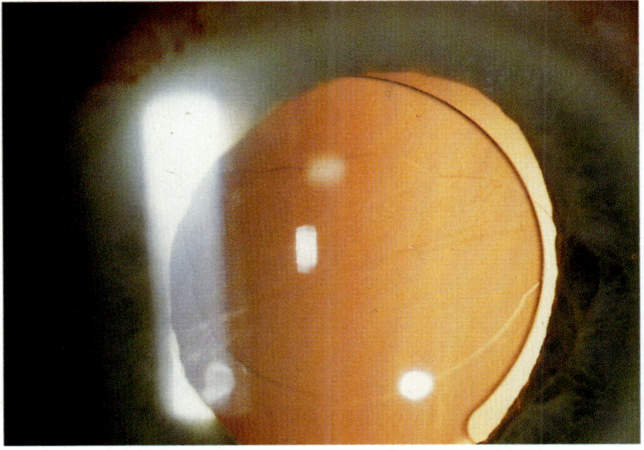

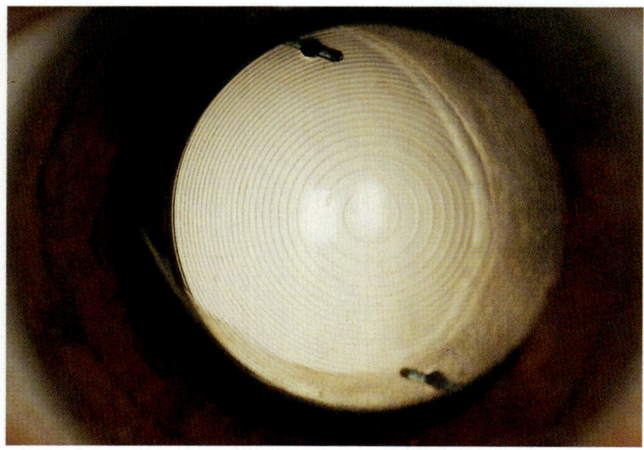

Figure 6.40 Multifocal lens in the posterior chamber. This artificial lens provides near and far vision. It can produce multiple foci using the diffractive properties of posterior, multiple, concentric structured surfaces.

Figure 6.41 Correction of aphakia with a hard contact lens. The hard contact lens lies on a thin tear film on the corneal surface and produces only a discrete, non-disturbing image enlargement. The correction of unilateral aphakia with a contact lens is therefore possible.

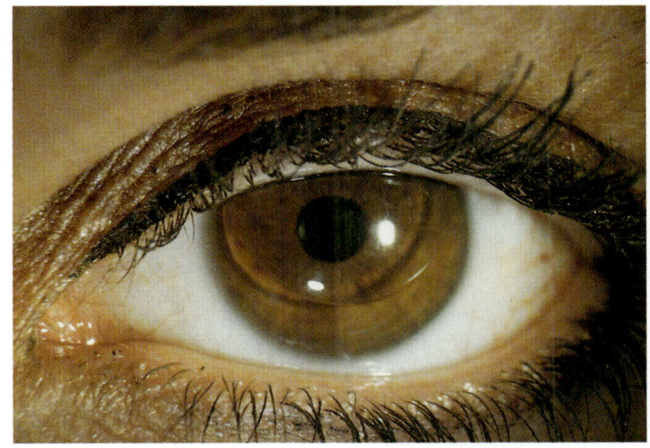

Figure 6.42 Correction of aphakia with spectacles. Spectacle correction of aphakia with high-density plus power lenses produces an enlargement of images on the retina as well as visual field constriction. The correction of unilateral aphakia with spectacles is not possible because of the difference in size of ocular images, so-called "aniseikonia" (compare with chapter 15).

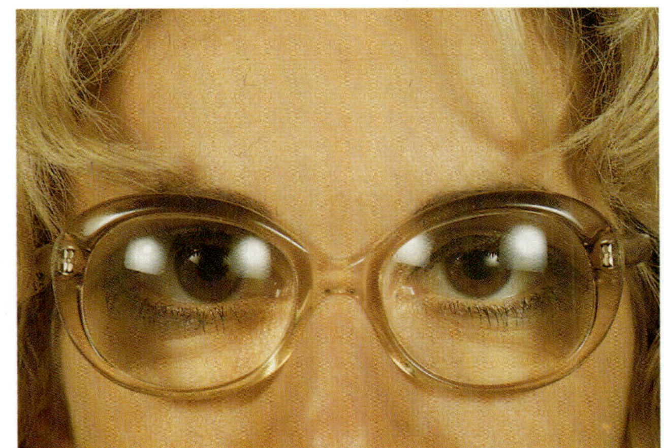

Uvea

7

7.1 Applied anatomy and examination techniques

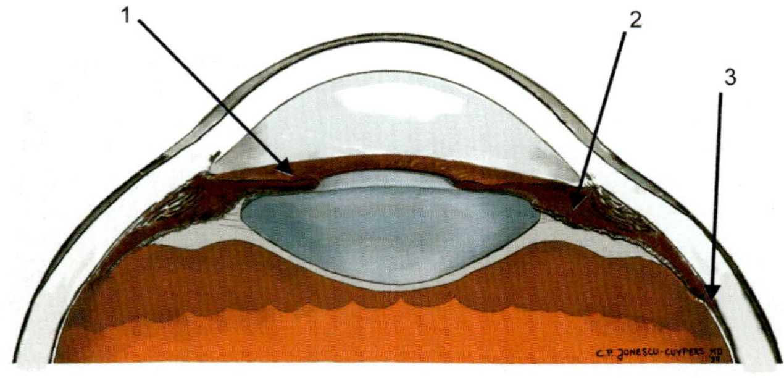

Figure 7.1   Scheme of the uvea. The uveal tract comprises the iris (1), the ciliary body (2) and the choroid (3, only anterior part is shown). These tissues are essential for the nutrition of the eye. The iris transmits oxygen to the aqueous humor, the ciliary body is responsible for the formation of aqueous humor (see chapter 9) and of hyaluronic acid (see chapter 10). The choroid supplies the outer retinal layers with blood.

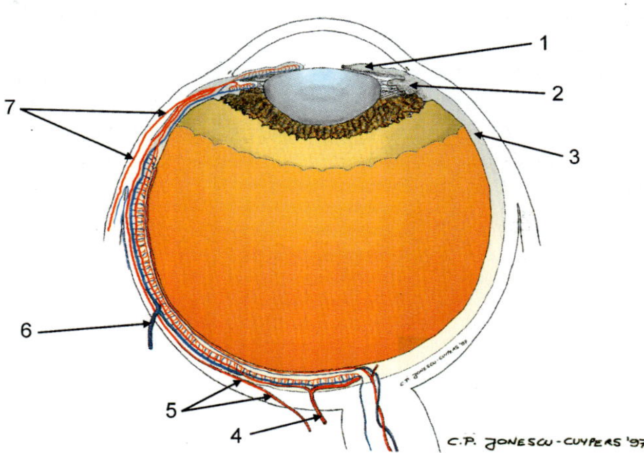

Figure 7.2   Vasculature of the iris (1), ciliary body (2) and choroid (3). The uvea is supplied in its posterior portion by the short posterior ciliary arteries (4) anteriorly by the long posterior and anterior ciliary arteries (5, 7). Anostomoses with the vasculature of the iris exist (see figure 7.3). The venous drainage is through the vortex veins (6).

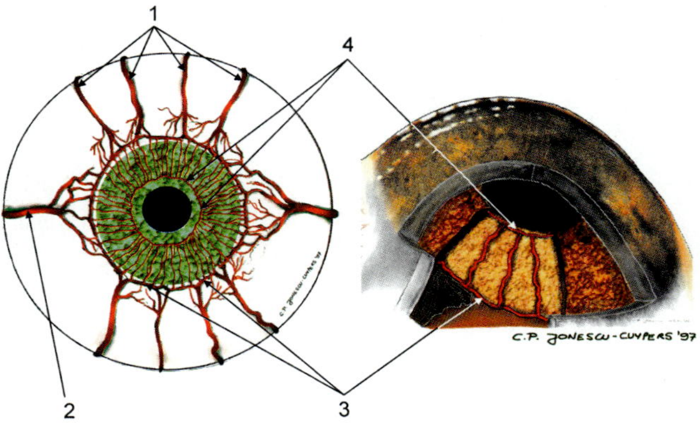

Figure 7.3   Vasculature of the iris. The iris consits of the iris stroma, that carries the melanocytes, the spincter and dilator muscle and the pigment epithelium. Blood is supplied via the major arterial circle (3), which is connected to the anterior and posterior ciliary arteries (1, 2) and anostomoses with the minor arterial circle. The endothelium of the vessels is non-fenestrated, maintaining the blood-aqueous-barrier when no inflammation is present.

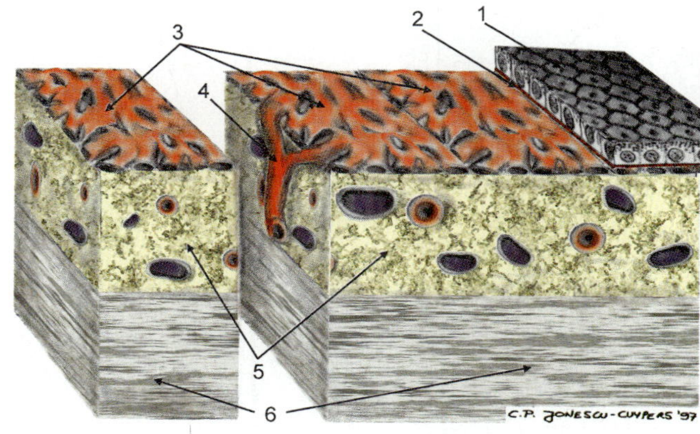

Figure 7.4 Choroid, scheme of structure and vasculature. The choroid is interposed between sclera (6) and retina . It is separated from the retinal pigment epithelium (1) by Bruch´s membrane (2). The blood supply is derived from the anterior and posterior ciliary arteries, the drainage is via the venae vorticosae (compare with figure 7.2). A layer of large and medium-sized choroidal vessels (5) can be distinguished from the choriocapillaris (3). The choriocapillaris is organized in lobules, that do not anastomose between each other. Each lobule is fed by a central arteriole (4). In contrast to the endothelium of the iris vessels, the choroidal vessels are fenestrated.

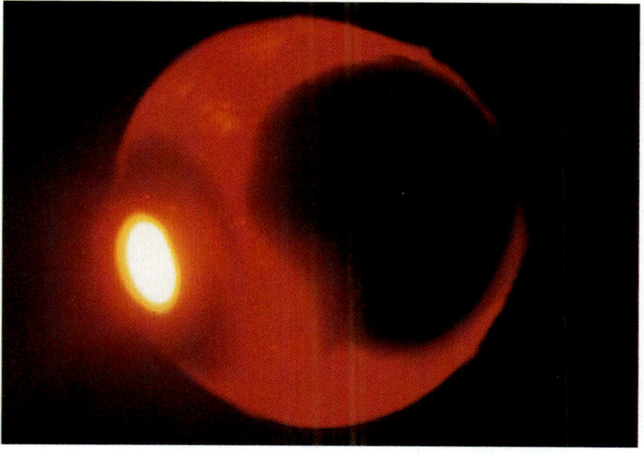

Figure 7.5 Transillumination. With the exception of the iris the uveal structures (ciliary body and choroid) are not visible. The pigment epithelium covers the choroid and obscures the direct view on the choroid. Consolidation of the structures - especially tumors - can be visualized by transillumination up to the equator. The eye is transilluminated with a powerful light-source. The figure shows the shadowing by a tumor.

7.1 Applied anatomy and examination techniques

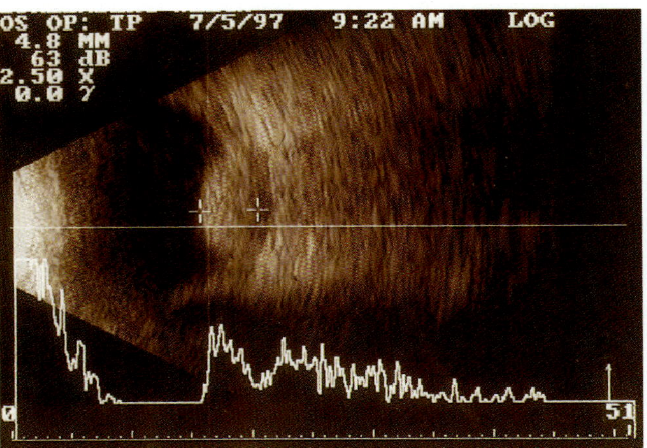

Figure 7.6 Ultrasonography. Ultrasonography is another technique suitable for the examination of the uvea besides slit-lamp biomicroscopy and diaphanoscopy. The sonogram provides information on the extension, thickness, density and vascularization of pathological processes (see chapter 5, posterior scleritis). The figure shows an elevated mass (pathologic elevation between the crosses).

Figure 7.7 Iris bicolor. The color of the iris is determined by the uveal melanocytes, which are located in the stroma. Physiologically, newborns have a blue iris with little pigment. The definite eye color develops later on. Irregularities in color can persist. The iris bicolor is tinted differently in one half or sector. It is considered an anomaly wihout clinical importance.

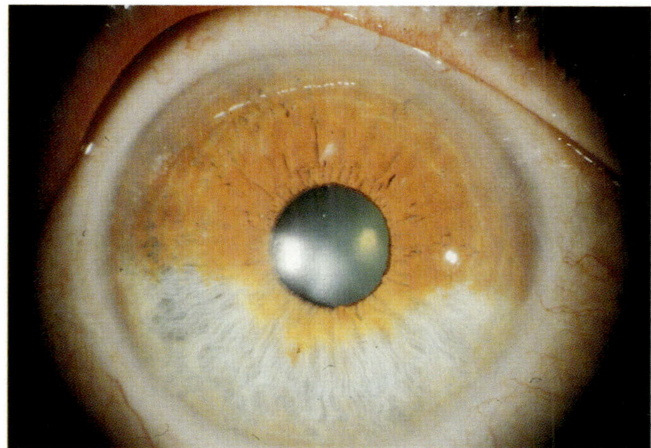

Figure 7.8 Bilateral heterochromia. The figure shows a different iris color on each side. It is considered an anomaly without clinical importance as well. Heredity may occur.

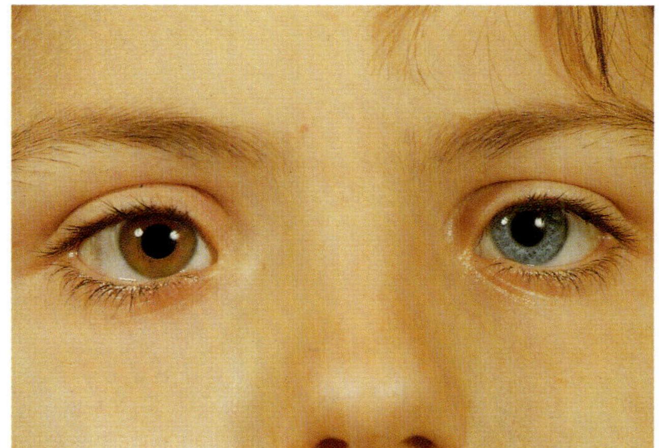

Figure 7.9 Multiple iris nevi. Iris nevi develop from the melanocytes of the iris stroma. The figure shows numerous brownish iris nevi. The lesions have ill-defined borders and are slightly elevated. It is considered a harmless finding and is frequent. Iris nevi have to be differentiated from tumorous, particularly malignant processes.

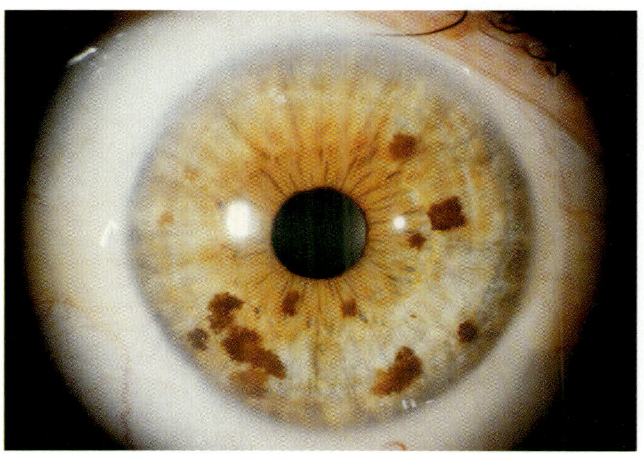

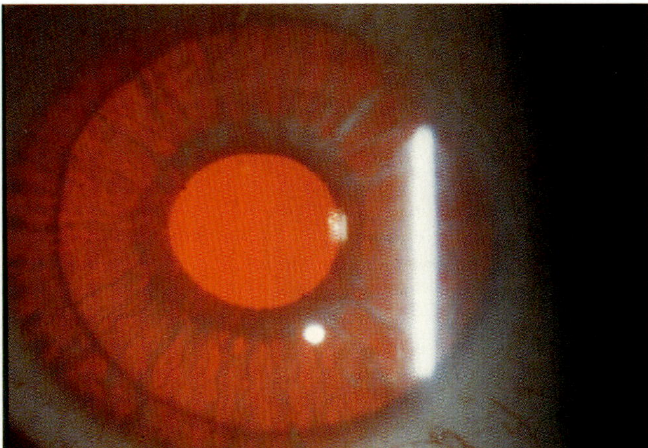

Figure 7.10 Albinism. View of the iris with retroillumination. The lack of pigment is caused by a defect in melanin synthesis. The ocular findings are a diaphanous iris, hypopigmentation of the fundus with visible choroidal vessels and hypoplasia of the fovea. Characteristic features are photophobia and poor visual acuity as well as an abnormal configuration of the chiasm (abnormal visual pathway).

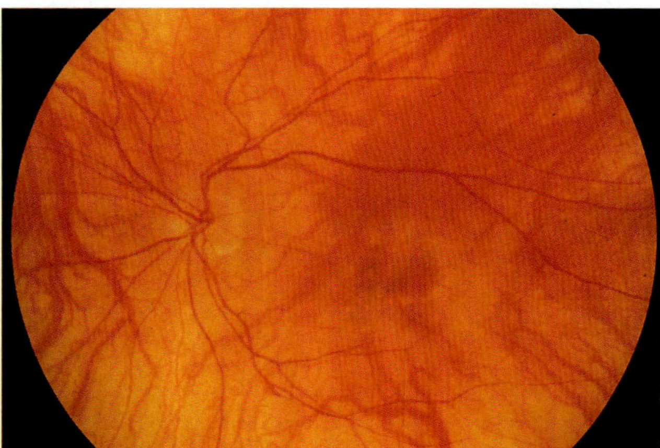

Figure 7.11 Fundus in albinism. The choroid is bared by lack of melanin in the retinal pigment epithelium. The normally invisible large choroidal vessels stand out.

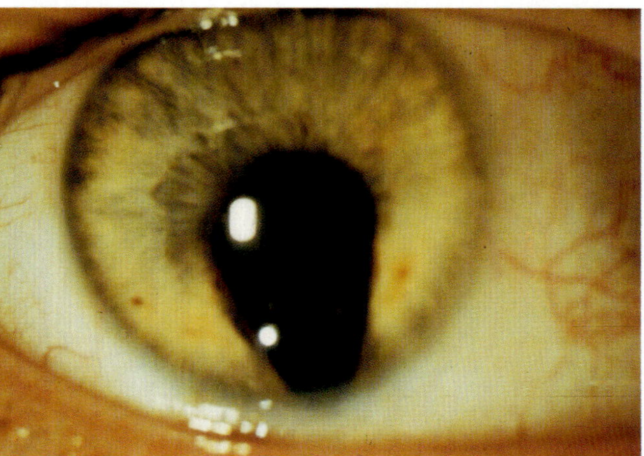

Figure 7.12 Coloboma of the iris. This congenital anomaly is caused by a maldevelopment in the 10. gestational week. The coloboma is typically located inferiorly. The stucture in the unaffected part of the iris is normal. An association with other anomalies, particularly colobomas of the fundus, may occur.

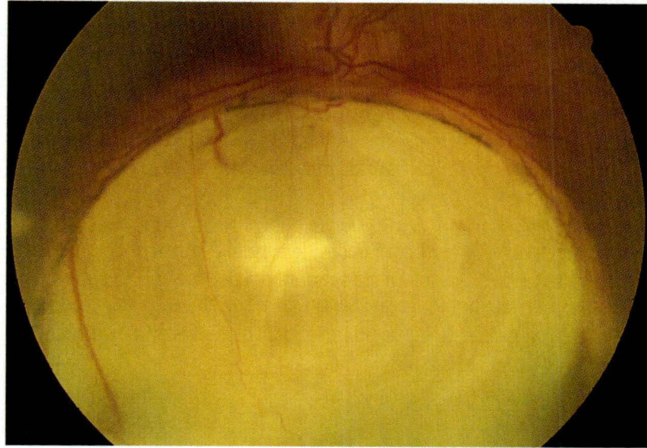

Figure 7.13   Coloboma of the choroid. The figure shows a large coloboma of the choroid just below the optic disc. In this area, the choroid and the retinal pigment epithelium are missing. Only abortive retinal vessels can be detected on the white sclera. An association with other colobomas or anomalies is frequently seen (same patient as in figure 7.12). The colobomas may reach from the papilla to the ciliary body. Sometimes the affected area may be subdivided by a streak of normal retina / choroid. Retinal detachment may develop from the margin of a fundus coloboma.

7.3 Inflammations

General: Visible signs of an inflammation of the iris are changes in the aqueous humor with increased protein content, suspension of cells, deposits on the corneal endothelium, secondary adhesions between the iris and the anterior lens surface and adhesions in the iridocorneal angle. Primary inflammations of the choroid lead to an involvement of the retina (chorioretinitis), while the choroid is secondarily involved in an inflammation of the retina (retinochoroiditis). The fact that often both structures are affected makes it difficult to differentiate. Anterior uveitis (iris, ciliary body) mostly causes severe pain and photophobia. Posterior uveitis may not cause complaints besides visual disturbance. Uveitis may be caused by infectious agents or immunoreactions. Systemic examination is important, but does often not reveal the causing agent. Therapy depends on the causing agent. In iritis, corticosteroids and mydriatic agents are always indicated.

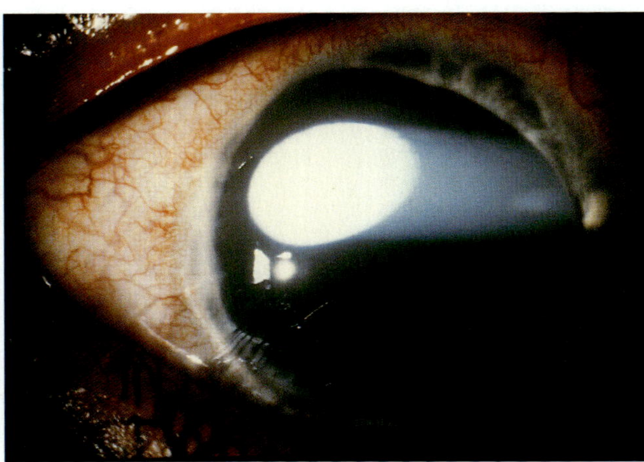

Figure 7.14   Aqueous flare. The aqueous humor is usually free of cellular elements and has a low protein content. A breakdown of the blood-aqueous barrier results in a leakage of proteins and suspension of cells of variable degree. Slitlamp examination reveals turbidity which is the result of the high protein content of the aqueous humor. Aqueous flare can be present long after the resolution of active inflammation.

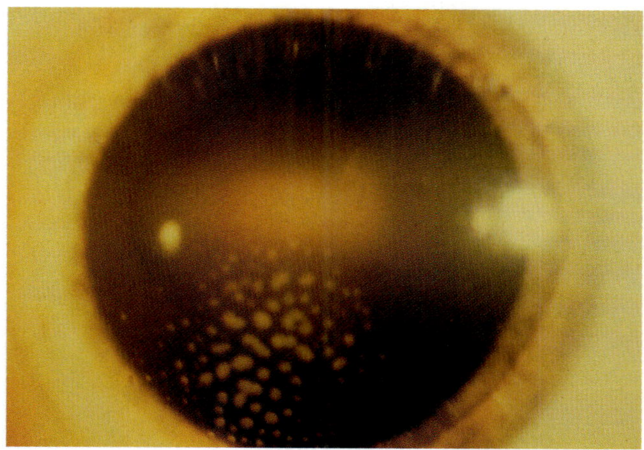

Figure 7.15 Keratic precipitates. Besides aqueous flare and cells in the anterior chamber, keratic precitptates are a sign of inflammation. The figure shows patchy deposits on the corneal endothelium in the inferior half. The precipitates represent a conglomeration of cells, which are present in almost all types of inflammation of the anterior segment. They vary in size and may be confluent. The thermal dynamics of the aqueous humor (temperature gradient between the iris and the corneal endothelium) lead to the deposition in the inferior zones of the cornea, characteristically in a triangular shape. Large keratic precipitates ("mutton fat") typically occur in granulomatous inflammations, e.g. sarcoidosis. The finding is not pathognomonic. Upon resolution of the inflammation, the precipitates become smaller with irregular margins.

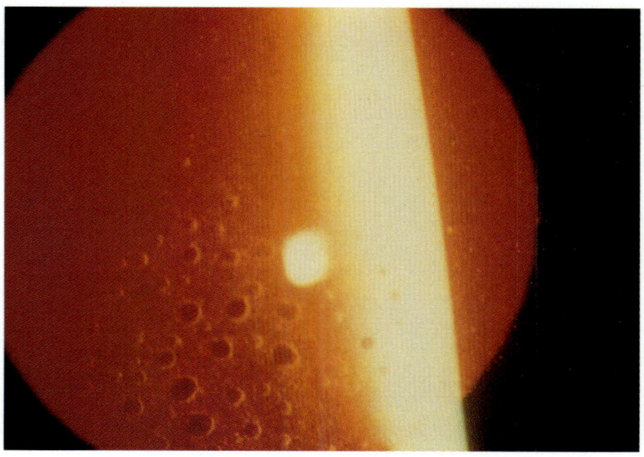

Figure 7.16 Keratic precipitates viewed with retroillumination. Same patient as in figure 7.15. The triangular constellation of the deposits is even better visible with retroillumination.

7.3 Inflammations

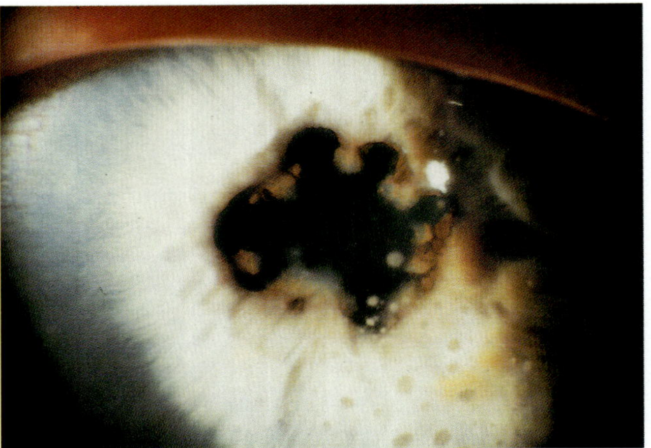

Figure 7.17 Keratic precipitates, posterior synechiae. The figure shows circumscribed adhesions between the iris and the anterior lens surface besides precipitates on the corneal endothelium *(bottom right)*. The pupil cannot be symmetrically dilated. In between the adhesions the pupil is retracted, allowing for the circulation of aqueous humor. The adhesions form with increased viscosity of the aqueous humor in inflammations. If the synechiae are extensive, the circulation of aqueous humor from the ciliary body into the anterior chamber is blocked (see chapter 9). The formation of synechiae can be prevented by early use of mydriatic agents.

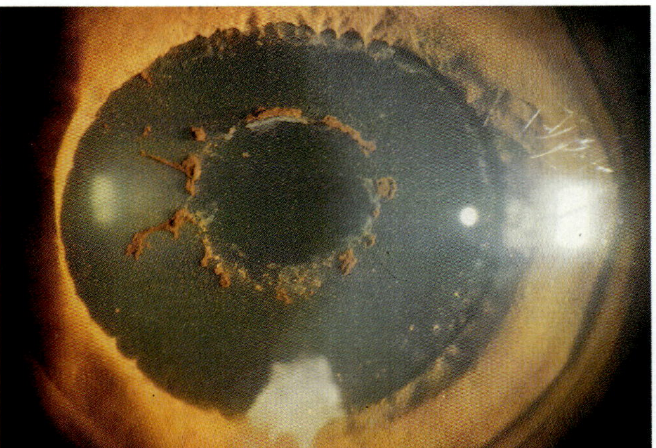

Figure 7.18 Status post iritis, pigment deposits on the anterior lens surface, fibrinous exsudation in the anterior chamber. The figure shows a status post severe irits. Fibrinous exudate (grey-white clot) remains in the lower iridocorneal angle. Centrally on the anterior lens surface is a ring of pigment. The finding indicates that in this area posterior synechiae had formed (see figure 7.17). The synechiae can be broken down by intensive use of topical mydriatics.

Figure 7.19 Keratic precipitates. The figure shows fine precipitates which are evenly spread over the corneal endothelium. They are very small in size and do not have the typical localization in the inferior zones of the cornea. The finding is characteristic of viral infections, e.g. cytomegalovirus and may also be present in heterochromia iritis (see figure 7.20).

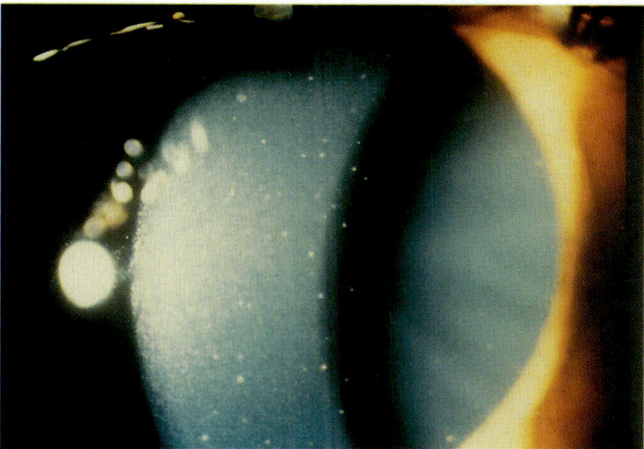

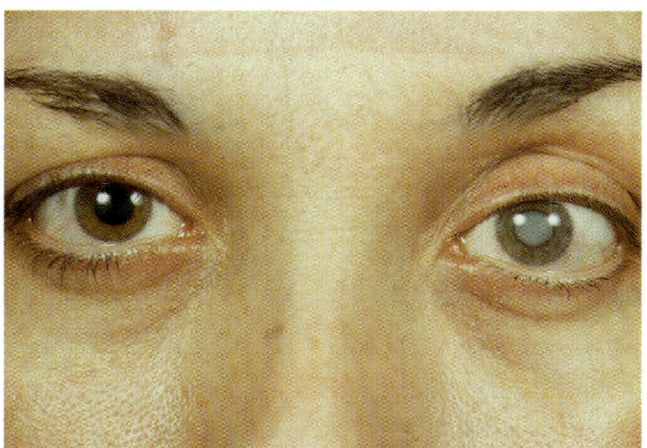

Figure 7.20 Heterochromia iritis of the left eye with cataract. Note the lighter iris color and the cataract in the affected eye. Heterochromia irits is usually unilateral, does not show signs of inflamma- tion or pain and is therefore often detected late. The keratic precipi- tates are small, star-shaped and may have fine processes. The hypo- chromia is associated with an atrophy of the stroma. A cataract often develops. The cause remains unclear, a viral infection is suspec- ted. Synechiae are not found. The inflammatory changes do not require treatment.

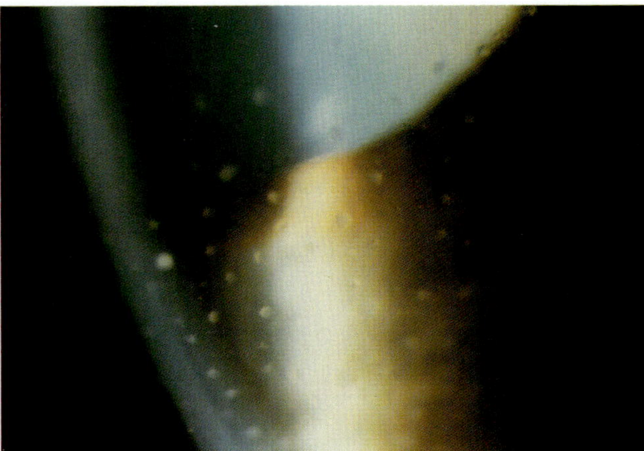

Figure 7.21 Keratic precipitates in heterochromia iritis, same patient as in figure 7.20. Small and medium-sized precipitates are present. The iris structure appears hazy, the lens opacity is homogenous.

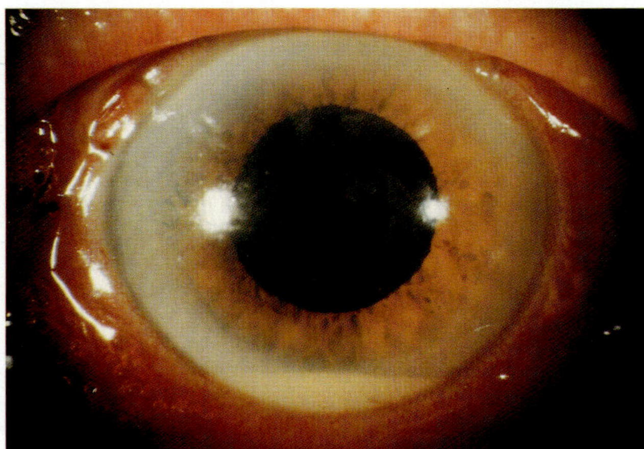

Figure 7.22 Hypopyon. In severe inflammations of the anterior segment, a deposition of inflammatory cells in the inferior part of the anterior chamber can occur. A marked hypopyon is macroscopically visible. Similar findings are associated with tumors or leukemia. Treatment depends on the underlying pathology.

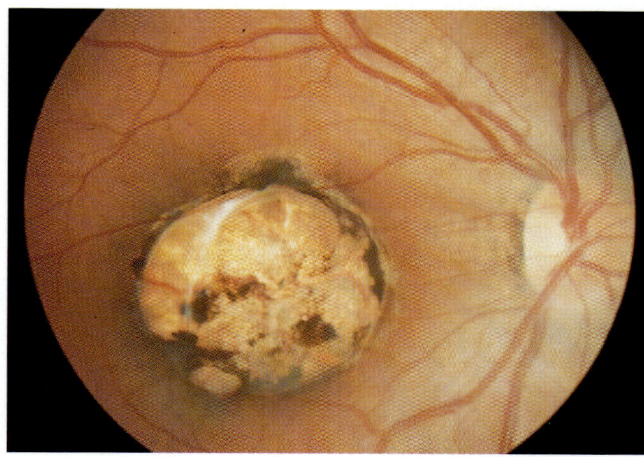

Figure 7.23 Chorioretinal scar in toxoplasmosis. The figure shows a sharply demarcated lesion in the posterior pole where the choroid is non existent and the sclera is bared. The area is surrounded by a hyperpigmented border. The inflammation has affected the retina and the choroid and led to a complete atrophy of both tissues. In most cases, the condition is congenital with infection of the mother during pregnancy. The scars are not susceptible to treatment. Recurrence at the margins of old scars is common (see figure 7.24).

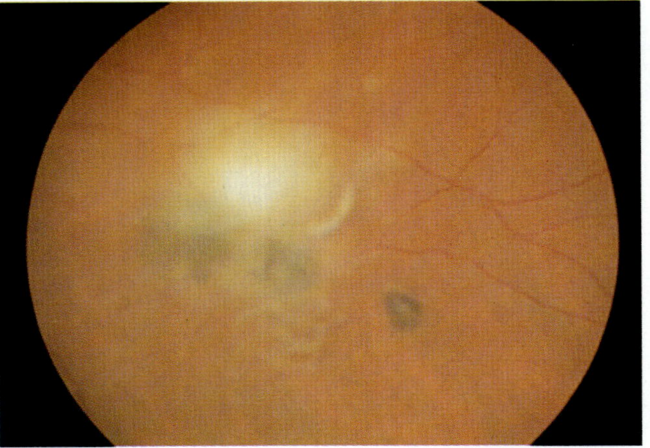

Figure 7.24   Active retinochoroiditis at the margin of a toxoplasma scar. The figure shows an active, ill-defined inflammatory focus at the superior margin of an old chorioretinal scar. It is a recurrence of congenital toxoplasmosis. The characteristic feature is the necrotizing retinitis at the margin of old scars. The recurrences are due to a reactivation of the parasites as well as immunologic processes. Therapy therefore includes antimicrobial agents as well as immunosuppressants (corticosteroids), which are recommended in vision-threatening lesions.

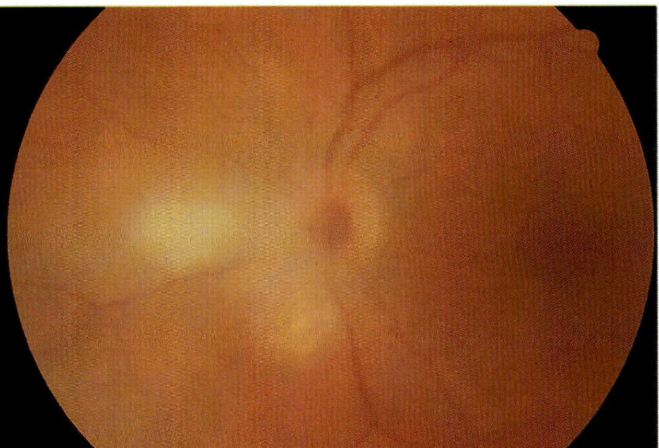

Figure 7.25   Juxtapapillar chorioretinitis . The figure shows two white-yellowish, ill-defined inflammatory foci adjacent to the nasal and inferior margin of the optic nerve head. The ocurrence of toxoplasmic chorioretinits outside of the macula is rare. The inflammation affects both choroid and retina and leads to a sectorial scotoma. Therapy see figure 7.24.

Figure 7.26 Status post chorioretinitis adjacent to the optic
nerve head. The figure shows a
white scar superior to the optic
nerve head. The choroid is completely atrophic, the overlying
retinal vessels are not attenuated.
In this case (figure), the cause for
the inflammation remains unclear.

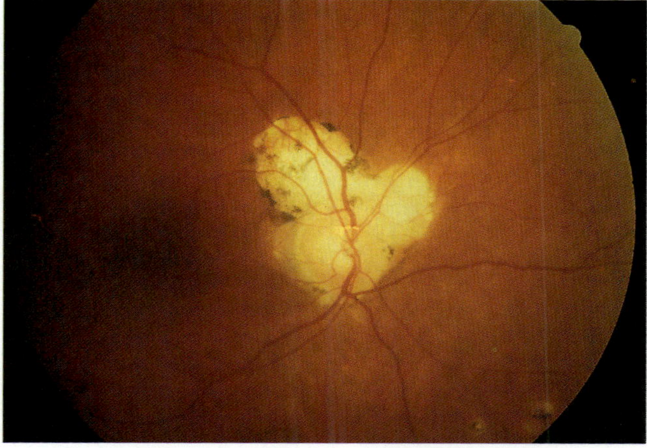

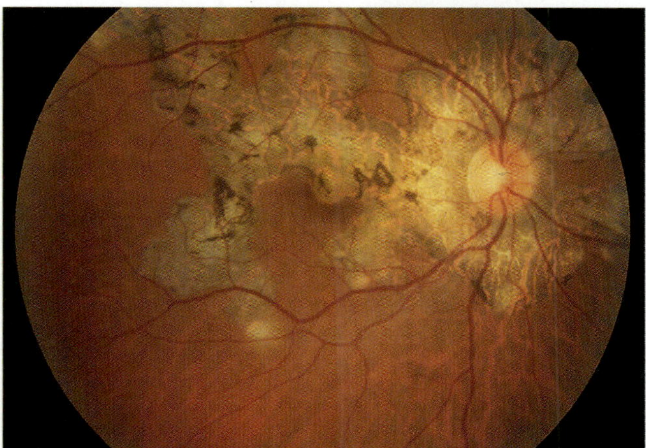

Figure 7.27 Peripapillary serpiginous choroiditis. The figure
shows a status post chorioretinitis
surrounding the optic nerve head
and in the midperiphery. The
retinal vessels are preserved, the
choriocapillaris and the retinal
pigment epithelium are atrophic.
The large choroidal vessels and the
sclera are bared. The margins of
the lesions are hyperpigmented.
The process affects mainly the
inner layers of the choroid and the
retinal pigment epithelium. The
inflammation spreads from the
peripapillary regions to the periphery within months to years. The
macula may remain unaffected
until late stages. The cause is unknown. Systemic steroids are
recommended in vision-threatening lesions.

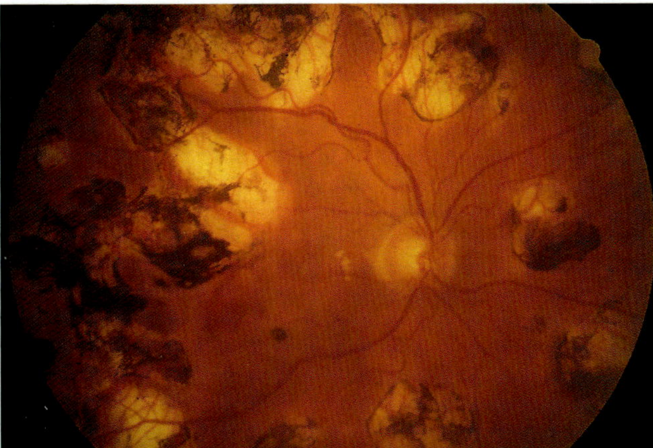

Figure 7.28 Status post choroiditis disseminata. Choroiditis may be multifocal in the entire fundus. The figure shows multiple healed lesions in multifocal choroiditis. The choriocapillaris and in places the whole choroid is atrophic. The white sclera is bared. The margins of the scars are hyperpigmented. The cause mostly remains unclear, systemic causes must be evaluated.

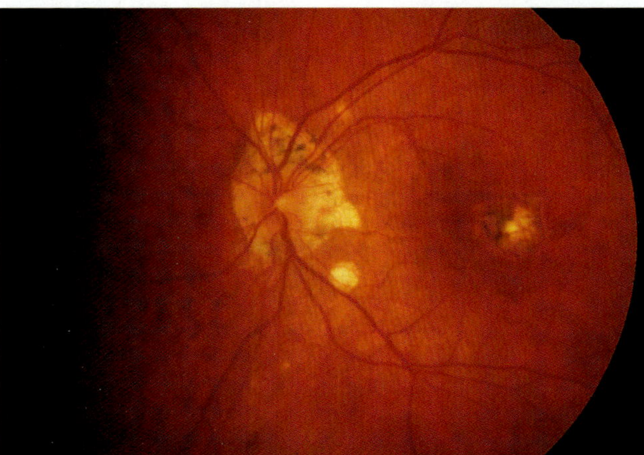

Figure 7.29 Presumed ocular histoplasmosis syndrome. The figure shows peripapillary atrophy and multiple sharply demarcated lesions in the posterior pole, which are the characteristic features of a syndrome of presumed infection with Histoplasma capsulatum. The scars are not susceptible to antifungal therapy. A complicating manifestation is subretinal choroidal neovascularization, which may lead to an impairment of vision. Follow-up is therefore important.

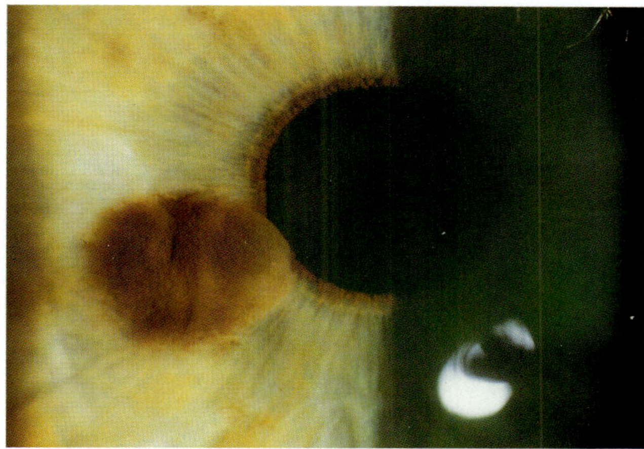

Figure 7.30 Iris nevus. The melanocytes of the iris stroma can be the origin of benign and malignant tumors. The figure shows an elevated brown tumor in the superficial layers of the iris, which is located at the pupillary margin.

This common benign tumor has to be differentiated from malignant processes. Signs of malignancy are growth and vascularization. A distortion of the pupil (see figure 7.36) may be present in benign tumors. Careful photographic documentation is important. Pupil size should be standardized. Surgical removal is required when features suggestive of malignancy are observed.

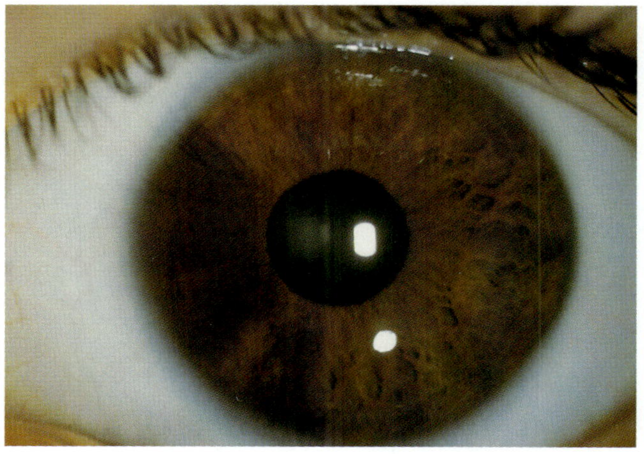

Figure 7.31 Iris nevus. In comparison to figure 7.30, this nevus is darker and larger. The process is considered benign, long-term observation did not display growth.

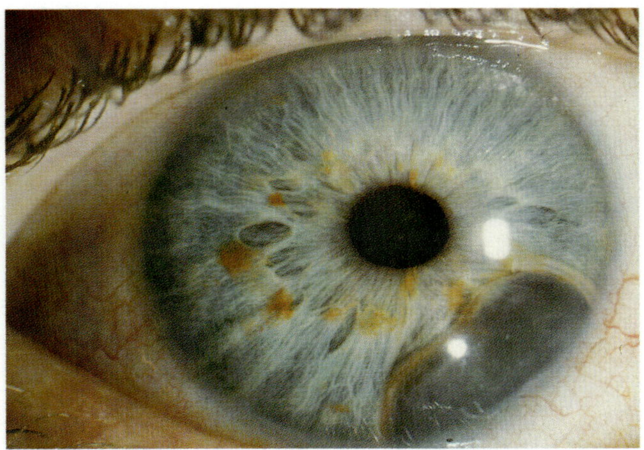

Figure 7.32 Iris cyst. Epithelial iris cysts are congenital. The clinical presentation may be confused with neoplasms. A differentiation can be made by transillumination. Complete surgical excision has to be considered if the cyst extends.

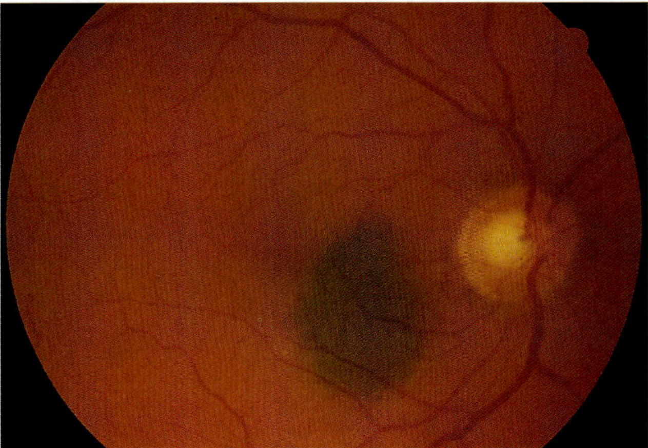

Figure 7.33 Choroidal nevus. The oval, grey-brown lesion in the posterior pole between the optic disc and the fovea is flat, the overlying retina and retinal vessels are unchanged. The flatness and the unchanged overlying retina are features that characterize benign nevi. Observation including photographic documentation is crucial for the early detection of growth, indicating malignant transformation.

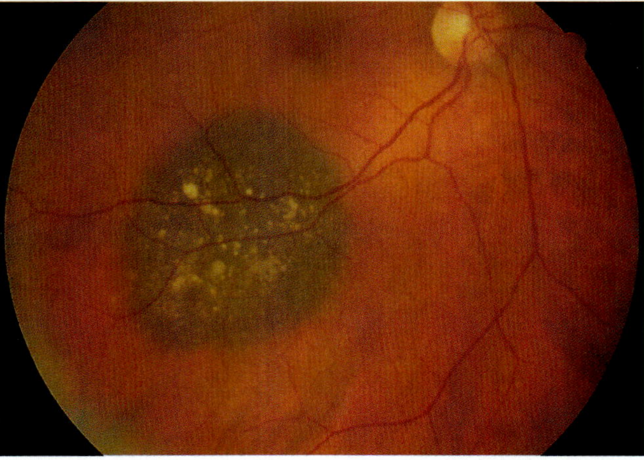

Figure 7.34 Choroidal nevus with secondary retinal changes. In comparison to the naevus in figure 7.33, yellowish drusen are found at the surface of this grey-brown lesion. The drusen are secondary degenerative changes of the overlying retina. The lesion is still considered benign, for it is not elevated and, as in figure 7.33, the retinal vessels are unchanged. Any change of the layers overlying the choroid demands frequent observation.

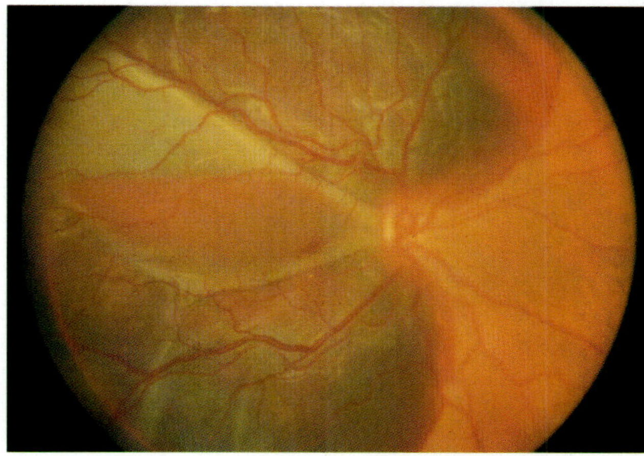

Figure 7.35 Subretinal hemorrhage. Grey elevation in the temporal quadrants with partly detached retina (light grey) and intraretinal hemorrhages at the margins. The extensive proportions and the intraretinal hemorrhages at the margins are suggestive for a subretinal hemorrhage rather than a neoplasm. A malignant tumor can be ruled out by ultrasonography (see figure 7.6). This type of choroidal hemorrage can be causally related to trauma, surgery with abrupt lowering of the intra-ocular pressure and systemic conditions with altered hemostasis as well as choroidal neovascularizations. Surgical removal of the blood can be considered, usually a spontaneous resorption is seen with partial visual restitution.

7.5 Malignant tumors

General: Malignant tumors can be found in the iris, the ciliary body
and the choroid. Processes in the iris are ususaly diagnosed in early
stages and are generally less malignant than those found in the posterior segment, irrespective of an early diagnosis. When surgical removal
of an iris tumor is indicated, a conservation of the globe can mostly be
achieved. Surgical procedures can be put off until the malignancy of a
process is verfied. An early intervention does not improve the prognosis.

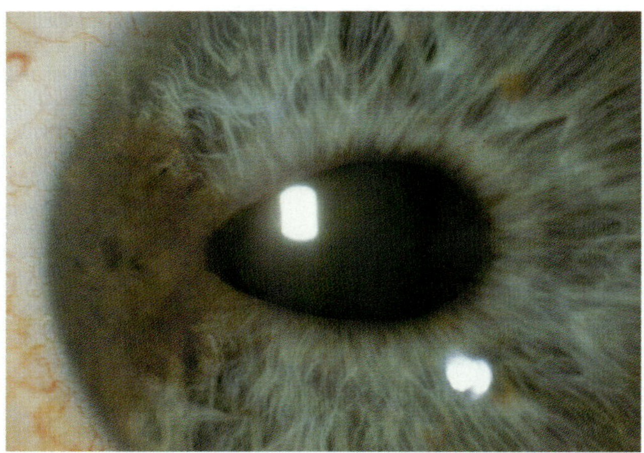

Figure 7.36   Iris melanoma
(spindle-cell). The figure shows a
pigmented tumor, which has
caused a distortion of the pupil.
The pupil distortion and even more
the documented growth were
suspicious features. The tumor was
excised. Histological evaluation
revealed a spindle-cell melanoma.
Local resection is usually sufficient
for the treatment of iris tumors.
Regardless of malignancy, the
growth is very slow and the prognosis is good. If the process is
restricted to the iris, a conservation
of the globe can be achieved.

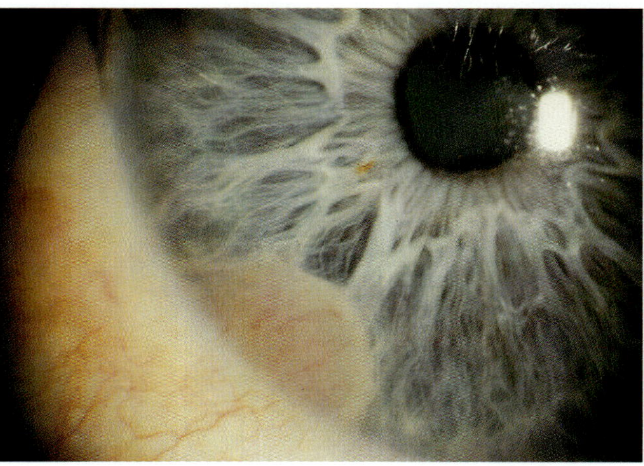

Figure 7.37   Iris / ciliary body
melanoma. In the inferior nasal
periphery of the iris a vascularized
tumor is found. Progressive growth
and extension into the ciliary body
had been noted. In this small
tumor the high degree of vascula-
rity is suggestive of malignancy. A
local resection was performed.

Figure 7.38 Status post en-bloc resection of an iris/ciliary body melanoma. Because of an invasion of the ciliary body an en-bloc resection had to be performed in addition to the iridectomy. The defect was covered with a corneal graft. Fair prognosis even with extension in to the ciliary body.

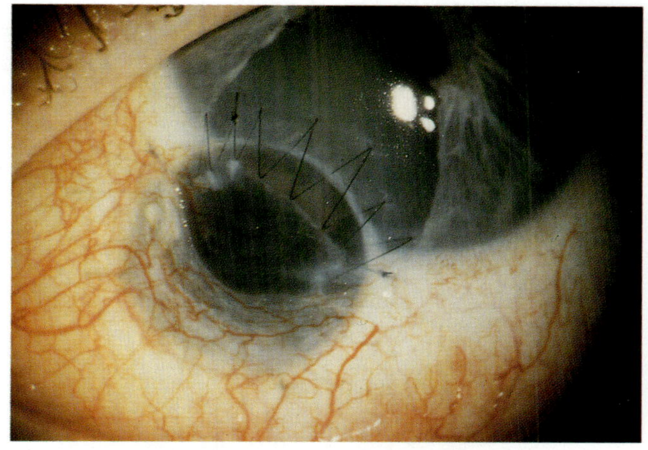

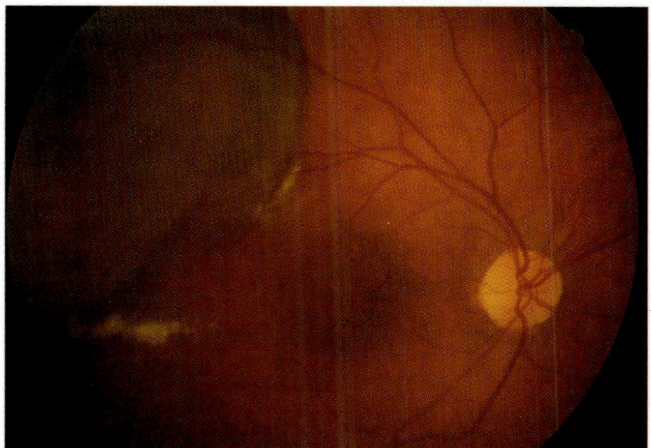

Figure 7.39 Choroidal melanoma. Typical picture of a choroidal melanoma with oval shaped elevation. The diagnosis is often late, for the patient does not notice the peripheral visual field defects. Its thickness differentiates the lesion from a benign nevus. The differen-tial diagnosis is subretinal hemor-rhage. The diagnosis is made by ultrasonography, transillumination (in anterior localization) and CT. A retinal detachment not adjacent to the tumor is highly suggestive for malignancy. Therapeutic options are irradiation, local resection and enucleation. The choice of manage-ment depends on the size, location and extent of the tumor. Metastatic disease may occur despite radical removal. The malignancy correlates with the histological classification.

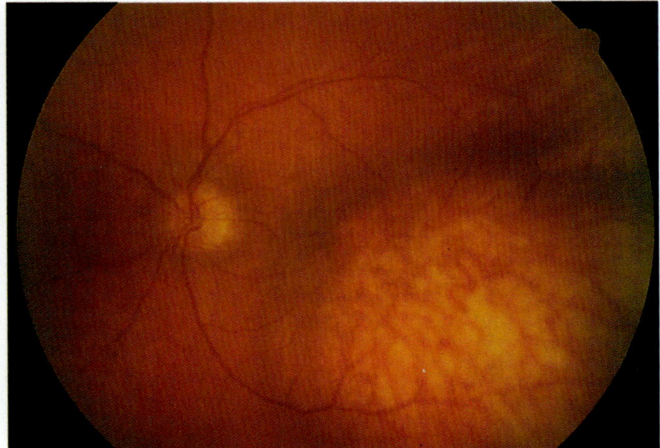

Figure 7.40   Amelanotic choroidal melanoma with perforation of Bruch´s membrane. The figure shows an elevated lesion in the lower temporal quadrant with markedly enlarged vasculature and hyperpigmented borders. It is a melanoma that has perforated Bruch´s membrane. Therefore the deeper strucures and the tumor vessels are visible. Diagnosis and therapy see figure 7.39.

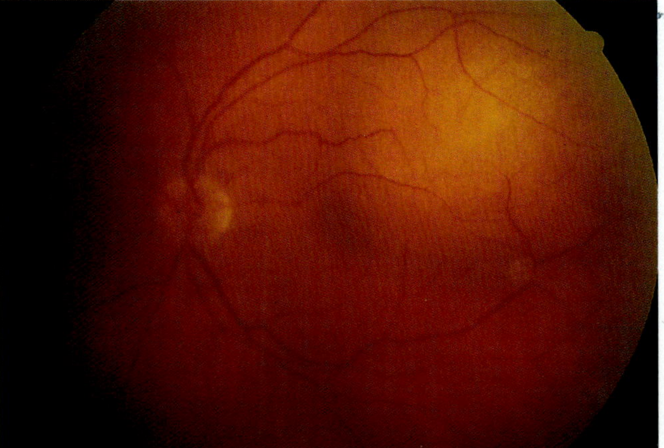

Figure 7.41   Choroidal metastasis. The figure shows a slightly elevated yellowish tumor below the superior temporal arcade. It is a metastatic tumor of a breast carcinoma. Metastases of malignant tumors in the eye are reltively common and may be the earliest manifestation. Primary neoplasms are mostly breast and lung carcinoma. In comparison to the primary malignant tumors of the choroid, the metastatic tumors exhibit a faster growth, are less elevated and have a superficial yellowish hue. The diffuse growth pattern and concomitant retinal detachment are features suggestive for a metastatic choroidal tumor. Prognosis and therapy depend on the type of primary neoplasm.

Figure 7.42   Central areolar choroidal dystrophy. The figure shows a circumscibed lesion with atrophic retinal pigment epithelium and choriocapillaris in the posterior pole. Dystrophies of the choriocapillaris can be hereditary (bilateral) or result from degenerative changes. Visual acuity is severly impaired.

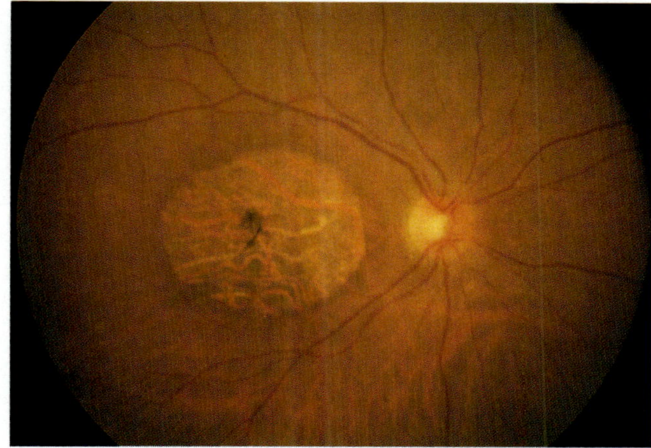

Figure 7.43   Choroideremia. Ophthalmoscopy shows an almost white fundus resulting from an atrophy of the choroid and the retinal pigment epithelium. The condition is hereditary and progressive. It develops first in the periphery and then spreads centrally, leaving the macula unaffected until last. The perfusion of the optic disc remains normal. Treatment is not available.

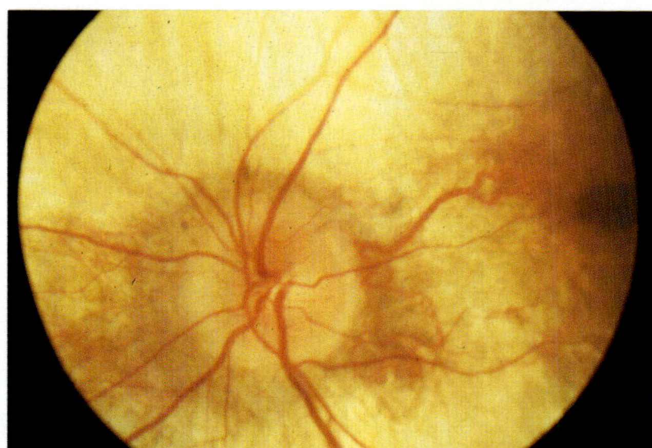

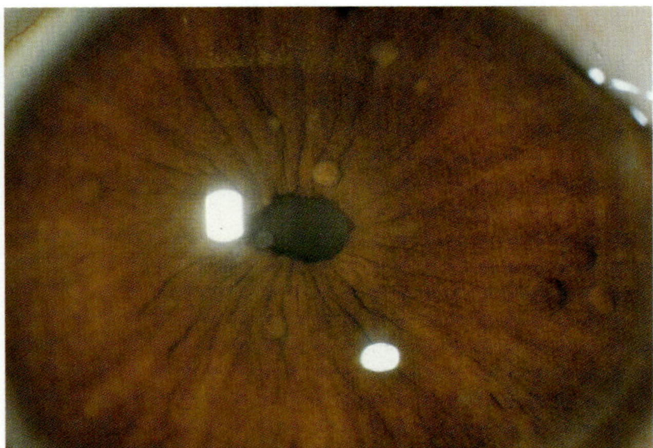

Figure 7.44 Lisch nodules. The darkly pigmented iris shows multiple, slightly elevated nodules. This finding is associated with neurofibromatosis type 1.

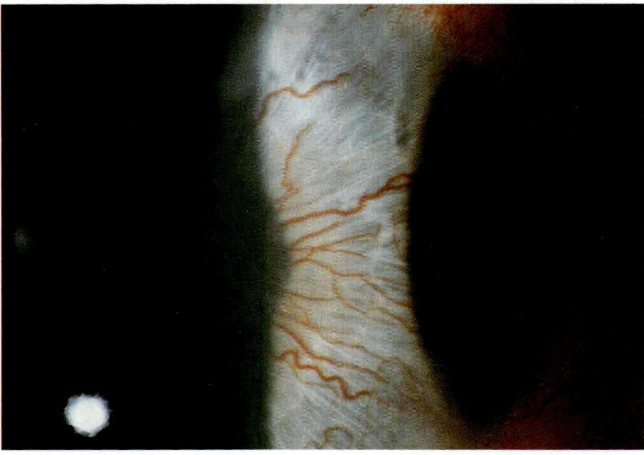

Figure 7.45 Rubeosis iridis. The condition occurs secondarily in the late stages of various ocular and systemic disorders with vascular pathology. The neovascularization in rubeosis iridis has to be differentiated from an atrophy of the iris stroma, in which the iris vessels become prominent. Closure of the iridocorneal angle (see chapter 9) is the most severe complication of rubeosis iridis besides hemorrhages. The condition requires careful ocular examination and systemic evaluation for vascular disease, such as diabetes mellitus and carotid artery occlusive disease. Therapeutic management depends on the underlying pathology.

Figure 7.46 Angioid streaks. The linear lesions can be found around the optic disc and in the mid-periphery. They are a result of dehiscences in Bruch´s membrane. Angioid streaks are associated with various systemic disorders, mostly pseudoxanthoma elasticum or Ehlers-Danlos syndrome. Visual impairment may be caused by choroidal neovascularization, which is a frequent complication.

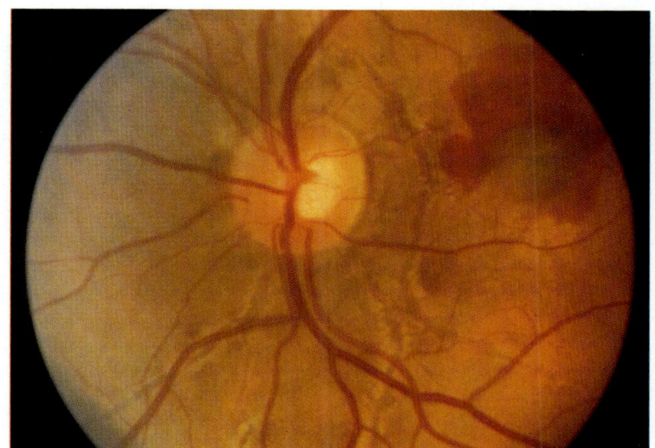

Pupil

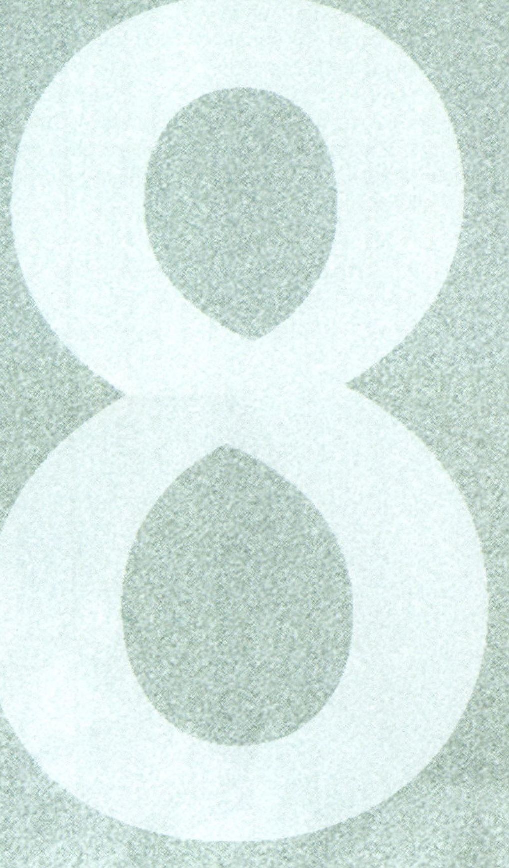

8.1 Pupillomotor pathway and examination techniques

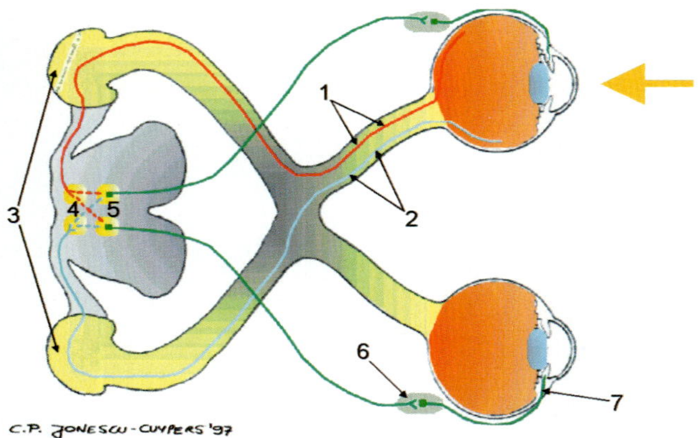

Figure 8.1 Pupillomotor pathway, schematic drawing. The afferent pupillary pathway originates in the retina and follows the optic nerve and the optic tract. The conduction from the temporal halves of the retinas is ipsilateral (1), the axons of the medial retinas (2) cross in the chiasma to the contralateral side. The afferent pupillomotor fibers bypass lateral geniculate nucleus (3) and terminate in the pretectal area (4), which projects to both Edinger-Westphal nuclei (5), from where the efferent pupillomotor pathway originates. The efferent pupillomotor fibers are synapsed in the ciliary ganglion (6) and innervate the pupillary sphincter muscle and the ciliary muscle (7). These parasympathetic fibers follow the oculomotor nerve into the orbit, the sympathetic fibers that innervate the pupillary dilator muscle originate from the ciliospinal center of the VIII. cervical segment and follow the internal carotid artery.

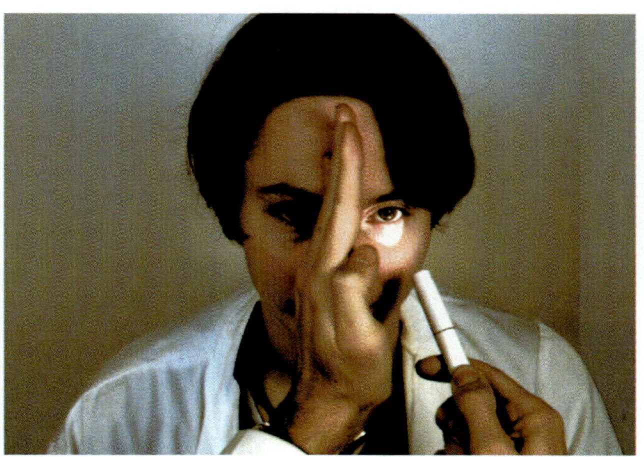

Figure 8.2 Testing for direct and indirect pupillary light reaction. Pupillary constriction develops with illumination of one eye (direct pupillary light rection). Observation of the contralateral eye, which is not illuminated, reveals a simultaneous pupillary constriction (indirect or consensual pupillary light reaction).

Figure 8.3   Testing for pupillary near reflex. When a subject fixates a near object, accomodative convergence occurs along with constriction of the pupils.

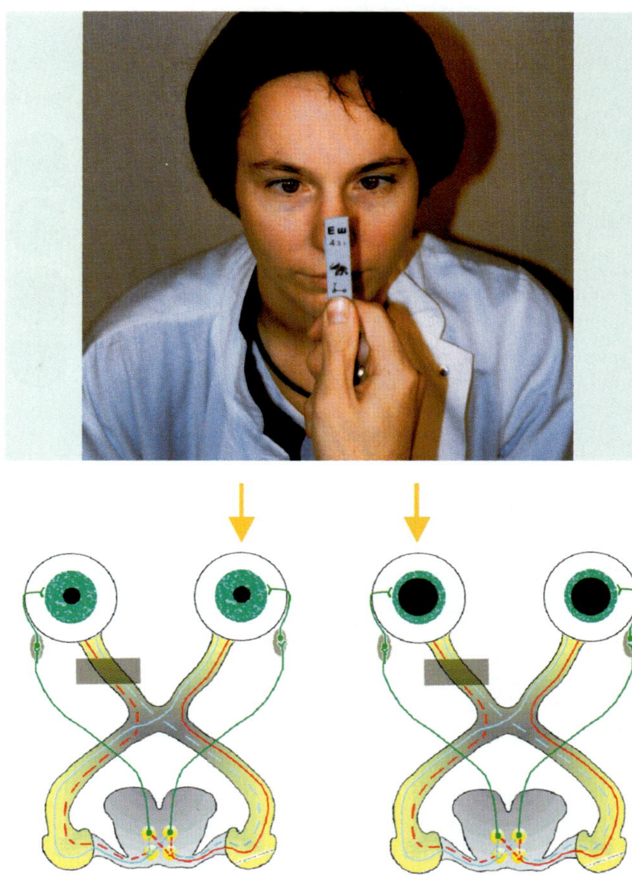

Figure 8.4   "Swinging flashlight test" for the detection of an afferent pupillary defect, schematic drawing. The illumination of the normal eye *(left figure,* right eye*)* leads to brisk pupillary constriction in both eyes. The illumination of the eye with the afferent pupillary defect *(right figure,* left eye*)* elicits only an incomplete pupillary constriction in the affected eye as well as the normal eye. The light is shone several times for a few seconds in each eye alternately. This alternate illumination test ("swinging flashlight") reveals a relative afferent pupillary defect. Following brisk pupillary constriction in the affected eye as a consensual light reaction (with illumination of the normal eye), the pupil is actually seen to dilate when light is shone directly in the affected eye.

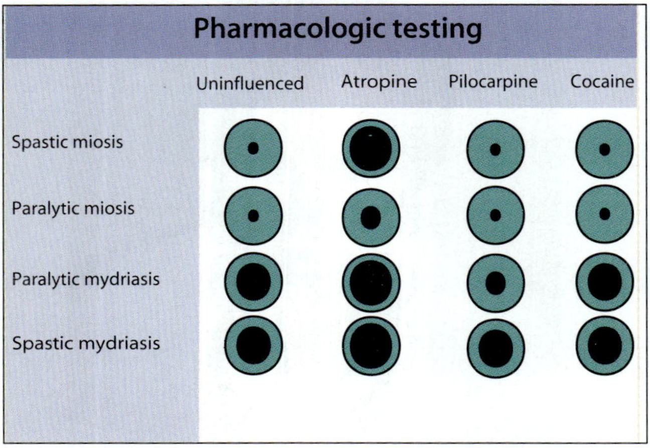

Pharmacologic testing

	Uninfluenced	Atropine	Pilocarpine	Cocaine
Spastic miosis				
Paralytic miosis				
Paralytic mydriasis				
Spastic mydriasis				

Figure 8.5 Pharmacologic pupillary testing, schematic overview. By applying different pharmacologic agents, which influence the pupil, a differentiation can be made between spastic miosis and spastic mydriasis (parasympathetic and sympathetic stimulation respectively), paralytic miosis (sympathoparesis) and paralytic mydriasis (parasympathoparesis).

Figure 8.6 Testing for Argyll Robertson pupil and pupillary paresis with illumination, with near effort and application of various pharmacologic agents, schematic overview.

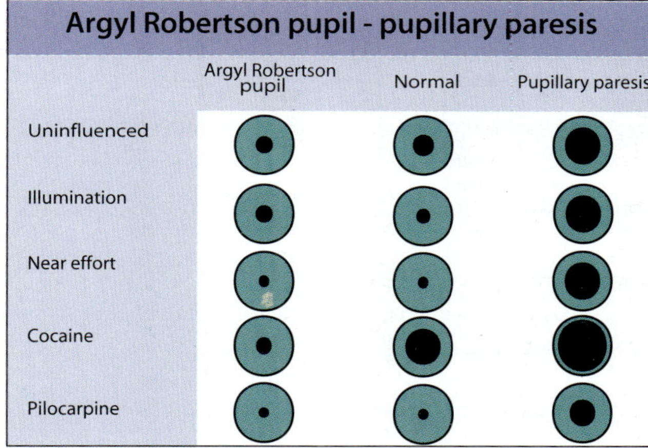

Figure 8.7 Right-sided Horner syndrome. A lesion of the sympathetic innervation of the right eye leads to pupillary constriction (miosis), due to the paresis of the pupillary dilator muscle, and to discrete ptosis by failure of the superior tarsal muscle of Müller. The comparison of both eyes gives the impression of apparent enophthalmos on the affected side. The clinical manifestations are summarized as: miosis, ptosis, enophthalmos.

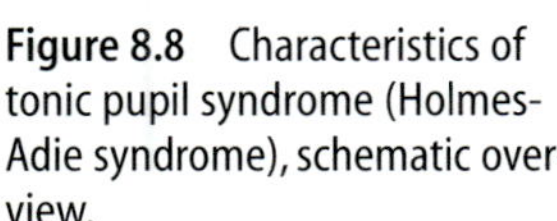

Figure 8.8 Characteristics of tonic pupil syndrome (Holmes-Adie syndrome), schematic overview.

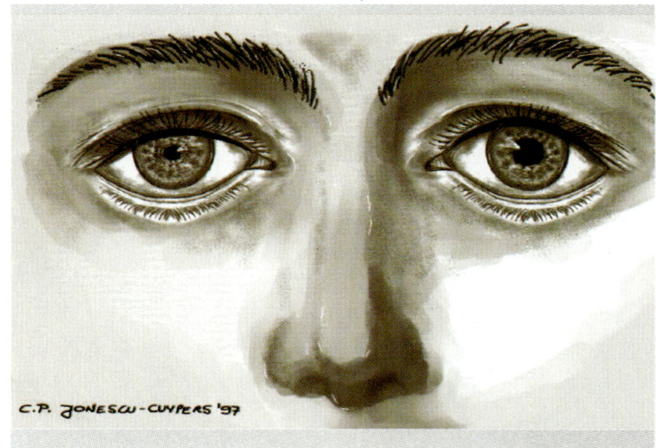

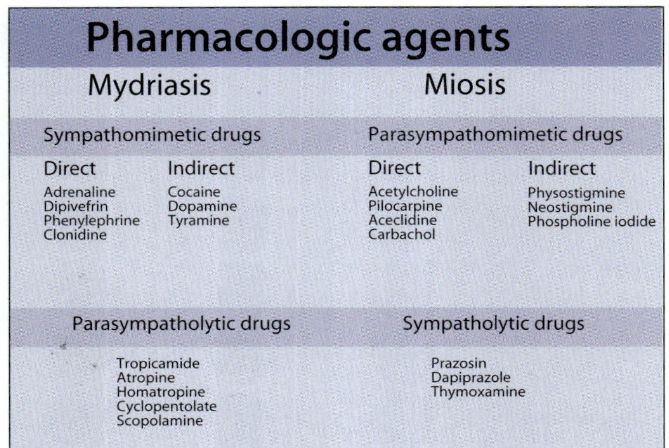

Figure 8.9 Overview of the various pharmacologic agents that influence the pupil.

Figure 8.10 Overview of the various causes of disturbances of accomodation.

Disturbances of accommodation

1. Physiologic with age
2. Diagnostic cycloplegia
3. Parasympatholytic (atropine, scopolamine, cyclopentolate)
4. Congenital defects of the ciliary muscle
5. Poisoning
   (ergot alkaloids, snake venom, lead)
6. Disorders involving the ciliary muscle (cyclitis)
7. Prolonged near-effort
8. Direct / indirect parasympathomimetic drugs
9. Orbital
10. Inflammatory disease
11. Oculomotor spasms

8 Pupil

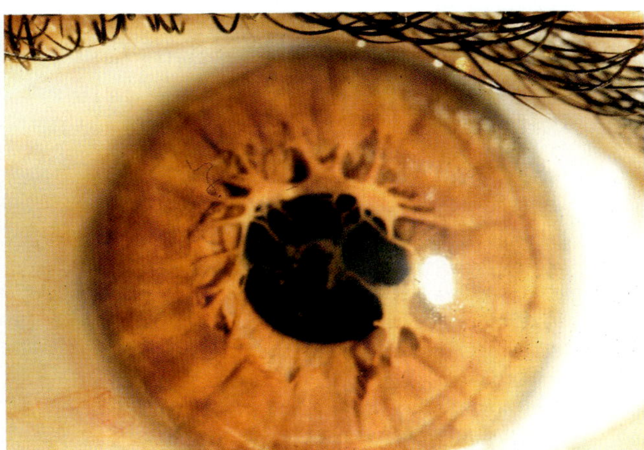

Figure 8.11 Persistent pupillary membane. The figure shows remnants of stromal iris tissue in the pupillary opening. This common finding is due to incomplete atrophy of the fetal pupillary membrane.

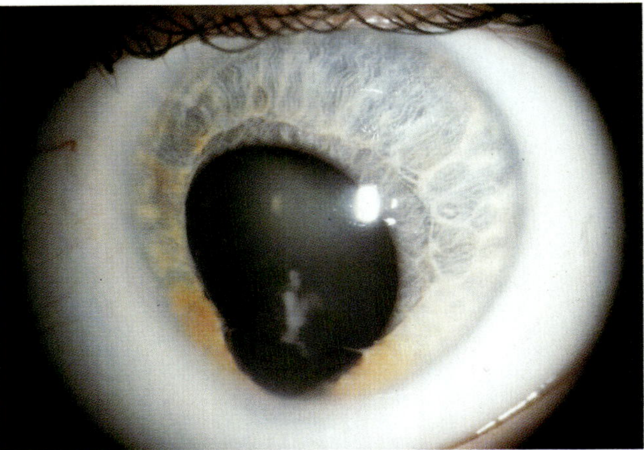

Figure 8.12 Coloboma of the pupil. This finding results from an incomplete fusion of the embryonic fissure of the optic cup. In accordance with the location of the embryonic fissure of the optic cup, the coloboma of the pupil is mostly located in the inferonasal quadrant. It presents as a characteristic notch in the pupillary margin. The pupillary sphincter muscle is absent in the area of the coloboma.

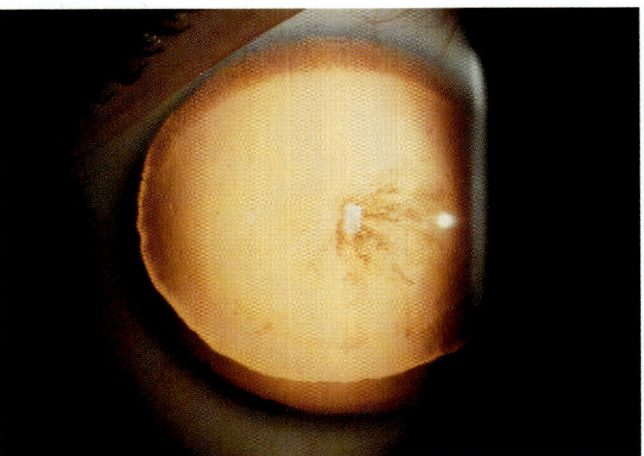

Figure 8.13 Congenital aniridia. In this condition, a large portion of the iris is absent, only a part of the iris root is present. With retro-illumination, the lens equator becomes visible *(inferior aspect)*. Aniridia is mostly associated with nystagmus and amblyopia.

Figure 8.14 Circular ectropion uveae at the pupillary margin. This dysgenetic iris finding is frequently associated with dysgenesis of the filtration angle and primary glaucoma.

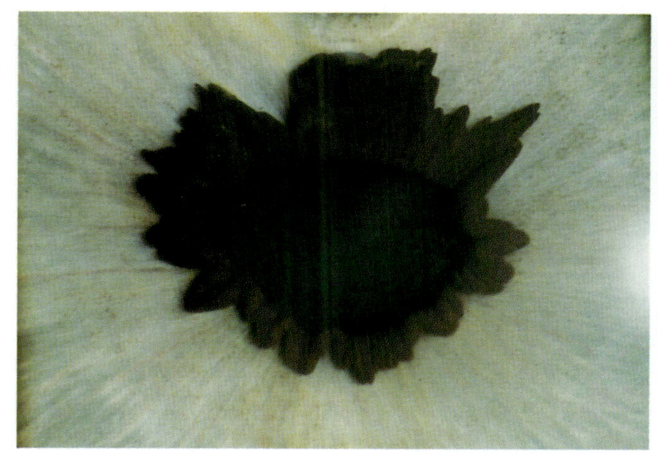

Figure 8.15 Irregular pupil and incomplete mydriasis in atrophic iris following acute glaucoma. Due to the extreme rise in intraocular pressure in acute glaucoma, a postischemic atrophy of the iris has developed with loss of marginal portions of iris tissue, pigment dispersion onto the iris stroma and baring of the underlying pigment epithelium.

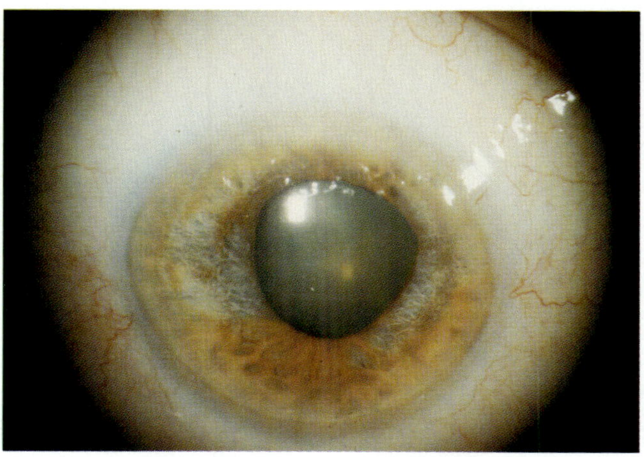

Figure 8.16 Atrophy of the iris in Rieger syndrome. In mesodermal dysgenesis of the anterior segment (Rieger syndrome), multiple holes in the iris may be present, resembling multiple pupils (polycoria). Characteristic features are the ectropion uveae at the oiginal pupillary margin and the irregularity of the pupil.

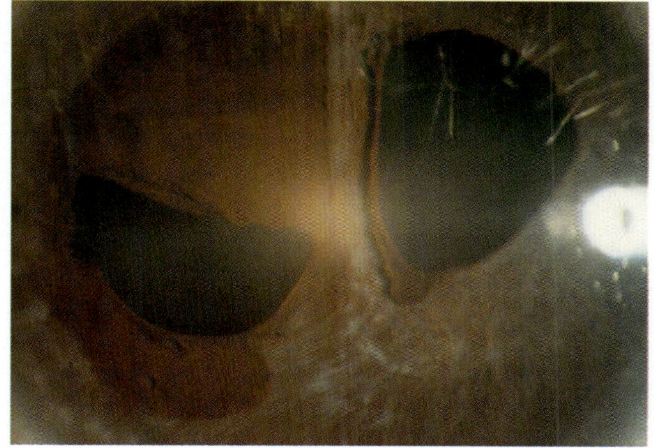

8.4 Congenital and acquired changes in shape of the pupil

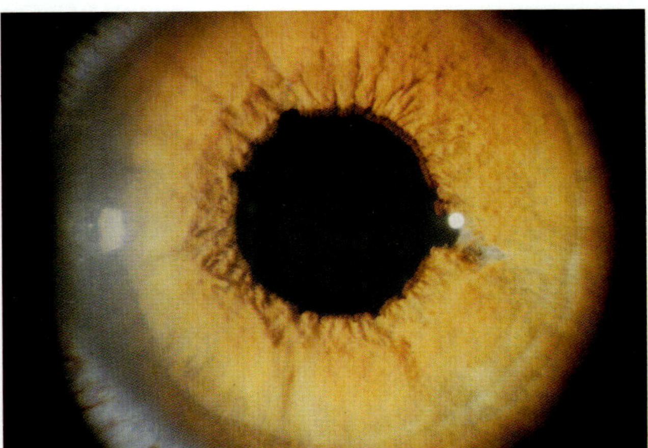

Figure 8.17 Rupture of the pupillary sphincter muscle at the 3 o´clock position following blunt trauma. The shock wave exerted on the globe has caused a localized tear of the pupillary sphincter muscle.

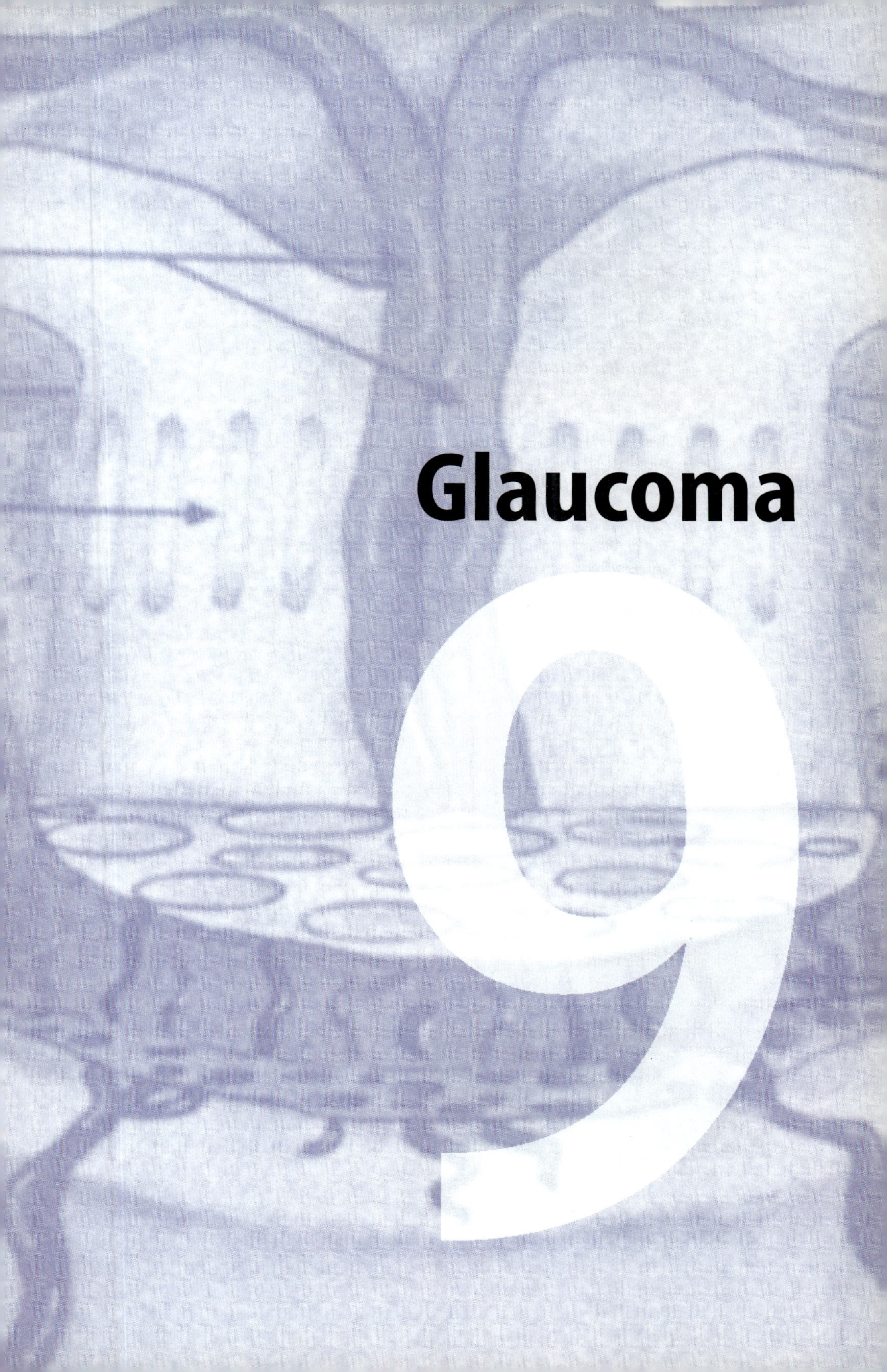

Glaucoma

9

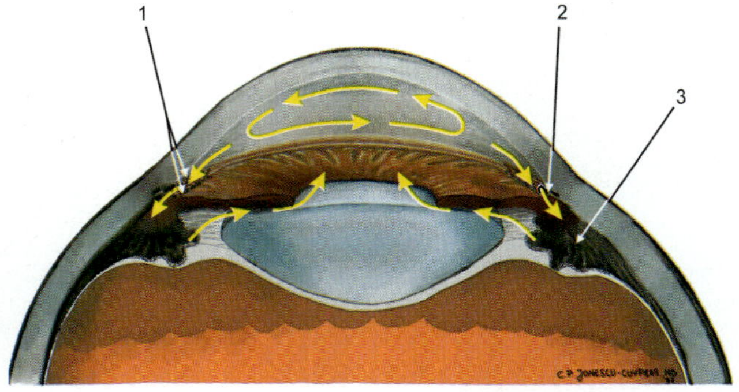

Figure 9.1 Hydrodynamics of the aqueous humor in the human eye, schematic drawing. Aqueous humor is produced in the non-pigmented epithelium of the ciliary body (3) in the posterior chamber. It then flows around the lens and through the pupil into the anterior chamber. In the anterior chamber it is subject to thermal convection, in which the aqueous humor flows downwards along the corneal endothelium (minor drop in temperature), while it rises in proximity to the warmer and well perfused iris. Most of the aqueous humor leaves the anterior chamber via the so-called conventional outflow pathway (trabecular meshwork, Schlemm´s canal, collector channels, episcleral veins) (1). A small portion of the aqueous humor is drained via the so-called unconventional outflow pathway across the ciliary muscle into the choroid and the suprachoroidal space (2).

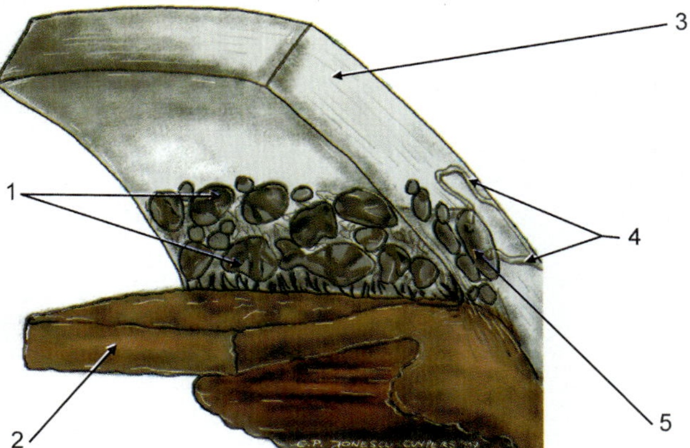

Figure 9.2 Schematic drawing of the outflow structures in the anterior chamber angle: (1) trabecular meshwork; (2) iris; (3) cornea; (4) collector channels; (5) Schlemm´s canal. The aqueous humor flows through the three layers of the trabecular meshwork into Schlemm´s canal and is then drained via approximately 20 collector channels, which perforate the sclera, into the episcleral veins.

Figure 9.3   Schematic drawing of the structure of the optic nerve and the blood supply of the optic disc. (1) central retinal artery and vein; (2) short posterior ciliary arteries; (3) sensory retina; (4) choroid; (5) arachnoid with pial blood vessels for the supply of the postlaminar optic nerve; (6) optic nerve sheath (dura mater); (7) lamina cribrosa. With myelinization of the nerve fibers, the optic nerve becomes thicker posterior to the lamina cribrosa.

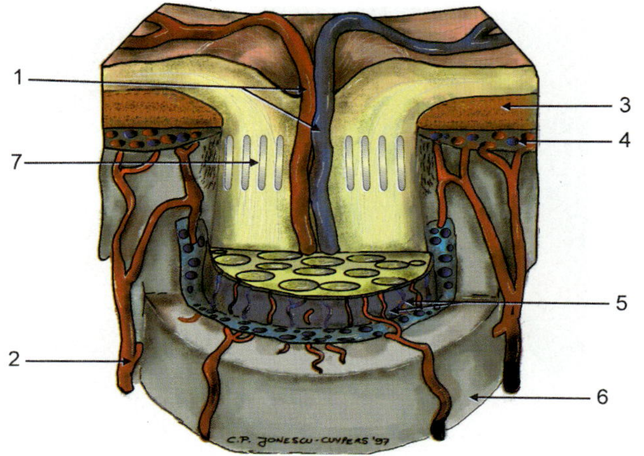

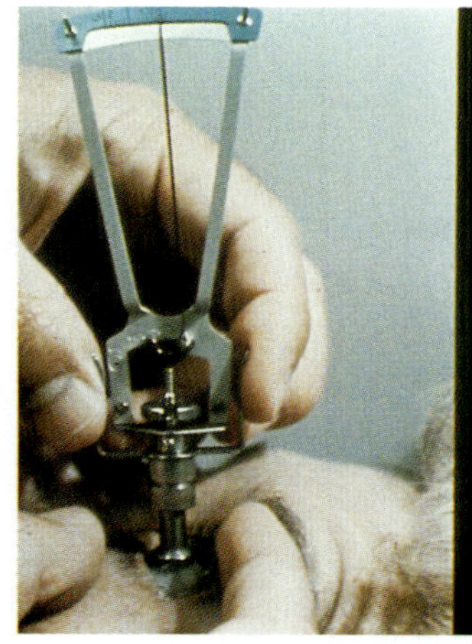

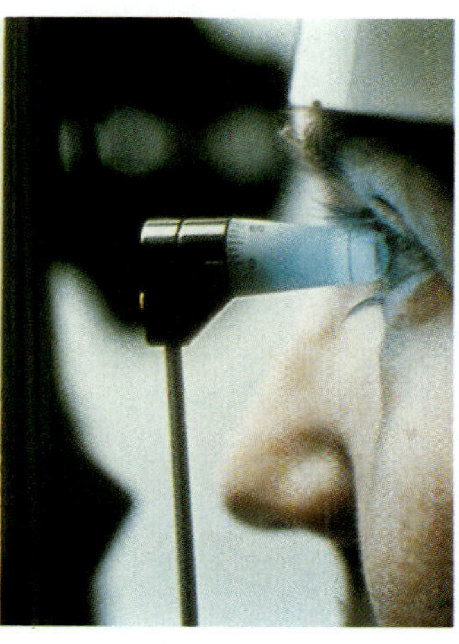

Figure 9.4   Measurement of intraocular pressure. The *left* part of the figure shows the so-called indentation tonometry, which is based on an assessment of intraocular pressure by measuring the variable indentation of the corneal dome with a defined weight. The metal plunger that indentates the central cornea is attached to a pointer, which rides along a scale. The *right* part of the figure shows the Goldmann applanation tonometry. An area of applanation of approximately 3 mm diameter is generated with a variable amount of force applied on a plastic cylinder, in which two prisms are incorporated. With an area of applanation of 3.06 mm diameter, 1 Pond of applanation force corresponds to 1 mmHg intraocular pressure. Both methods require local anesthesia of the ocular surface. In applantion tonometry, the tear film is stained with fluorescein vital dye. The applanation of the corneal surface produces a ring of fluorescence viewed under blue light at the slit lamp.

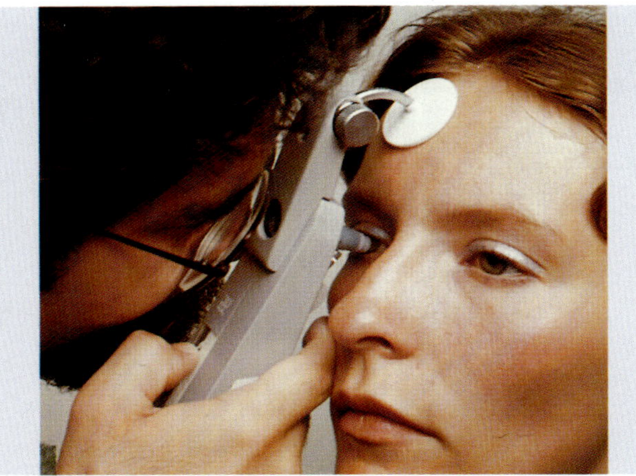

Figure 9.5 Hand-held tonometry with the Perkins tonometer. Hand-held applanation tonometry applies the priciple of Goldmann tonometry. It does not require defined positioning of the patient and can be performed at the bedside or in infants under general anesthesia.

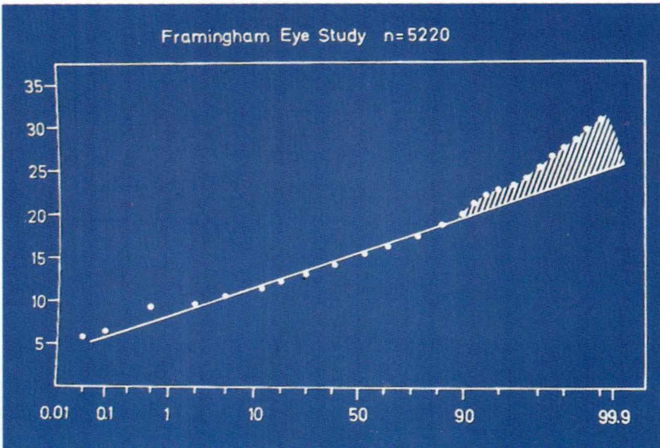

Figure 9.6 Graph of the cumulative frequency of intraocular pressure values measured in a population of 5220 subjects in the Framingham Eye Study. The *ordinate* gives the intraocular pressure (IOP; mmHg), the *abscissa* gives the cumulative frequency (%). 90% of the adult population therefore have an IOP of up to 20 mmHg. An IOP higher than 20 mmHg is determined ocular hypertension and is considered the most important risk factor for glaucoma.

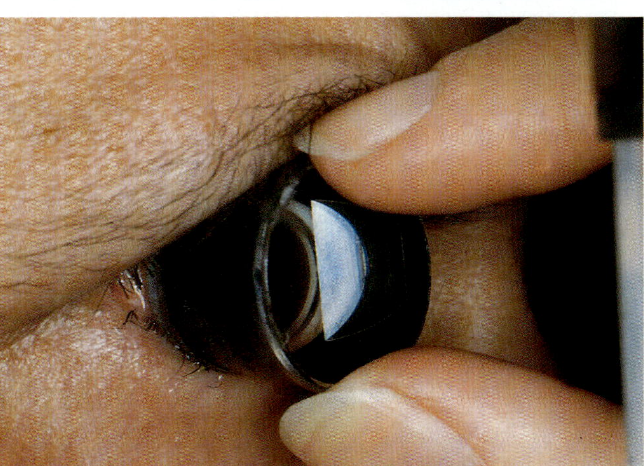

Figure 9.7 Gonioscopy with the Goldmann lens. For the examination of the anterior chamber angle (gonioscopy) a contact lens is placed on the eye, in which an inclinated mirror is incorporated in a such way that a view of the chamber angle on its opposite side is provided. The entire circumference of the angle can be viewed by turning the contact lens. Anesthetic eye drops are given prior to the examination.

Figure 9.8 Gonioscopic appearance of a wide, open anterior chamber angle. The mirror of the gonioscopic contact lens is at the 12 o´clock position, so that the chamber angle at the 6 o´clock position is viewed. The limitation of the dark pigmentation towards the cornea corresponds to Schwalbe´s line. The area of most intense pigmentation marks the position of Schlemm´s canal. The anterior chamber angle is wide, the outflow structures are almost entirely visible. There is no anatomic disposition to angle-closure glaucoma. ·

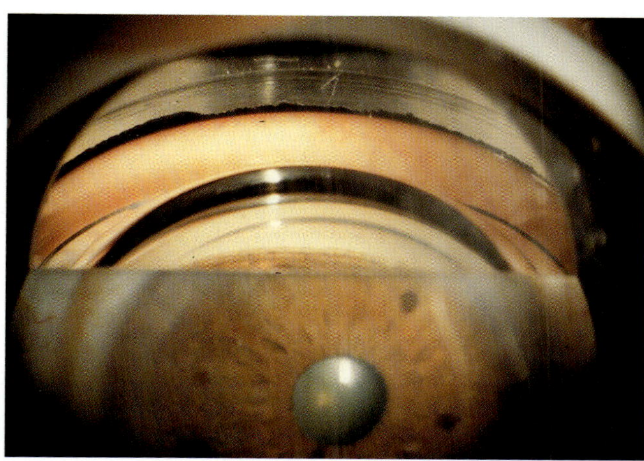

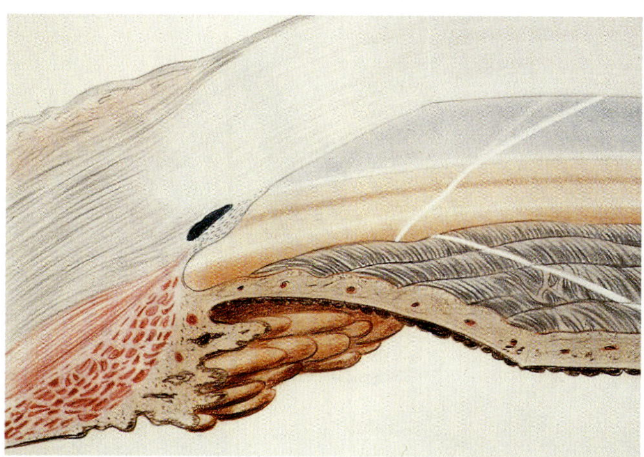

Figure 9.9 Section through a wide, open anterior chamber angle. Schwalbe´s line lies at the point where the narrow light beams reflected from the epithelial and endothelial corneal surfaces meet. The adjoint darkly pigmented band marks the position of Schlemm´s canal. The white band below corresponds to the scleral spur, the only area of firm attachment between the choroid and the sclera. In between the peripheral iris and the scleral spur lies the ciliary body band, which is the anterior surface of the ciliary body. If the structures in between Schwalbe´s line (anterior limitation of the outflow structures) and the scleral spur (posterior limitation of the outflow structures) are visible for the most part of the circumference upon gonioscopy, the anterior chamber angle is determined wide and open, without risk of closure.

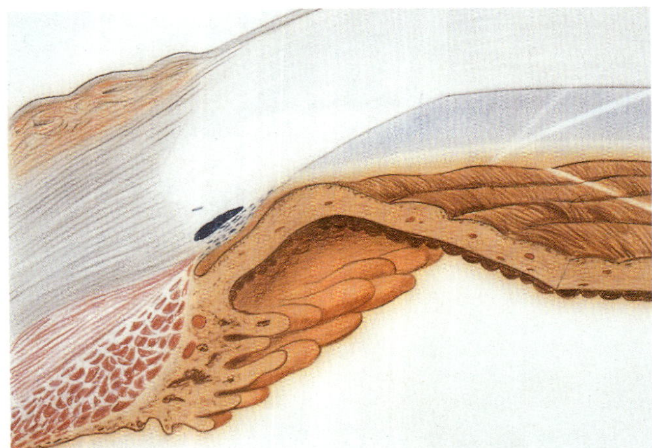

Figure 9.10 Section through a narrow anterior chamber angle. Only the anterior portions of the outflow structures are gonioscopically visible. There is an anatomic disposition to acute angle-closure glaucoma.

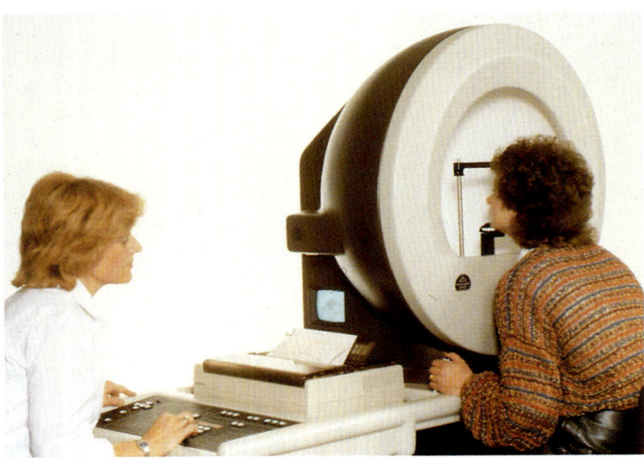

Figure 9.11 Examination of a glaucoma patient with a computer perimeter. The patient´s head lies on a headrest. She looks into a white hemisphere, in which light stimuli of variable location and intensity are projected. The patient is asked to fixate a central point and document the perception of a light stimulus by operating a switch. With this so-called computerized automated static threshold perimetry, the threshold of light perception at variable points of the visual field is determined using a special bracketing strategy. The result is presented numerically or graphically as gray scale or pattern printouts.

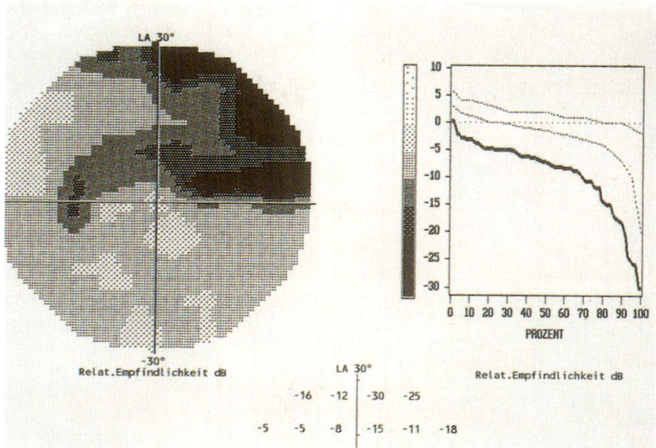

Figure 9.12 Printout of glaucomatous visual field defect, *(left)* grey scale *(right)* cumulative defect curve. The grey scale printout shows an arcuate scotoma that starts at the blind spot and lies horizontally between 12 and 18 degrees. The arcuate scotoma arches into the periphery and merges with a nasal step defect. The darkness of the color correlates with the density of the scotoma. Homogenous black color represents an absolute defect, different shades of grey a relative defect. The *right* part of the figure shows the cumulative defect curve, i.e. a graphic ranking of the defect for each point in the visual field. The *thick line* shows the measured values, the two *thin lines* the age-corrected normal range. Cumulative defect curves are helpful in differentiating between a localized absolute defect and a diffuse depression of the visual field.

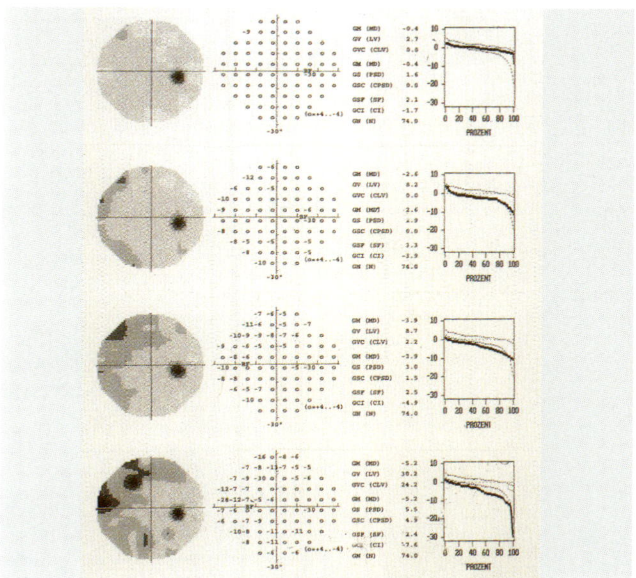

Figure 9.13 Progression of glaucomatous visual field defects with time *(from top to bottom).* On the *left* side is the grey scale printout, in the *middle* is the numeric difference plot, displaying the difference between the measured threshold and the normal value in dezibel, on the *right* side are the cumulative defect curves.

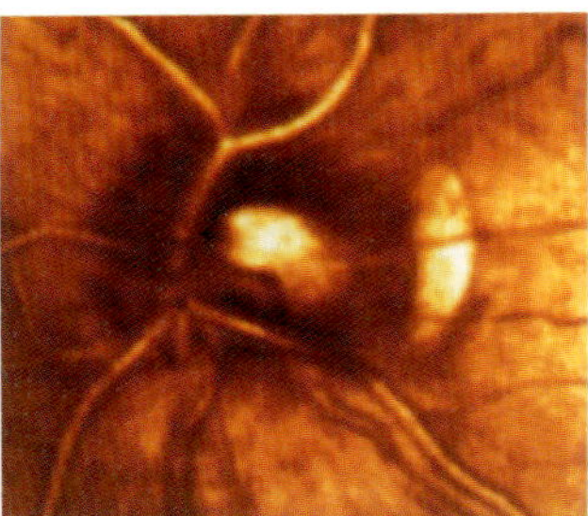
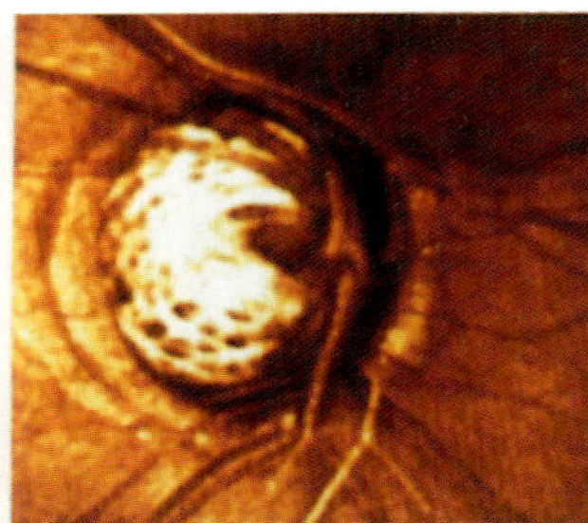
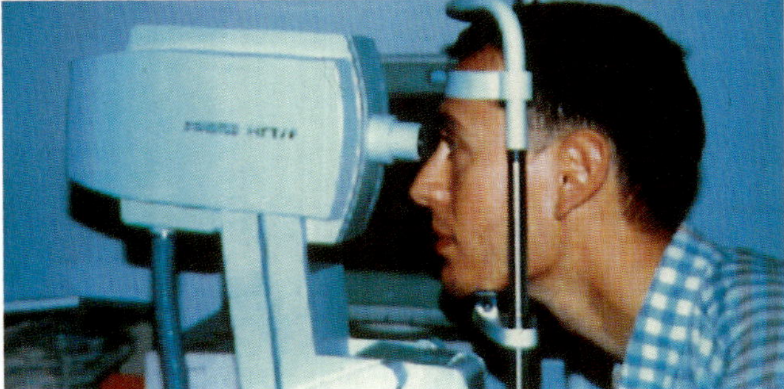

Figure 9.14 Modern examination technique for biomorphometric evaluation of the optic disc using the Heidelberg retinal tomograph (laser scanning tomography). The morphology of the optic disc is quantified with confocal laser beams scanning different image plains. Scanning-tomography is performed with the patient sitting in the same position as in slit lamp examination. The *top* frames show the laser scanning tomogram of a normal optic disc (*left*) and of an optic disc with glaucomatous cupping (*right*).

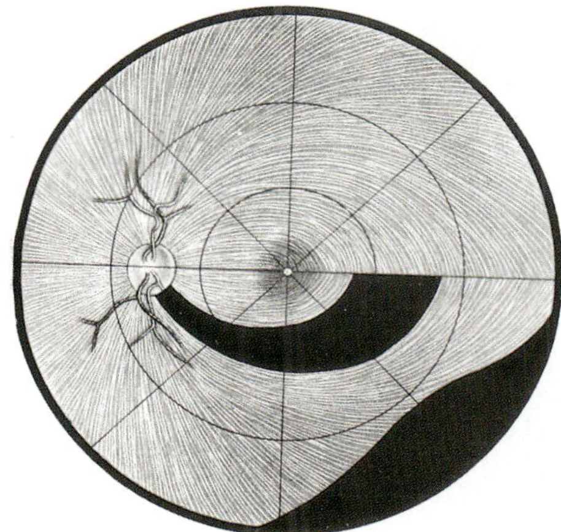

Figure 9.15   Diagram of a characteristic glaucomatous nerve fiber defect. The nerve fiber layer is ophthalmoscopically visible, especially with red free light. The inferior pole of the optic disc is particularly vulnerable. If only the superficial nerve fiber layer (which extends to the periphery) is damaged, a nasal peripheral scotoma results. An impairment of the deeper portions of the nerve fiber layer produces an arcuate scotoma. With damage to the entire thickness of the nerve fiber layer at the inferior pole of the optic disc, an arcuate scotoma, extending to the periphery, results.

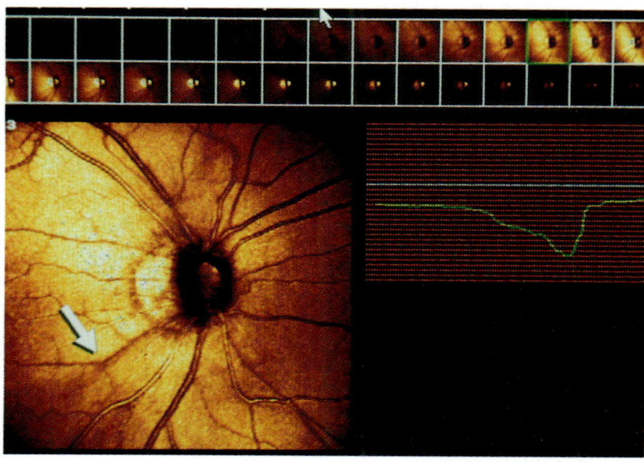

Figure 9.16   Wedge-shaped defect (*arrow*) of the nerve fiber layer in a glaucoma patient, depicted with the laser scanning tomograph. The *left* frame shows a three-dimensional reconstruction of the nerve fiber layer with the wedge-shaped defect (*arrow*), the *right* frame represents the cross-sectional profile of the cupped optic disc. The *top* frames show a series of scans at sequential tissue depths.

9.2 Chronic open-angle glaucoma

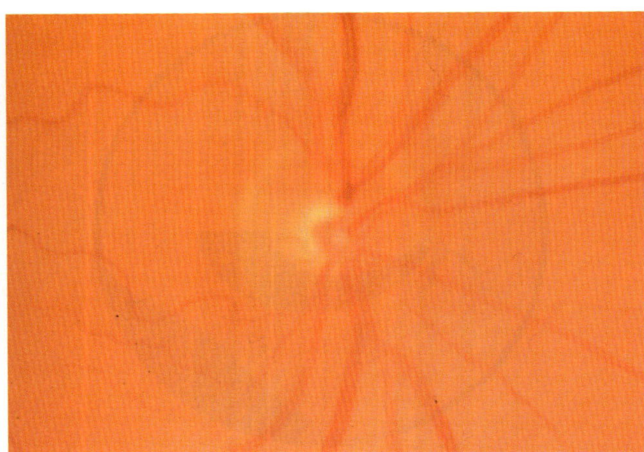

Figure 9.17 Normal, non-glaucomatous optic disc. The optic disc is pink, it has a small central cup, the retinal vessels emerge centrally. The neuoretinal rim (tissue between the edges of the disc and the cup) is evenly wide and well perfused.

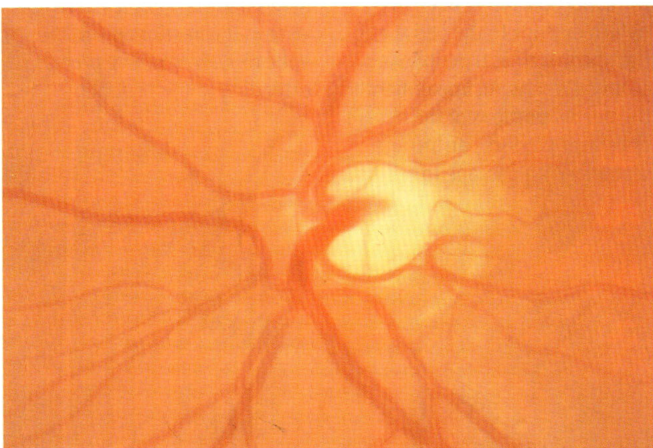

Figure 9.18 Early glaucomatous cupping of the optic disc. The cup area is larger than in figure 9.17. The retinal vessels follow the edge of the cup (so called circumlinear vascular pattern). The cup is very deep and has a punched-out appearance. The neuroretinal rim is still intact.

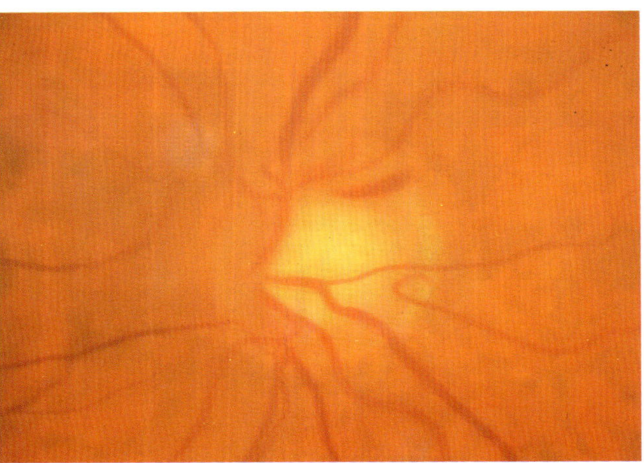

Figure 9.19 Glaucomatous splinter hemorrhage on the disc margin. Note the wedge-shaped splinter hemorrhage on the disc margin at the 2 o´clock position. Marginal hemorrhages of this kind are pathognomonic for a hemorrhagic nerve fiber bundle infarct. Subsequently, a wedge-shaped defect of the nerve fiber layer develops, which produces an arcuate scotoma in the later course.

Figure 9.20   Glaucomatous nerve fiber bundle defect at the inferior pole of the optic disc. The cup is vertically oval and asymmetrically enlarged. The neuroretinal rim of the disc is markedly narrowed at the 6 o´clock position in comparison with the superior pole of the disc. The fenestrated lamina cribrosa is visible in the optic nerve cup.

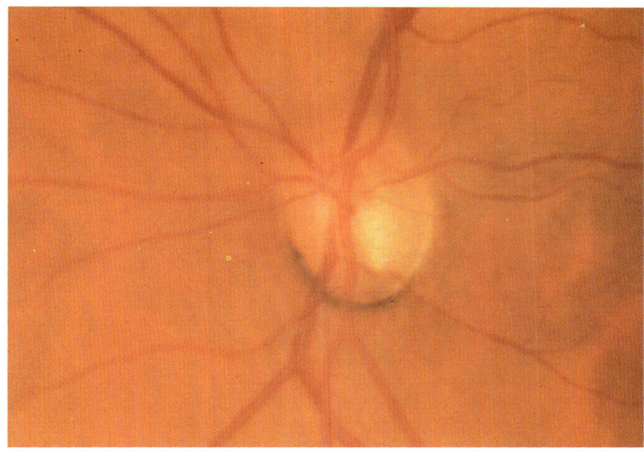

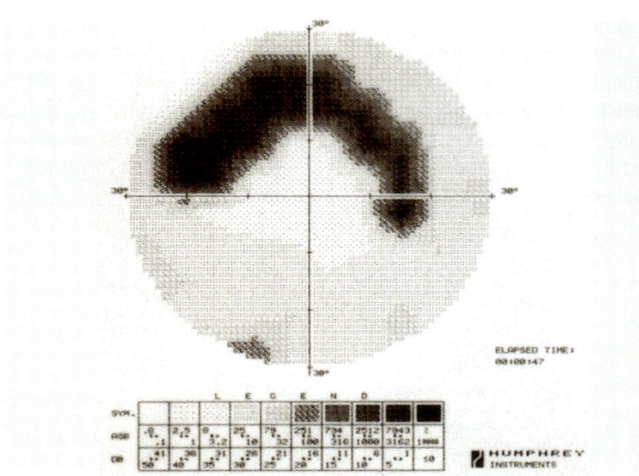

Figure 9.21   Arcuate, glaucomatous scotoma, so called Bjerrum scotoma. The grey-scale graphical depiction of the central 30 degree visual field shows an arcuate defect within the so-called Bjerrum area between 10 and 25 degrees, starting from the blind spot in the temporal half of visual field. In accordance with the nerve fiber pattern, the arcuate scotoma ends at the horizontal meridian, the so-called raphe. This arcuate scotoma corresponds to a nerve fiber bundle defect at the inferior pole of the optic disc, similar to figure 9.20.

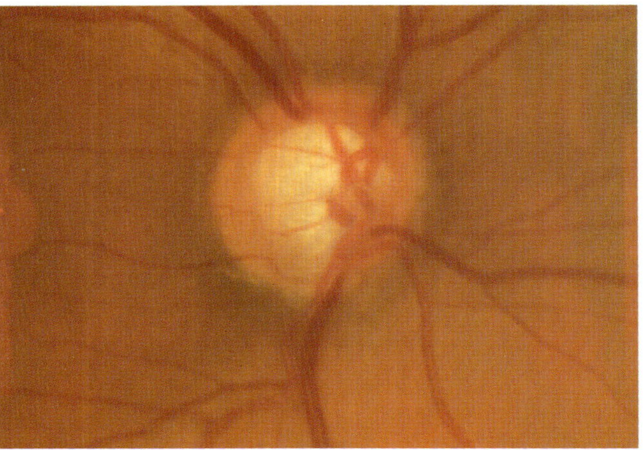

Figure 9.22 Advanced glaucomatous cupping with broad nerve fiber bundle defect (so-called "rim notch") at the inferior pole of the optic disc. There is a loss of neuroretinal rim tissue at the inferior pole of the disc. As the nerve fibers at the superior and inferior poles of the disc are thicker than they are nasally and temporally, the width of the neuroretinal rim is physiologically greater at the poles. In the present case, the ophthalmoscopic picture of the optic disc suggests visual field defects in the superior and inferior Bjerrum areas. The relative size of the cup is about 80% vertically and 60% horizontally. The structures of the lamina cribrosa are visible in the optic nerve cup.

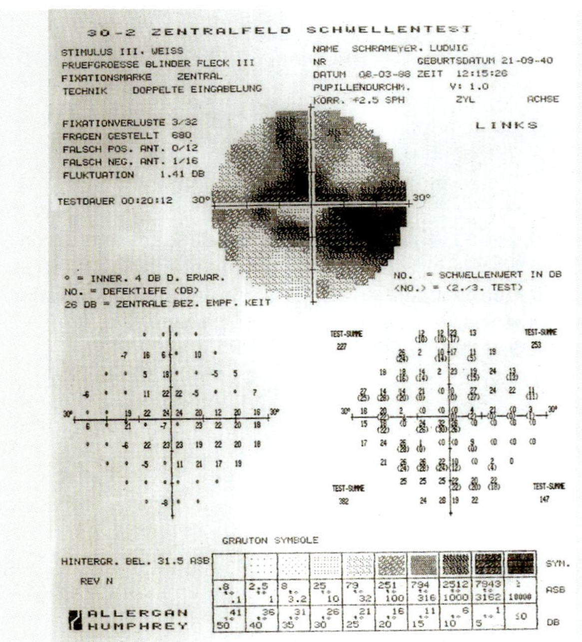

Figure 9.23 Visual field test corresponding to the optic disc shown in figure 9.22. The grey-scale printout shows arcuate Bjerrum scotomas superiorly and inferiorly, spreading towards the periphery in the inferior half of the visual field. Since the superior as well as the inferior pole of the optic disc are affected, almost a ring scotoma results, combined with a nasal step. Below the grey-scale printout is the numeric plot of the differences to normal threshold values (*bottom left*) and the numeric plot of the measured retinal thresholds (*bottom right*).

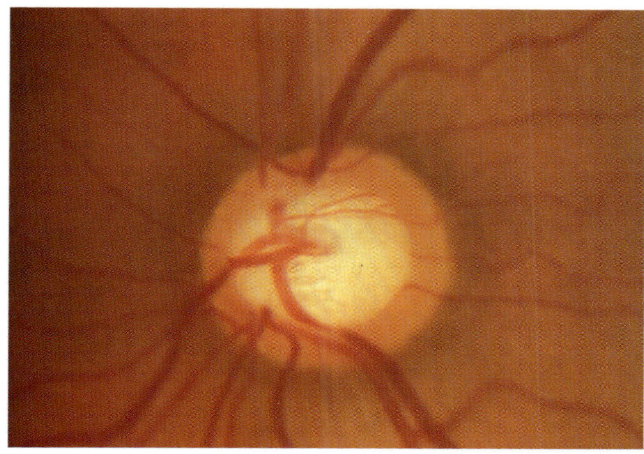

Figure 9.24 Advanced glaucomatous cupping. Note the general enlargement of the cup in all meridians and the kink in the course of the retinal vessels as they cross the edge of the cup. The central retinal vessels emerge nasally, the lamina cribosa is exposed at the bottom of the cup. The vessels at the temporal aspect of the disc disappear underneath the edge of the cup, a phemomenon that results from the undermining of the neuroretinal rim by the glaucomatous atrophy.

Figure 9.25 Glacomatous cupping with broad nerve fiber bundle loss inferorly and hemorrhage on the superotemporal neuroretinal rim. In glaucoma patients with systemic or ocular vascular abnormalities, recurrent hemorrhages at the disc margin frequently occur in the course of glaucomatous cupping. These splinter hemorrhages are signs of episodic infarctions of nerve fiber bundles.

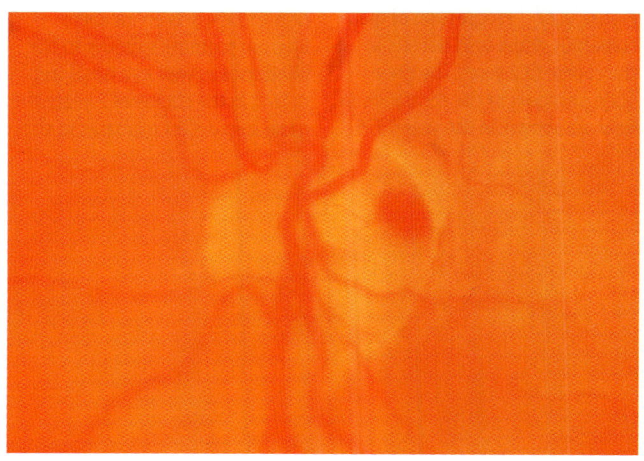

9.2 Chronic open-angle glaucoma

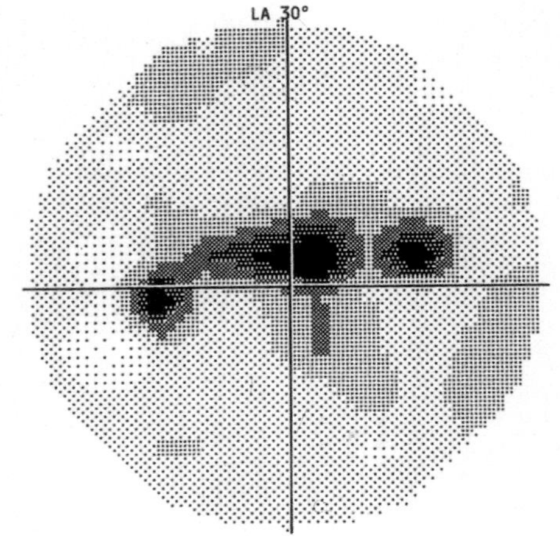

Figure 9.26 Glaucomatous arcuate scotoma, grey-scale graphical depiction of the central 30° visual field corresponding to the optic disc shown in figure 9.25. The blind spot lies in the temporal field, it merges with two Bjerrum scotomas, which are connected to a relative visual field defect. The Bjerrum scotomas shown here correspond to the glaucomatous optic disc lesion at the inferior pole shown in figure 9.25.

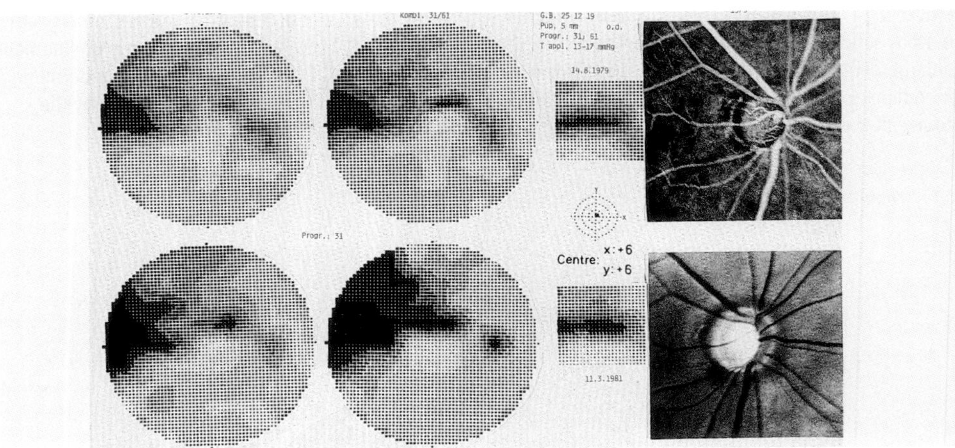

Figure 9.27 Progression of glaucomatous visual field defects in the course of 2 years. The grey-scale printouts of the central visual field are shown. In the year 1979 *(top left)* there is an incipient Bjerrum scotoma superior to the blind spot as well as a nasal step defect. In the course of 2 years, the nasal step defect increases in size and merges with the initial Bjerrum scotoma around the blind spot (order: *top left, top right, bottom left, bottom right*).

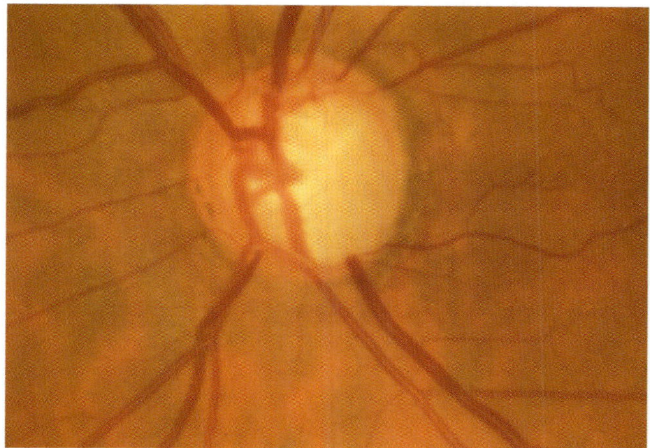

Figure 9.28 Advanced glaucomatous atrophy of the optic disc. The ophthalmoscopic picture of this glaucomatous disc shows a pronounced loss of the neuroretinal rim in the inferior pole. In the superior pole and nasally, there is still some neuroretinal rim tissue remaining. This glaucomatous damage to the optic disc results in an almost complete loss of the visual field.

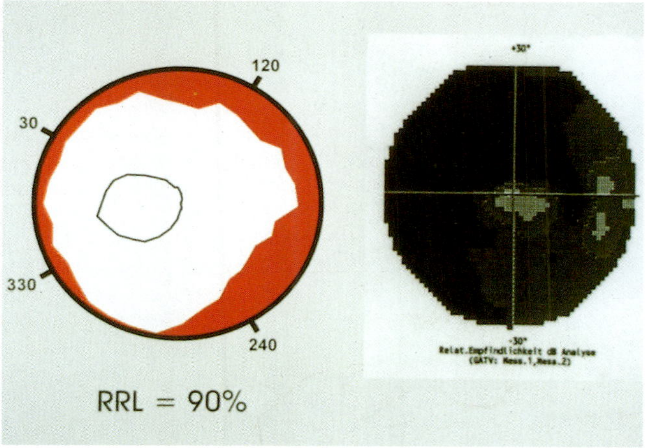

Figure 9.29 Comparison of optic disc cup and visual field using biomorphometry with the laser scanning tomograph. In the *left* frame, the loss of neuroretinal rim tissue is depicted as the difference between what would be the physiologic cup of the disc *(central circle)* and the red area. The right frame shows an advanced glaucomatous visual field defect with small residual central and temporal islands of vision. The biomorphometric analysis of the optic disc with the laser scanning tomograph gives the possibility to relate the loss of neuroretinal rim tissue to the physiologic variability of the disc size.

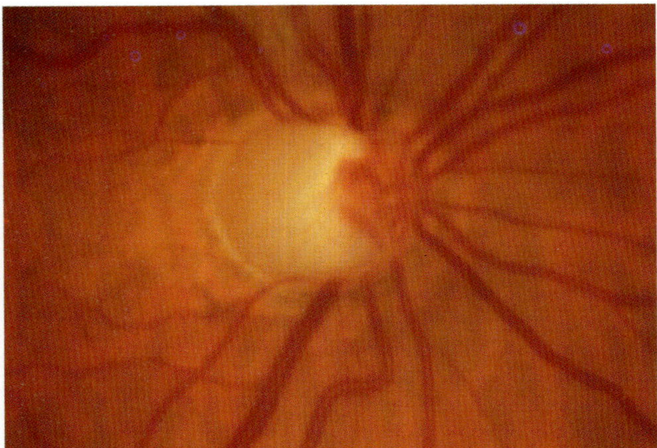

Figure 9.30 Advanced glaucomatous optic disc damage. The neuroretinal rim tissue in the temporal aspect of the disc is practically nonexistant. The cup extends temporally to the edge of the disc. The central retinal vessels are displaced nasally. In the temporal portion of the circumference, the retinal vessels seem to disappear as they cross the edge of the cup (severe kinking of radial vessels).

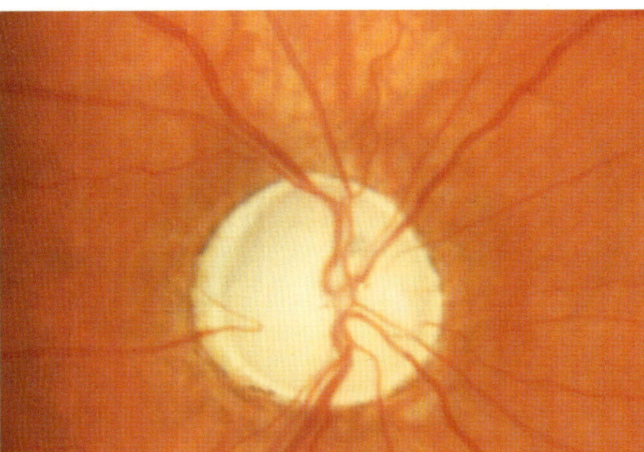

Figure 9.31 Glaucomatous atrophy of the optic disc in absolute glaucoma. Note the total cupping in the entire circumference. The optic disc is pale, there is no neuroretinal tissue remaining. The eye has become blind from glaucoma (absolute glaucoma).

Figure 9.32 Classification of glaucomatous visual field defects by Aulhorn with traditional, kinetic perimetry. An isolated, peripheral scotoma supero- or inferonasally corresponds to stage I, a peripheral scotoma in combination with a Bjerrum scotoma would be stage II. If the Bjerrum scotoma spans over two quadrants or spreads to the periphery, the defect would be classified as stage III. Stage IV is characterized by the loss of at least an entire quadrant of the visual field, stage V corresponds to a remaining central island or temporal crescent of vision.

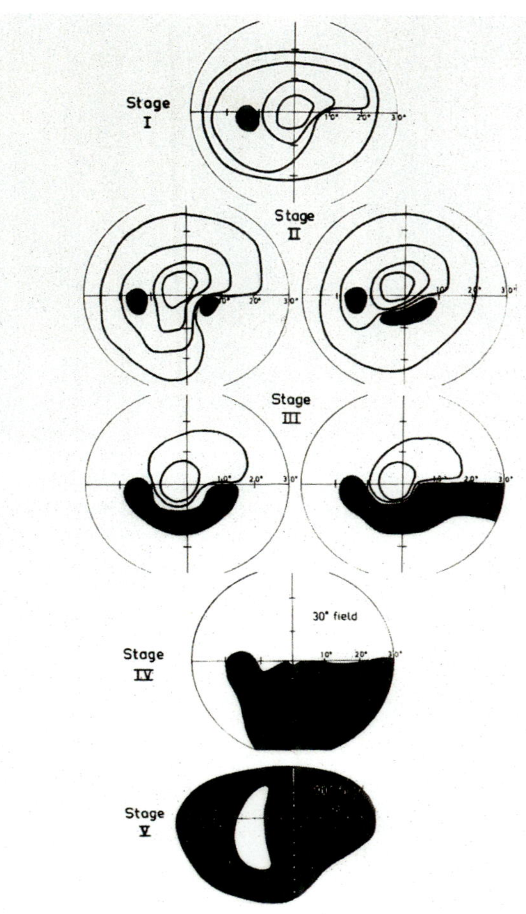

9.3 Acute angle-closure glaucoma

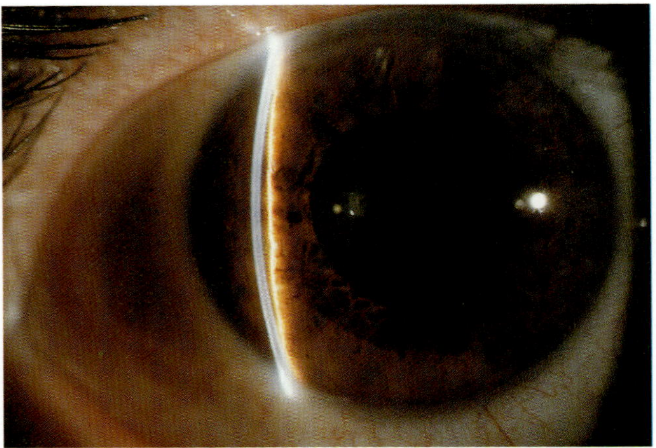

Figure 9.33 Anterior chamber depth, slit lamp photograph of a hyperopic eye with very shallow peripheral anterior chamber. With the narrow beam of the slit lamp illuminating the corneal thickness and the anterior surface of the iris, the shallowness of the peripheral anterior chamber becomes visible. There is an anatomic disposition for an acute angle-closure glaucoma. If the depth of the peripheral anterior chamber (estimated with the narrow beam of the slit lamp at an oblique angle) is less than the corneal thickness, this is a sign of an anterior chamber angle at risk of closure.

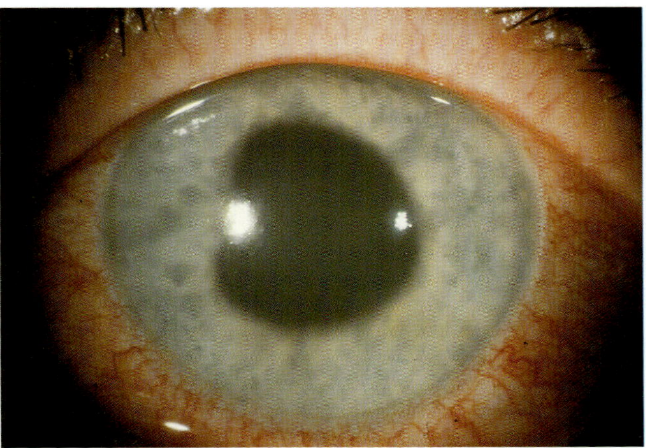

Figure 9.34 Attack of acute glaucoma. Note the discrete velvety opacification of the cornea representing corneal edema, which developed as a consequence of very high intraocular pressure. The paretic, irregularly dilated pupil also results from high intraocular pressure. The eye is red, painful and rock-hard to palpation. The vascular injection is mainly conjunctival. In prolonged attacks, there is ciliary injection as well.

Figure 9.35 Status post pharmacologic treatment of acute angle-closure glaucoma. Corneal edema develops following the drop of intraocular pressure to normal levels, due to impaired endothelial function. Note the broad folds in Descemet´s membrane a well as the discrete edema of the central stroma.

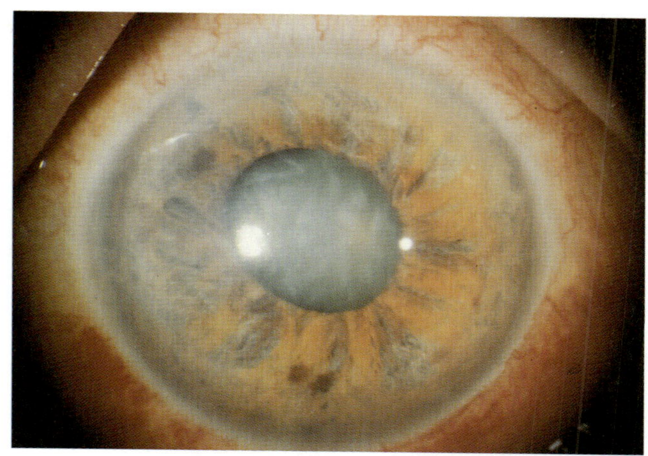

Figure 9.36 Ophthalmoscopic picture of the central fundus following an attack of acute glaucoma. Due to the speedy drop of intraocular pressure following medical treatment in acute glaucoma, a hemorrhage inferior to the optic disc has developed. The hemorrhage results from decompression of the retinal circulation when breaking the attack of acute glaucoma.

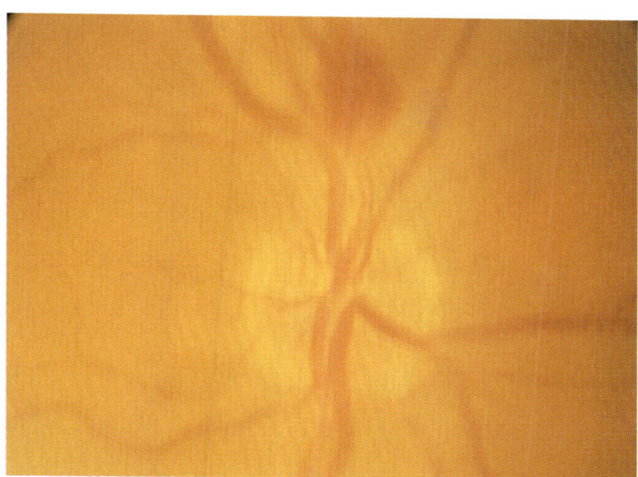

Figure 9.37 Subepithelial necrosis of the lens, so-called "glaukomflecken". Morphologically, they consist of epithelial, subcapsular necroses, which develop due to high intraocular pressure during an attack of acute glaucoma. Through appositional growth to the epithelial surface, with time, the sucapsular lens opacities seem to move inwards.

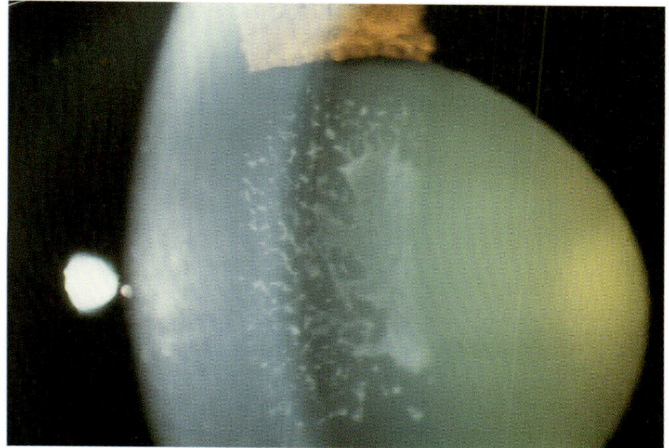

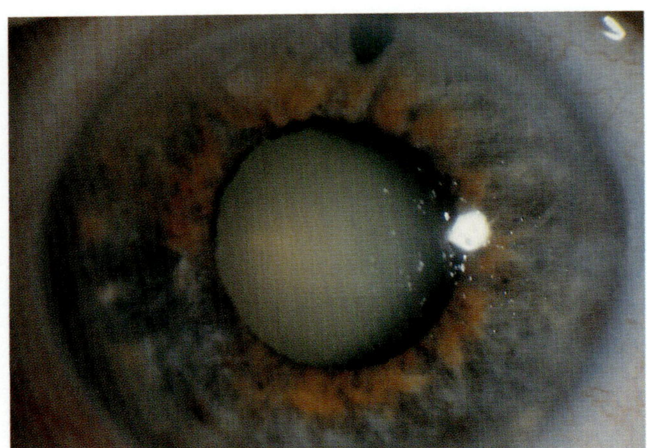

Figure 9.38 Iris atrophy following recurrent acute glaucoma. The iris stroma is atrophied in three quadrants due to ischemic iritis as a consequence of the attacks of acute glaucoma. Normal iris stroma remains at the pupillary border and in the superonasal quadrant. At the 12 o´clock position, there is a peripheral iridectomy, which was implemented as surgical treatment of the acute glaucoma.

Figure 9.39 Bilateral congenital glaucoma in a 3 month-old infant. Note the bilateral discrete corneal clouding. The corneal diameter is enlarged in comparison to other children of this age. In this very early manifestation of glaucoma, the elevated intraocular pressure leads to opacification of the corneal stroma.

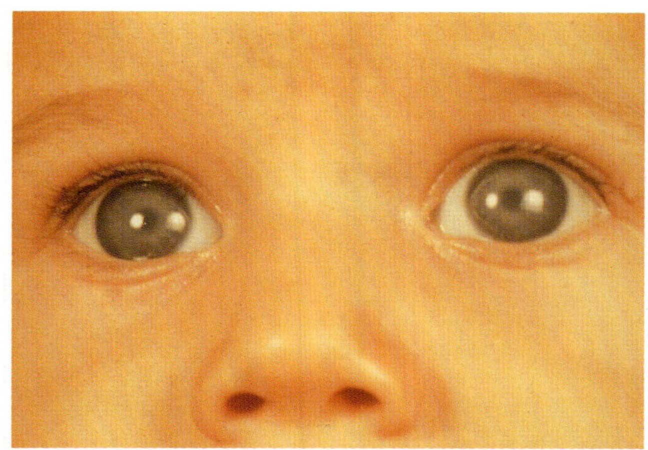

Figure 9.40 Infant with bilateral congenital glaucoma. An elevation of intraocular pressure within the first years of childhood causes an enlargement of the globe (buphthalmos), due to the connective tissue which forms the outer coat of the eyeball being still very elastic. An enlargement of the corneal diameter is a pathognomonic sign of an early elevation of intraocular pressure and thus of congenital glaucoma.

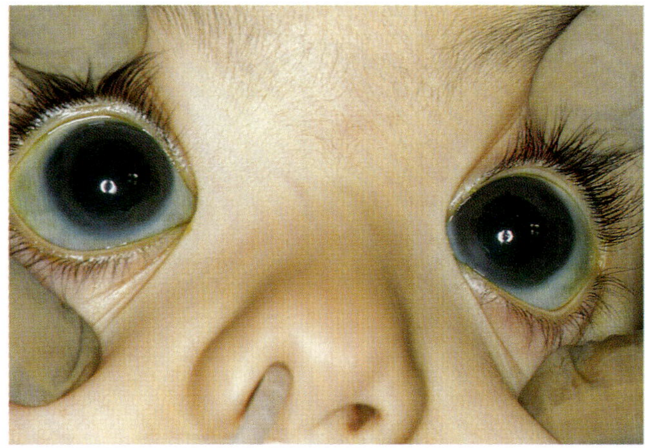

Figure 9.41 Congenital glaucoma in the left eye of a 5 year-old girl. Note the enlarged corneal diameter in the left eye as a result of elevated intraocular pressure in unilateral congenital glaucoma.

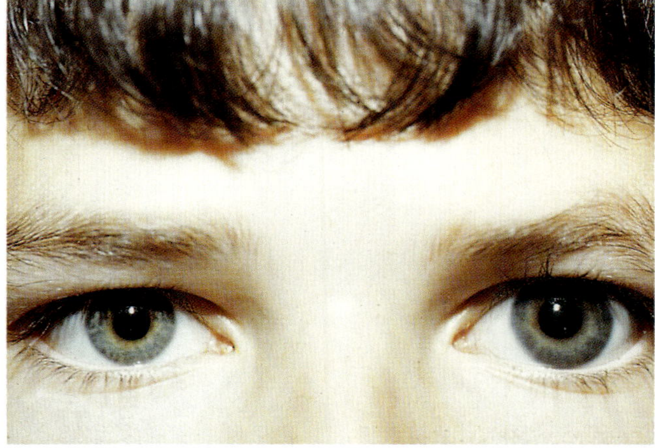

9.4 Congenital glaucoma

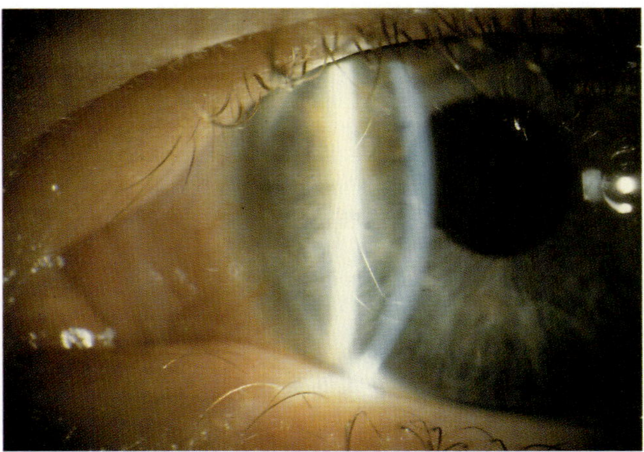

Figure 9.42 Haab´s striae in the midperipheral cornea in congenital glaucoma. Stretching of the cornea by elevated intraocular pressure in congenital glaucoma causes ruptures of Descemet´s memrane. Scarring of these defects results in transpartent, elevated striae at the midperipheral posterior corneal surface, so called „Haab´s striae", which are a pathognomonic finding, indicating pathologic stretching of the cornea in early childhood in the course of congenital glacoma. Once the connective tissues forming the outer coat of the eyeball have developed a certain firmness after the sixth year of childhood, buphthalmos, megalocornea or Haab´s striae do not occur any more.

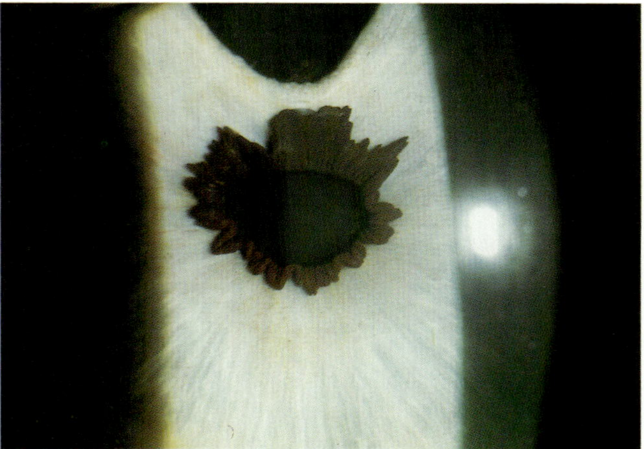

Figure 9.43 Ectropion uveae at the pupillary margin in congenital glaucoma. The ectropion of the iris pigment layer at the pupillary margin is a pathognomonic finding, indicating the presence of iridodysgenesis, which is frequently associated with goniodysgenesis, being the cause for developmental glaucoma (termed congenital glaucoma with manifestation in the first year of life).

Figure 9.44 Anomalous iris vessels. Note the enlarged, anomalous vessels at the pupillary border at the 9´o clock position extending to the peripheral iris. Vascular anomalies of the iris are a sign of embryonal dysgenesis of the anterior segment. They are frequently associated with dysgenetic, congenital glaucoma.

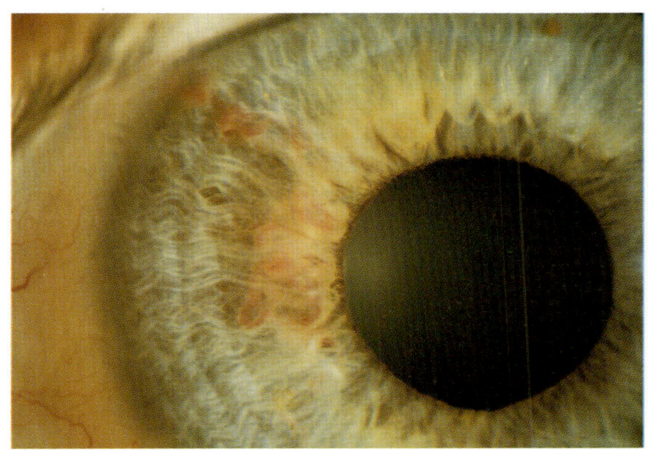

Figure 9.45 Mesodermal dysgenesis. Dysplasia of the iris stroma with attachment of embryonal iris tissue in the anterior chamber angle is often seen in mesodermal dysgenesis of the anterior segment. The embryonal iris tissue causes goniosynechiae and blockage of the outflow pathways. This kind of mesodermal dysgenesis is termed Axenfeld´s disease.

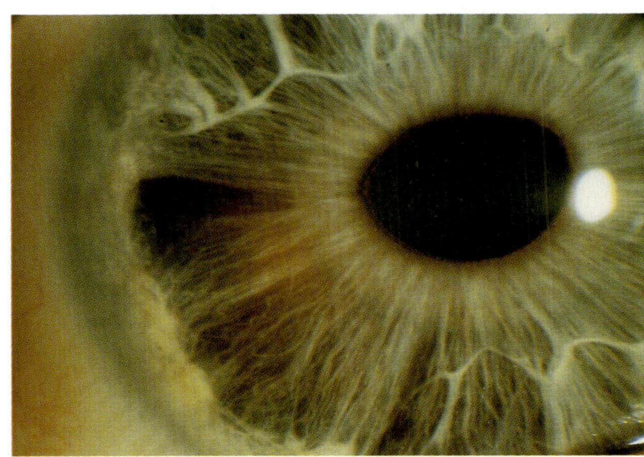

Figure 9.46 Iridodysplasia Rieger´s anomaly. This entity, which is a variation of to the iridocorneal endothelial (ICE) syndrome, is characterized by slow atrophy of the iris stroma due to traction caused by proliferative corneal endotheliopathy with consecutive distortion of the pupil, development of "stretch" holes (pseudopolycoria) and almost always early-onset glaucoma.

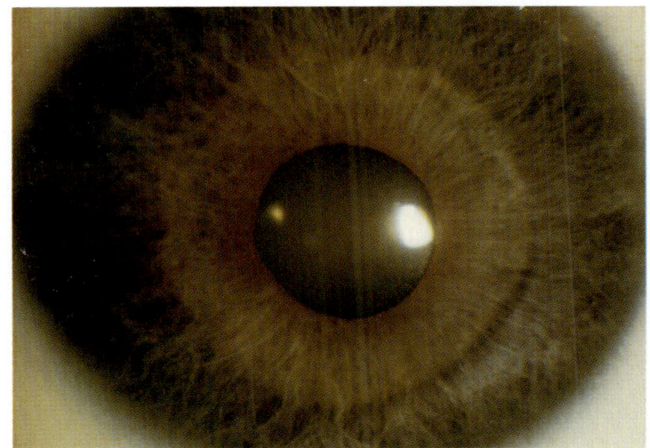

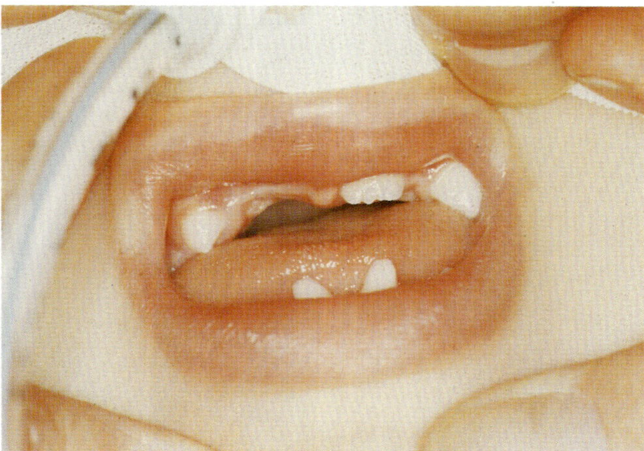

Figure 9.47 Dental abnormalities in Rieger´s syndrome. Apart from anterior chamber anomalies Rieger syndrome includes dental anomalies (abnormally small teeth, so-called microdontia).

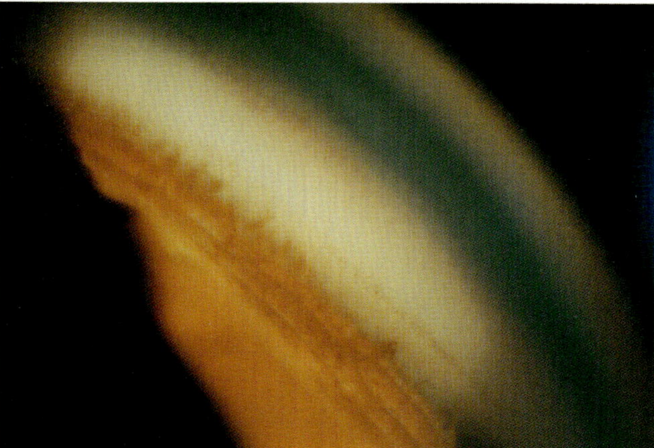

Figure 9.48 Gonioscopic appearance of dysgenetic, congenital glaucoma. During embyogenesis, the iris stoma has not recessed from the trabecular meshwork and obscures the anterior chamber angle entrance. Small strands of iris stroma insert on the trabecular meshwork. Typically described are a posterior insertion of the iris on the posterior meshwork and an anterior insertion on the anterior meshwork or on Schwalbe´s line.

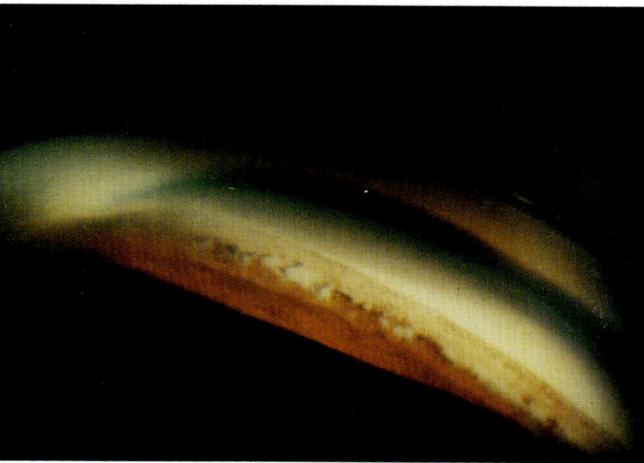

Figure 9.49 Gonioscopic appearance of congenital glaucoma with insertion of remaining embryonal iris tissue on the trabecular meshwork.

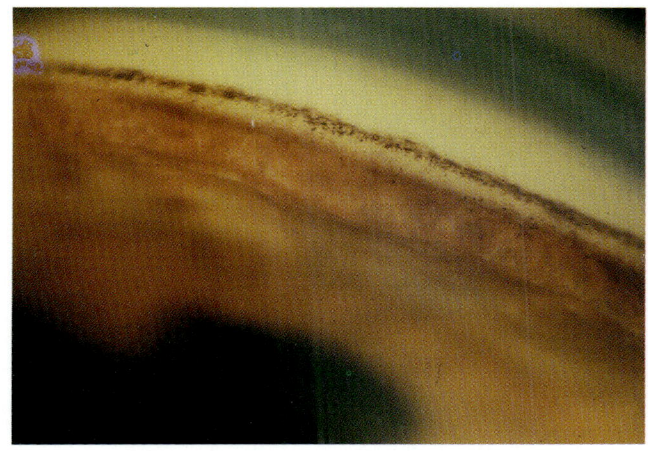

Figure 9.50 Gonioscopic appearance of the anterior chamber angle in congenital glaucoma. The iris lines the entrance of the anterior chamber angle, the outflow structures are obscured. Anterior to the high insertion of the iris a broad band of pigment is visible, where the outflow pathways are originally located. Unlike in the healthy eye, this pigment band does not mark the position of Schlemm´s canal.

9.5 Secondary glaucomas

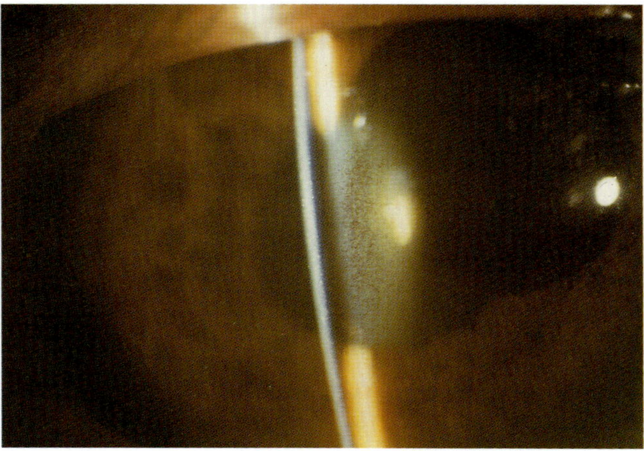

Figure 9.51 Deposition of pigment on the central corneal endothelium in the shape of a spindle, so-called "Krukenberg´s spindle". This finding is pathognomonic of pigment dispersion syndrome, which frequently causes glaucoma with delayed onset. The arrangement of the pigment on the posterior corneal surface marks the thermal convection of the aqueous humor in the anterior chamber. The aqueous humor flows downwards along the corneal endothelium and leaves deposits of suspended pigment granules in a spindle shape on the corneal endothelium.

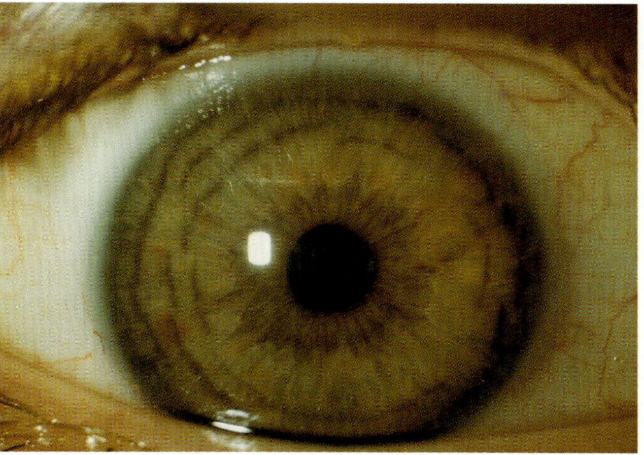

Figure 9.52 Pigment dispersion on the iris stroma in pigmentary glaucoma. Note the wavelike deposits of pigment ganules on the peripheral and midperipheral iris – a typical finding of pigmentary glaucoma.

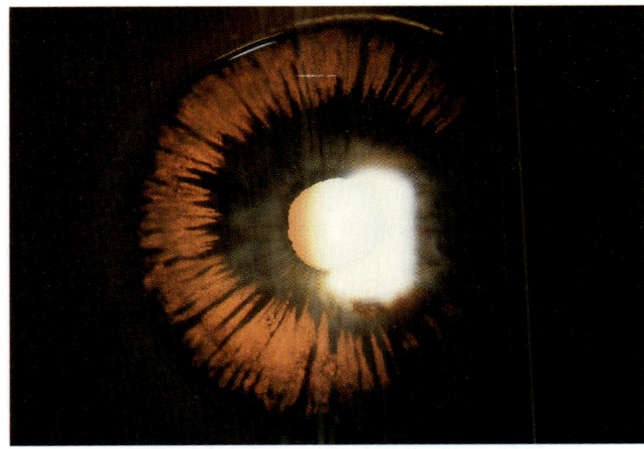

Figure 9.53 Increased iris transillumination in pigmentary glaucoma. With retroillumination, the increased transillumination of the iris pigment epithelial layer becomes visible. This picture arises from the loss of pigment due to the rubbing action of the zonules. Owing to an increaesed depth of the anterior chamber angle, the zonules cause mechanical irritation of the peripheral iris. This results in the loss of pigment from the pigment layer of the iris.

Figure 9.54 Pigment deposits in the posterior chamber in pigmentary glaucoma. Note the small lumps of pigment in the superior circumference of the lens equator viewed with maximal pupillary dilation. Since pigment dispersion is caused by rubbing of the zonules against the peripheral iris, pigment deposits are also found in the posterior chamber.

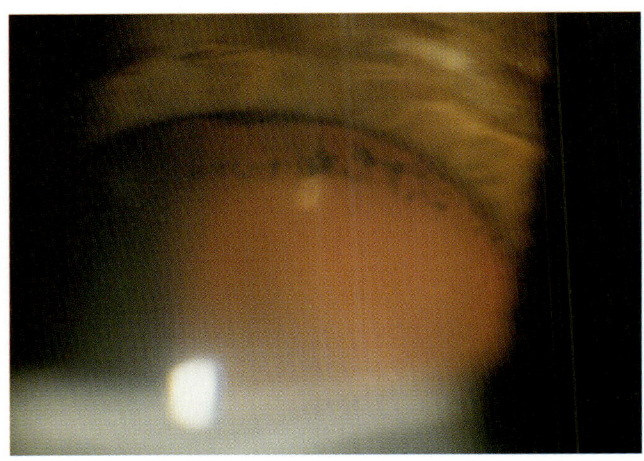

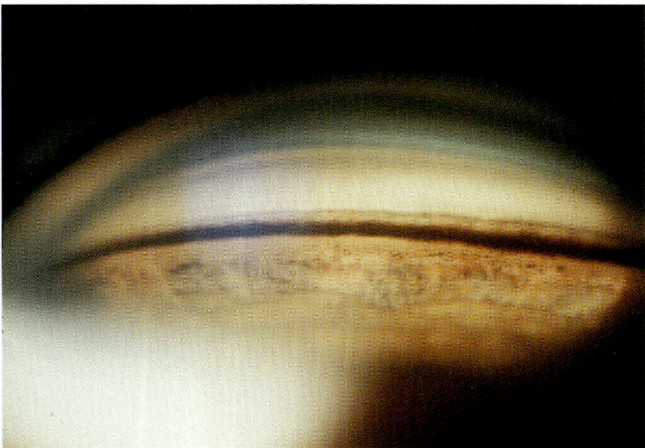

Figure 9.55 Gonioscopic appearance of an anterior chamber angle in pigmentary glaucoma. Note the dark-brown band of pigment over the circumference of the trabecular meshwork, resulting from deposition of pigment granules. The excessive pigment in the trabecular meshwork leads to obstruction of aqueous outflow and thereby to an elevation of intraocular pressure.

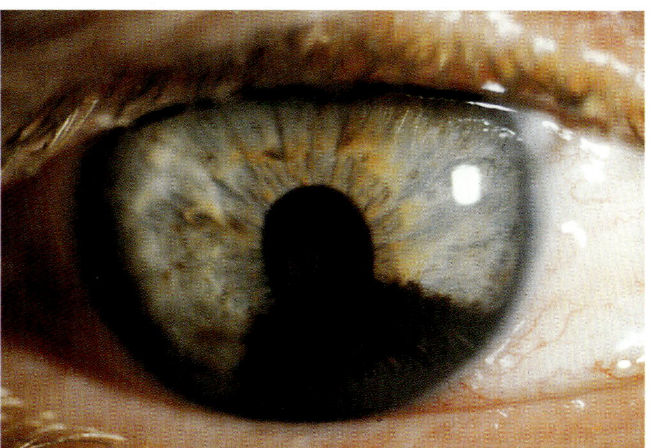

Figure 9.56 Melanolytic secondary glaucoma in iris melanoma. There is an advanced iris melanoma in the anterior chamber between the 4 and 7 o´clock position with distortion of the pupil towards the tumor. The disintegration of tumor cells leads to an obstruction of the aqueous outflow pathways by melanin granules and invading melanoma cells.

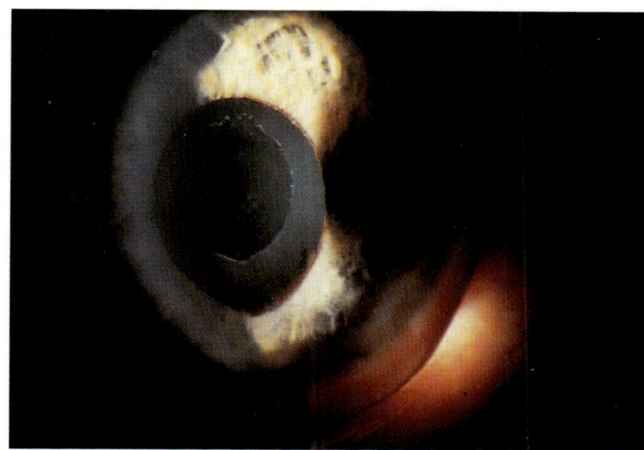

Figure 9.57 Secondary glaucoma associated with pseudoexfoliation syndrome. In pseudoexfoliation syndrome, a defect in the biosynthesis of extracellular matrix leads to the release of amyloid-like paraprotein. This material accumulates on the iris, the corneal endothelium, typically on the midperipheral anterior lens surface and in the outflow structures, accounting for the development of secondary glaucoma. The frost-like deposition of pseudoexfoliative material can be seen with pharmacologic mydriasis at the pupillary margin as well as on the anterior lens surface, mostly sparing the central area.

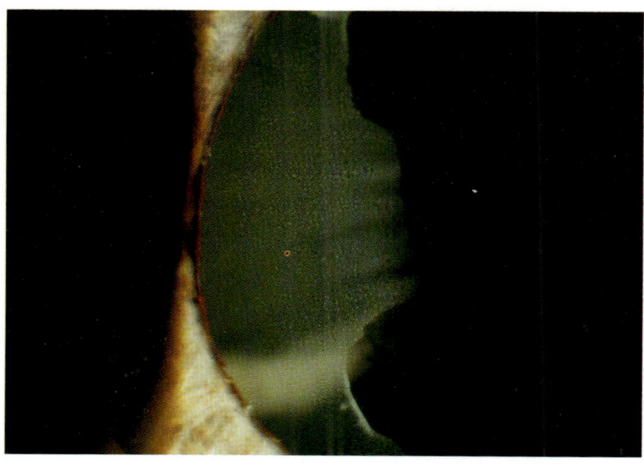

Figure 9.58 Extensive deposition of pseudoexfoliative material on the anterior lens surface, appearing in the present case as a semitransparent membrane. Very pronounced pseudoexfoliation syndrome.

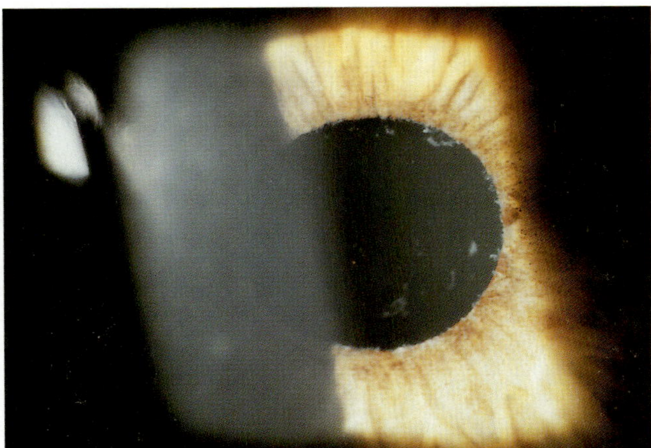

Figure 9.59 Deposition of small flakes of pseudoexfoliative material on the pupillary margin. Note the characteristic deposition of pigment granules on the pupillary margin and the defects in the pupillary ruff. The loading of the iris pigment layer with pseudoexfoliative material reduces the elasticity of the iris. The release of pigment increases with the rigidity of the iris.

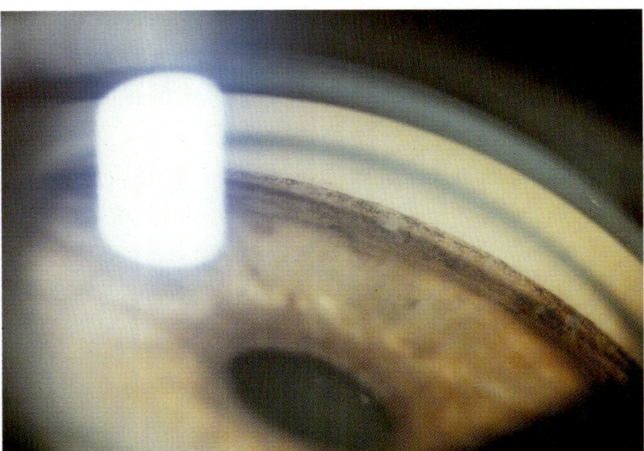

Figure 9.60 Goniscopic appearance of the anterior chamber angle in pseudoexfoliation syndrome. Note the increased pigmentation of the outlflow structures and the deposition of flaky pseudoexfoliative material. The pigmentation in pseudoexfoliation syndrome is more pronounced in the inferior portion of the angle circumference and tends to be more coarse-grained and inhomogenous, while the trabecular pigmentation in pigmentary glaucoma is more dense, homogenous and equally pronounced in the entire circumference.

Figure 9.61 Gonioscopic appearance of the anterior chamber angle following blunt trauma. Note the blood on the aqueous outflow structures. A traumatic recession of the angle has occured, it appears deeper in the affected area.

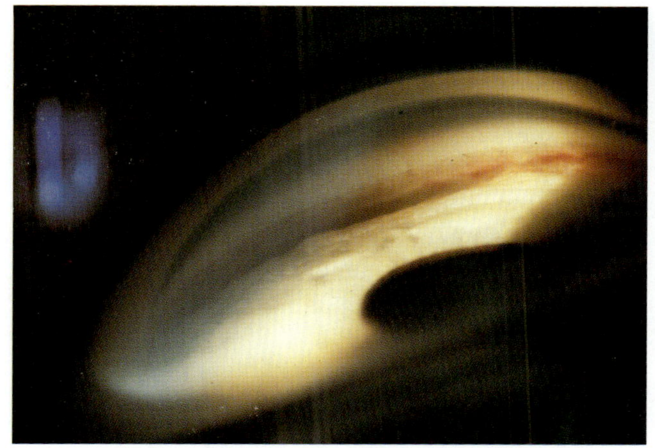

Figure 9.62 Gonioscopic appearance of the anterior chamber angle following blunt trauma with posttraumatic secondary glaucoma. The tearing of the ciliary body causes a disinsertion of the ciliary muscle at the trabecular meshwork as well as direct damage to the outflow structures. As a result, the aqueous outflow facility is decerased and secondary posttraumatic glaucoma develops.

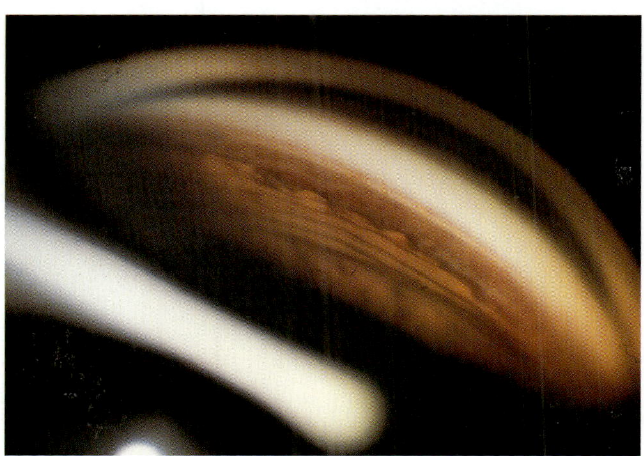

Figure 9.63 Secondary inflammatory glaucoma in chronic iritis. Note the signs of anterior uveitis: central posterior synechiae and extensive keratic precipitates (conglomerates of inflammatory cells). Consolidation of inflammatory cells and debris in the aqueous outlow structures leads to the development of secondary inflammatory glaucoma.

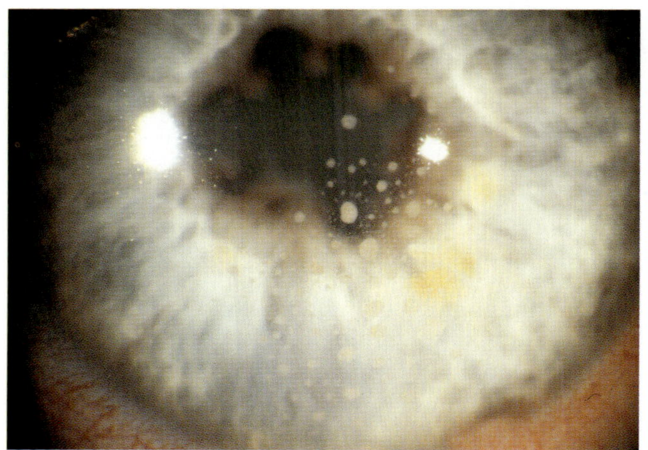

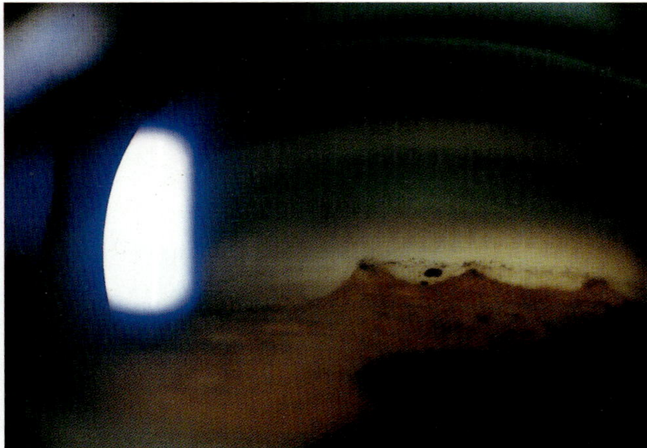

Figure 9.64 Gonioscopic appearance of an eye with secondary inflammatory glaucoma with goniosynechiae and deposition of pigment in the drainage angle in the form of small lumps. The gradual formation of synechiae in the anterior chamber angle (permanent apposition of the peripheral iris to the trabecular meshwork induced by chemotactic inflammatory mediators) leads to closure of the anterior chamber angle and formation of postinflammatory, chronic angle-closure glaucoma.

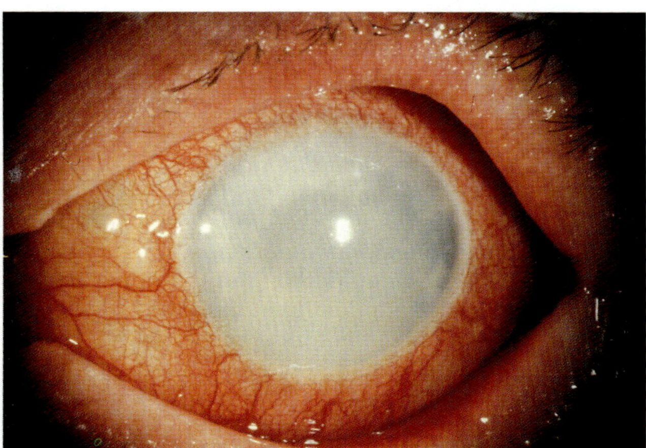

Figure 9.65 Akute, phacolytic glaucoma. Note the hypermature cataract with swelling of the opaque lens cortex. The release of lens proteins from the intumescent cataract into the aqueous humor causes an acute inflammatory reaction in the anterior chamber with acute inflammatory glaucoma, so-called phacolytic glaucoma.

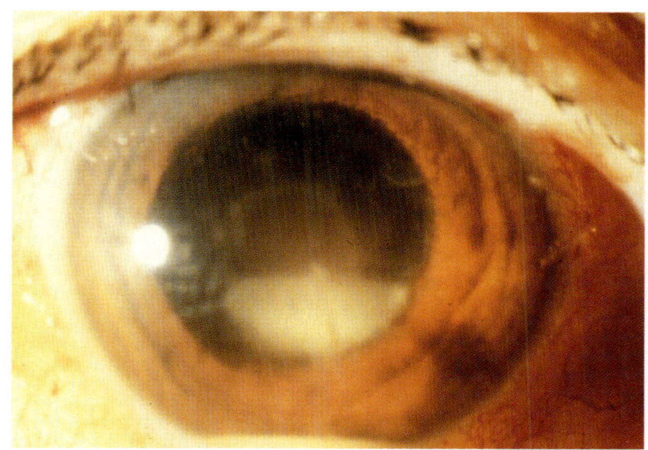

Figure 9.66 Pseudophakic secondary glaucoma due to chronic endophthalmitis. Facultative pathogens like Staphylococcus epidermidis can cause bacterial endophthalmitis and secondary inflammatory glaucoma following intraocular lens implantation. The figure shows an intraocular lens implanted into the capsular bag. Note the sedimentation of inflammatory cells in the peripheral anterior chamber (hypopyon) as well as in the capsular bag posterior to the artificial lens. Surgical posterior capsulotomy via pars plana and irrigation of the posterior chamber has to be peformed in combination with vitrectomy and lavage of the vitreous cavity with antibiotic agents.

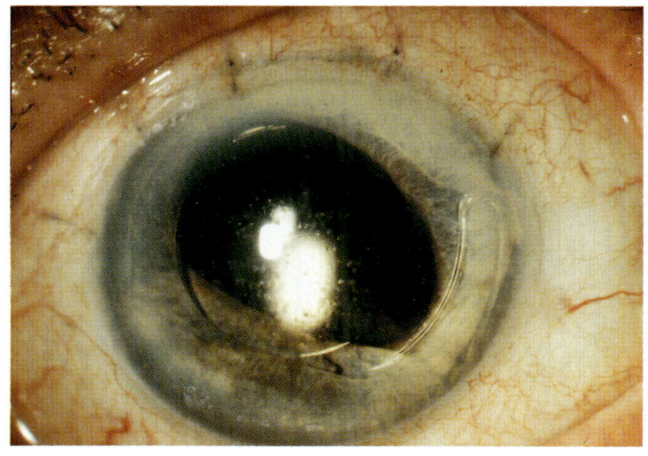

Figure 9.67 Pseudophakic glaucoma following implantation of a flexible anterior chamber lens. The implanted lens has caused a pseudophakic pupillary block, in which the lens pushes the iris posteriorly with subsequent development of iris bombé. The presence of keratic precipitates indicates a chronic inflammatory reaction due to irritation of the anterior uvea by the implanted anterior chamber lens. Surgical iridectomy or laser iridecromy is required to resolve pupillary block, occasionally combined with lens explantation.

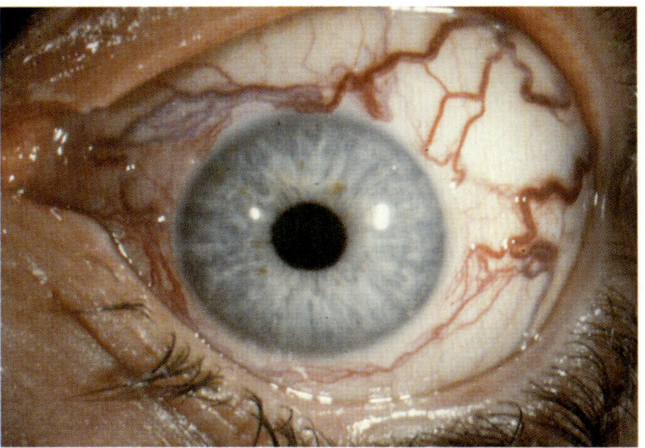

Figure 9.68 Pronounced episceral venectasias due to orbital arteriovenous fistula. The pathologically elevated episcleral venous pressure due to an arteriovenous shunt in the orbita leads to elevated intraocular pressure and development of secondary glaucoma. There is a cascade of pressure along the posterior chamber, anterior chamber, Schlemm´s canal and episcleral veins. A pathologic elevation of episcleral vein pressure is transmitted retrogradely to the inside of the globe. The adequate treatment for this kind of secondary vascular glaucoma is repair of the orbital arteriovenous fistula by vascular surgery.

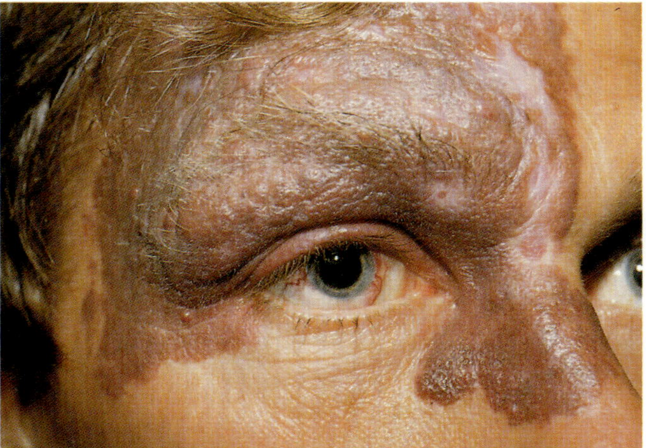

Figure 9.69 Hemangioma of the right upper face with segmental extension in Sturge-Weber disease. The facial hemangioma in Sturge-Weber disease, one of the phakomatoses, is frequently associated with conjunctival hemangioma, choroidal hemangioma as well as intracranial hemangioma with calcification. The epibulbar hemangioma leads to an elevation of episcleral venous pressure and to secondary vascular glaucoma.

Figure 9.70 Perilimbal, epibulbar hemangioma in the affected eye of the patient with Sturge-Weber disease shown in figure 9.69.

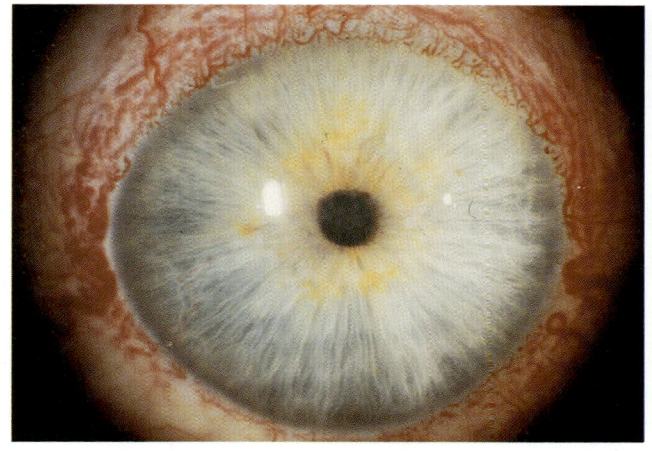

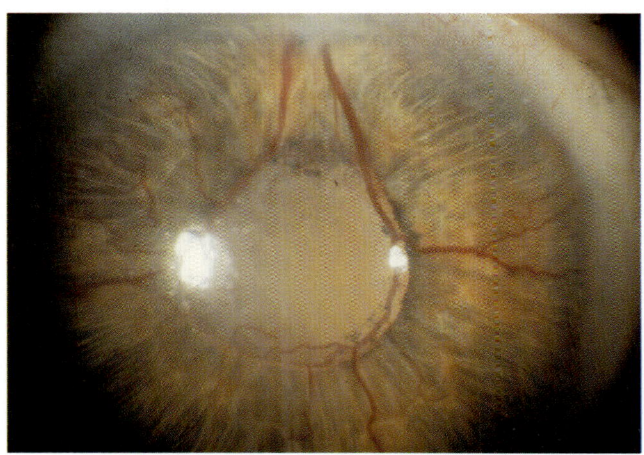

Figure 9.71 Secondary rubeotic, neovascular glaucoma with total posterior synechiae in the pupillary area and mature complicated cataract. In various disorders associated with retinal ischemia, vasoproliferative mediators are released, which induce neovascularization of the iris. The so-called rubeosis iridis, concurrently with a descemet-like membanous structure, expands until the anterior chamber angle is lined with fibrovascular tissue, resulting in secondary glaucoma. Treatment has to be directed towards the underlying retinal ischemia, since regression of rubeosis only occurs as the biosynthesis of vasoproliferative factors stops

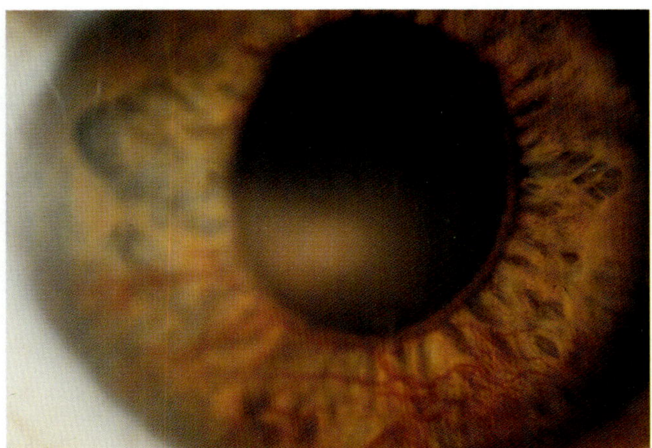

Figure 9.72 Rubeosis iridis and secondary neovascular glaucoma following central retinal vein thrombosis with ischemic retinopathy. The epiiridial, fibrovasular tissue, due to its contractile properties, causes ectropion of the pupillary margin and pupillary distortion.

Figure 9.73 Medical therapy of glaucoma. Overview of the pharmacologic agents that lower intraocular pressure for topical application.

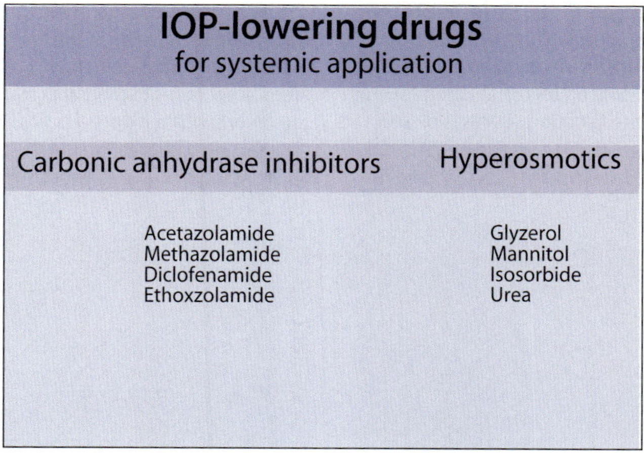

Figure 9.74 Medical therapy of glaucoma. Overview of the pharmacologic agents for systemic (intravenous or peroral) application, used for immediate lowering of intraocular pressure in acute angle-closure glaucoma or preparation for surgery. Hyperosmotic agents have only temporary effects. Long-term use of systemic carbonic anhydrase inhibitors is justified only in exceptional cases, owing to the numerous side-effects of these agents.

IOP-lowering drugs
for systemic application

Carbonic anhydrase inhibitors	Hyperosmotics
Acetazolamide	Glyzerol
Methazolamide	Mannitol
Diclofenamide	Isosorbide
Ethoxzolamide	Urea

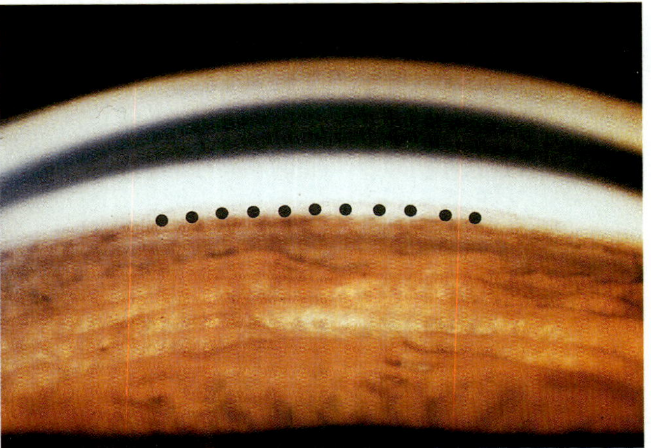

Figure 9.75 Technique of laser trabeculoplasty, laser surgical treatment of open angle glaucoma under certain morphologic preconditions. In cases of well accessible trabecular meshwork, lowering of intraocular pressure can be achieved by argon-laser trabeculoplasty. The *black dots* mark the sites of placement of argon-laser burns in the trabecular meshwork, which induce a cicatricial reaction with traction to the adjacent trabecular meshwork, this way increasing aqueous outflow facility. The therapeutic effect of laser trabeculoplasty is confined to a limited period of time, other surgical measures are thereby often only postponed.

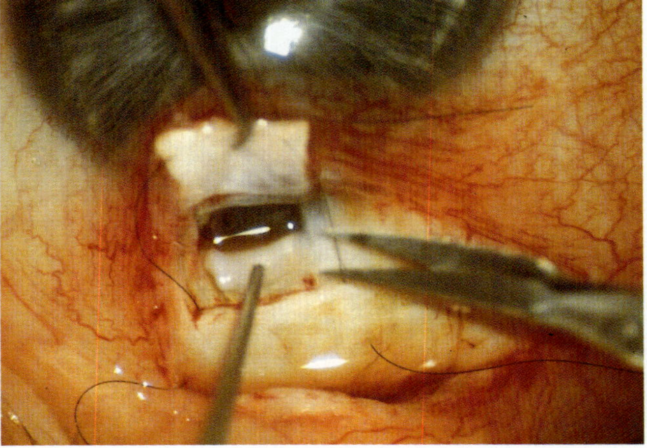

Figure 9.76 Intraoperative photograph of trabeculectomy, a filtering procedure for treatment of chronic open-angle glaucoma. Following conjunctival incision, a limbus-based lamellar scleral flap is created (the lamella is grasped with a forceps by an assistant) a 1.5 mm wide and 3 mm long block of corneoscleral tissue is excised. This block of tissue contains trabecular meshwork and Schlemm´s canal. At the site of filtration, an iridectomy is made. The scleral lamella is sutured in place to protect the filtering aperture and the conjunctiva is closed above it.

Figure 9.77 Functional filtering bleb following trabeculectomy in the superonasal quadrant of a right eye. The site of the filtration procedure is recognizable by the small peripheral iridectomy. Owing to the filtration of aqueous humor, the conjunctiva is diffusely lifted over the filtering site, a filtering bleb forms. Drainage of aqueous humor underneath the conjunctiva compensates for the functional deficiency of the genuine outflow structures, intraocular pressure is surgically regulated.

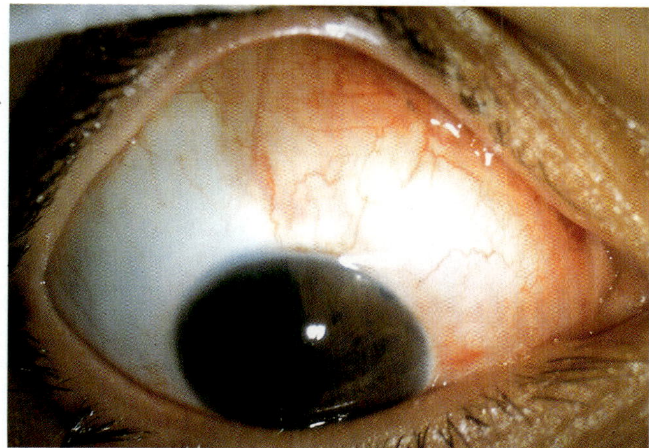

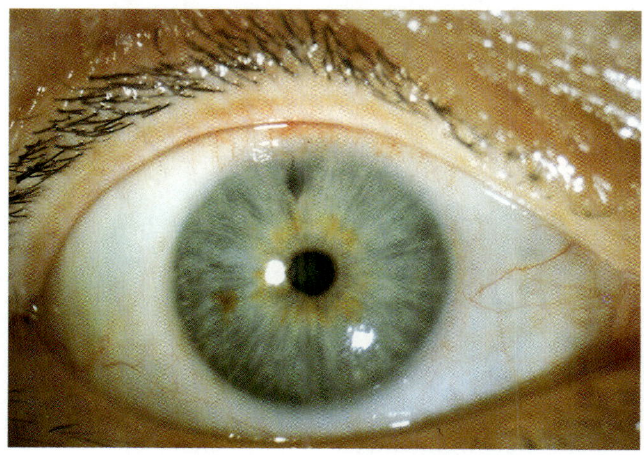

Figure 9.78 Status post peripheral iridectomy at the 12 o´clock position following angle-closure glaucoma. In eyes with shallow anterior chamber and large sagittal diameter of the lens, the pupillary margin is pressed onto the anterior lens surface, resulting in increased pressure in the posterior chamber relative to the anterior chamber and thereby in an elevation of the peripheral iris with apposition to the aqueous ouflow structures (so-called pupillary block mechanism). The iridectomy eliminates this pressure gradient between the anterior and posterior chamber, the peripheral anterior chamber deepens and the filtration angle becomes wider. This way, the risk of acute angle-closure glaucoma is eliminated.

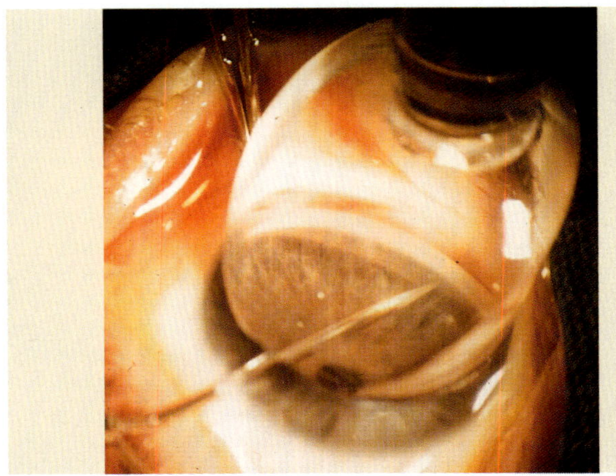

Figure 9.79 Goniotomy in congenital glaucoma. Goniotomy is a proven procedure for the treatment of congenital glaucoma. The anterior chamber angle is visualized with a gonioscopic prism and the abnormal embryonal tissue, which creates the restriction to aqueous outflow, is incised with a sharp knife. Lowering of intraocular pressure results, provided that the genuine outflow structures that lie underneath gain a certain functionality as a result of the procedure.

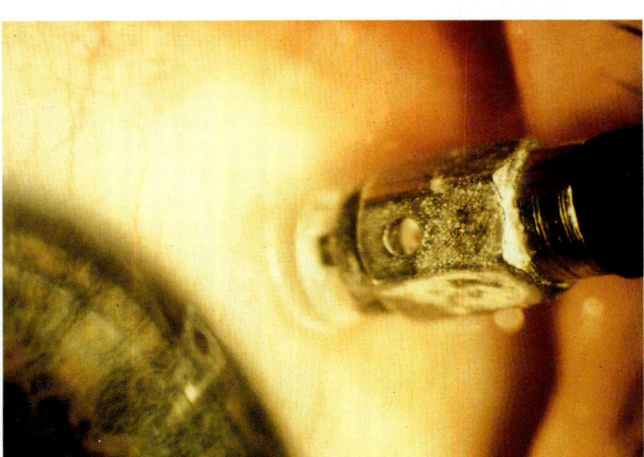

Figure 9.80 Transscleral cyclophotocoagulation. A contact fiberoptic probe is placed posterior to the limbus, transscleral application of laser light results in coagulative necrosis of the ciliary body. Cyclophotocoagulation is a cyclodestructive procedure, which reduces the secretion of aqueous humor. It is indicated when filtration surgery is not possible or with contraindications for intraocular surgery.

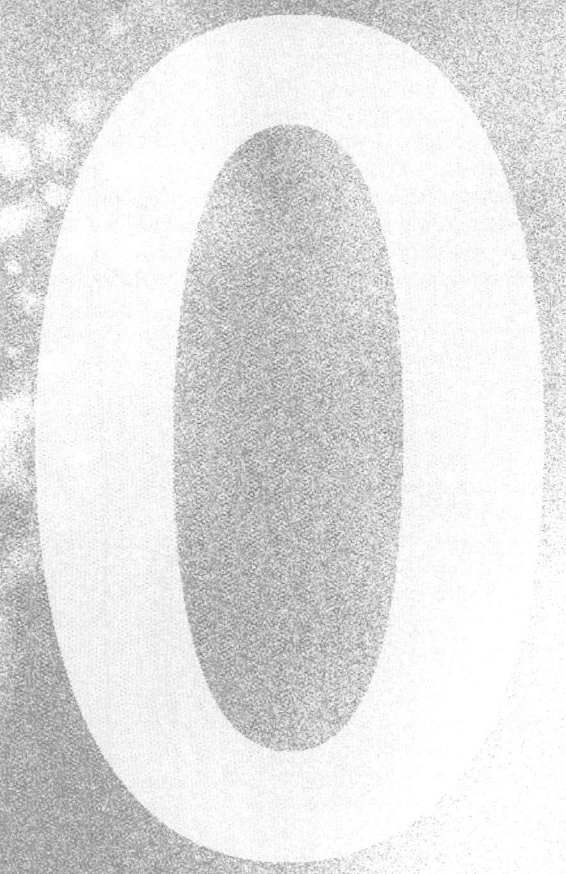

Vitreous

10

10.1 Applied anatomy and examination techniques

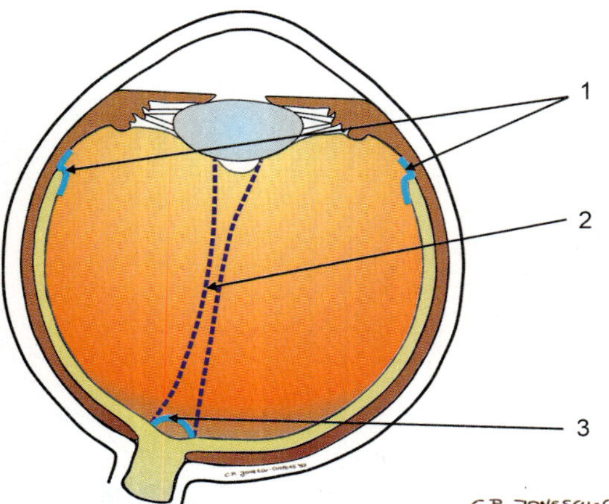

Figure 10.1 Horizontal section through the eye with vitreous body, schematic drawing. The vitreous body fills the space between the uvea (choroid and ciliary body) and the lens, sparing only small areas posterior to and besides the lens. The vitreous body of the postnatal eye is termed secondary vitreous, which arises from the vascular primary vitreous during fetal development. It is a transparent gel with high water content (99%). Unlike the primary vitreous, the secondary vitreous is completely avascular and contains very fine collagen fibrils. In between these fibrils lie molecules of hyaluronic acid with high water-binding ability. The peripheral vitreous body (vitreous cortex) contains an increased amount of collagen fibrils, mucopolysaccharides, proteins and hyalocytes. The vitreous body is normally only attached to the retina at the 2 mm broad vitreous base (1) and the posterior pole (ring of Martegiani) (3). Retinal breaks frequently occur at the posterior limitation of the vitreous base or in areas with atypical attachments between the vitreous and the retina. Cloquet´s canal (2) is an optically empty space, which courses from the lens to the optic disc, it may contain remnants of the primary vascularized vitreous, e.g. the hyaloid artery.

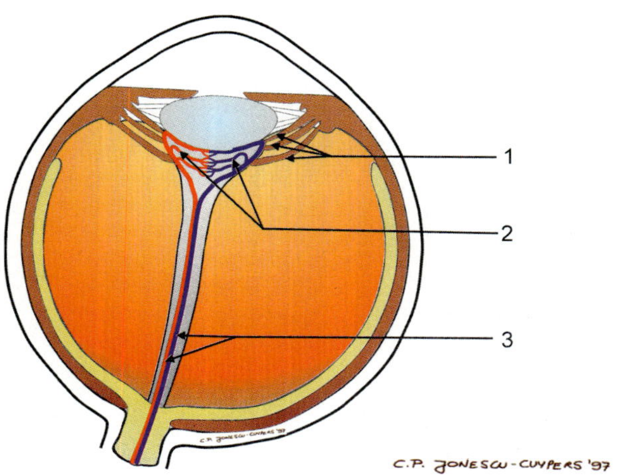

Figure 10.2 Persisitent primary vitreous, schematic drawing. The primary, highly vascularized vitreous normally regresses completely. Hyperplastic remnants, which may persist in the retrolental space (2) and may be connected to atypically elongated ciliary processes and vessels in Cloquet´s canal derived from the hyaloid artery (3), may have pathologic significance.

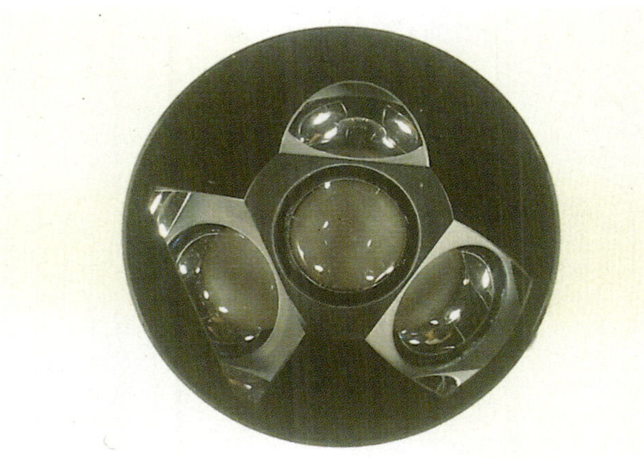

Figure 10.3 Three-mirror contact lens used for the examination of the vitreous. A clinical examination of the vitreous can be performed with the three-mirror contact lens. The contact lens consists of a central lens with concave surface and three peripheral mirrors, which are arranged at different angles of inclination. The lens is placed onto the cornea on a layer of methylcellulose. The arrangement of the mirrors allows for examination of the entire vitreous and retina (compare with figure 10.4). In case of poor visibility (opacities within the anterior optic media or vitreous hemorrhage), the examination is performed with ultrasonograhy.

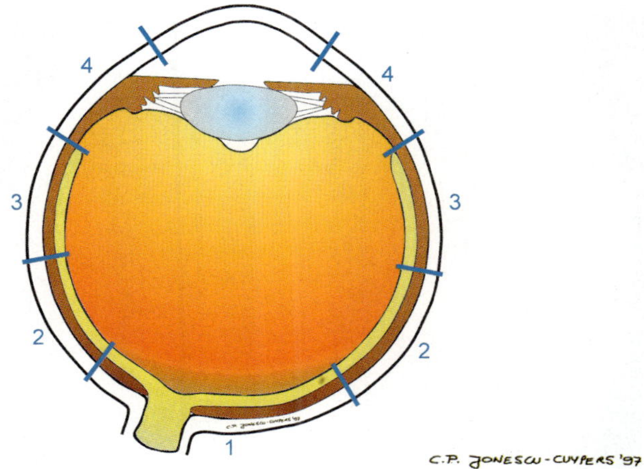

Figure 10.4 Areas of examination of the three-mirror contact lens, schematic drawing. The mirrors in the three-mirror contact lens are arranged at different angles of inclination. In this way, different areas of the peripheral fundus and the vitreous can be visualized. The area 1 is viewed through the center of the lens, areas 2,3 and 4 are viewed through the differently inclined peripheral mirrors.

10 .2 Developmental anomalies

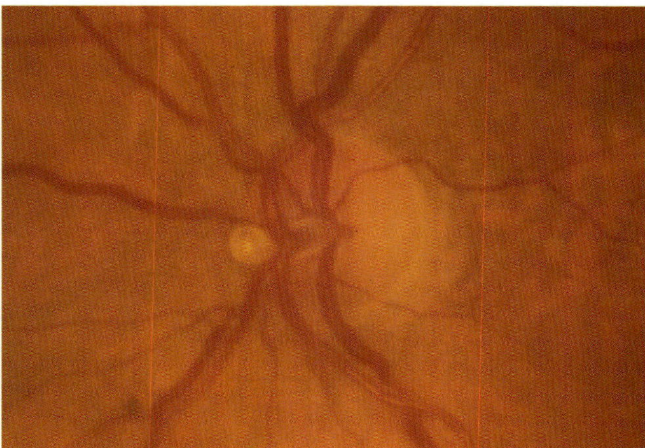

Figure 10.5 Prepapillary vascular loop, remnant of the hyaloid artery. Remnants of the hyaloid artery can perisist as prepapillary vascular loops. This finding has no pathologic significance.

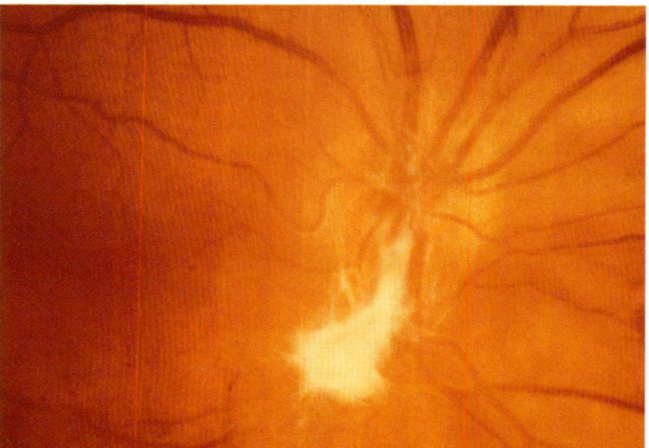

Figure 10.6 Persistent posterior primary vitreous. With incomplete regression of the primary vitreous, whitish tissue may extend into the vitreous from the optic disc. This so-called "Bergmeister´s papilla", which may be more or less pronounced, usually has no pathologic significance.

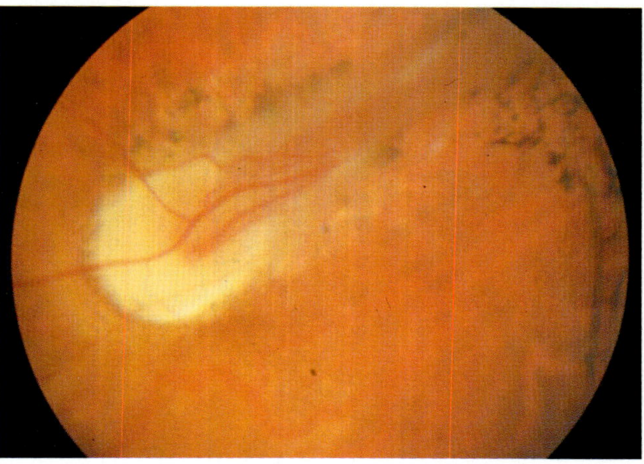

Figure 10.7 Falciform retinal folds. Any contraction of the vitreous can cause traction to the retina and retinal detachment. The picture of falciform retinal folds is typically associated with persistent posterior primary vitreous. Traction of the incompletely regressed posterior primary vitreous causes retinal detachment. In this case, a congenital radial retinal fold is found. Visual acuity is usually diminished, concomitant abnormalities are possible.

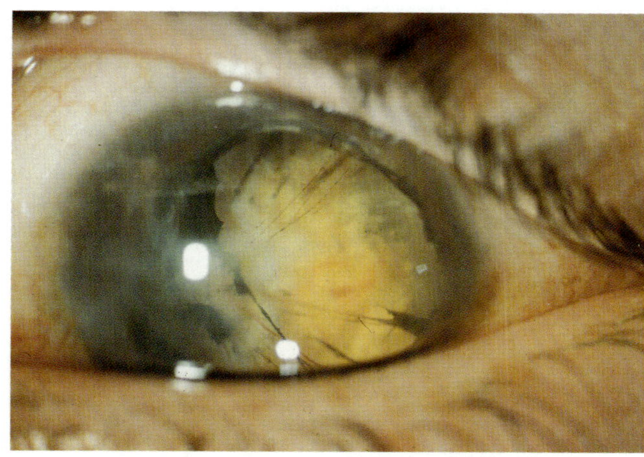

Figure 10.8 Anterior persistent hyperplastic primary vitreous. The anterior portions of the primary vascularized vitreous can persist in the retrolental space (compare with figure 10.2). In such cases, the retrolental fibrovascular tissue frequently causes concomitant cataract formation. With or without cataract the obsever sees a white pupillary reflex (leucocoria). The differential diagnosis of leucocoria includes inflammatory disorders and retinoblastoma in particular. Persistent hyperplastic primary vitreous is frequently associated with microphthalmia.

10.3 Degenerative changes

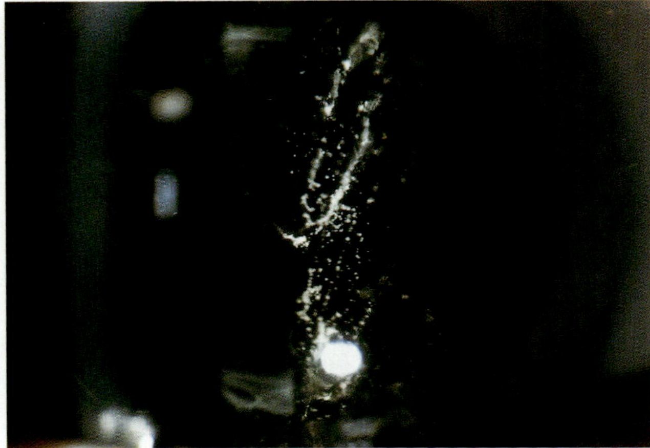

Figure 10.9 Synchisis scintillans. The vitreous opacities consist of glistening, freely mobile cholesterol crystals, which are not associated with collagen fibrils and therefore setlle in the inferior portions of the vitreous body. They are related to vitreous hemorrhage or inflammatory processes. Visual acuity is mostly only slightly impaired. Surgical removal (vitrectomy) is therefore not indicated.

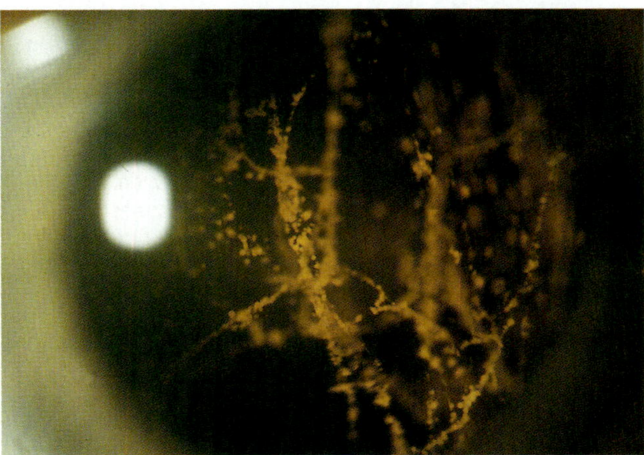

Figure 10.10 Asteroid hyalosis (synchisis nivea). As in synchisis scintillans, this condition is characterized by multiple opacities throughout the vitreous body, which, in this case, appear spheric, white and more dense. Unlike synchisis scintillans, the opacities are strongly associated with collagen fibrils and are therefore less mobile. Visual acuity is usually only slightly impaired in this condition as well. The asteroid bodies consist of calcium salt crystals. Their etiology remains unclear, an association to diabetes mellitus is discussed. If the patient is severly disturbed, surgical removal by means of vitrectomy can be considered.

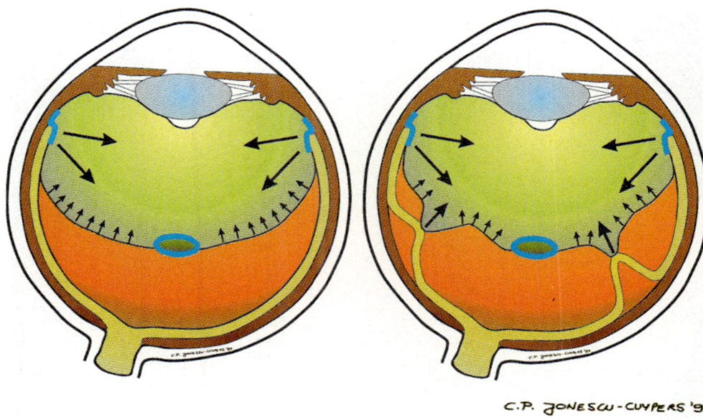

Figure 10.11 Posterior vitreous detachment (PVD), schematic drawing. *Left* complete, *right* incomplete with atypical vitreoretinal adherences. PVD frequently occurs in old age. Etiologic factors apart from normal involution can be inflammation, trauma and surgery. The complete detachment is usually a rather harmless event, while the incomplete detachment can be associated with retinal traction, preceding retinal breaks and retinal detachment. Retinal breaks typically occur at the posterior limitation of the vitreous base (compare with figure 10.1) and in areas of atypical vitreoretinal adhesion *(right)*. The involutional changes of the vitreous structure include aggregation of vitreous collagen fibrils, which the patient perceives as mobile, fine opacities (so-called "mouches volantes"). This finding is essentially benign. Photopsias, on the other hand, are an important symptom of vitreoretinal tractions. In these patients, repeated fundus examinations should be performed in order to rule out retinal breaks. Prophylactic measures aimed at the production of firm retinal adhesions such as laser therapy or cryotherapy may be considered.

Figure 10.12 Status post complete posterior vitreous detachment, including tear of the peripapillary vitreoretinal adhesion (ring of Martegiani). An annular opacity is visible superior to the optic disc, which corresponds to the torn posterior vitreortinal adhesion around the optic disc. This finding is a visible sign of posterior vitreous detachment. Careful fundus examination should be performed in order to rule out vitreoretinal tractions, retinal tears or hemorrhages. With early diagnosis of retinal breaks, prophylactic surgical procedures, which carry a good prognosis, can be applied.

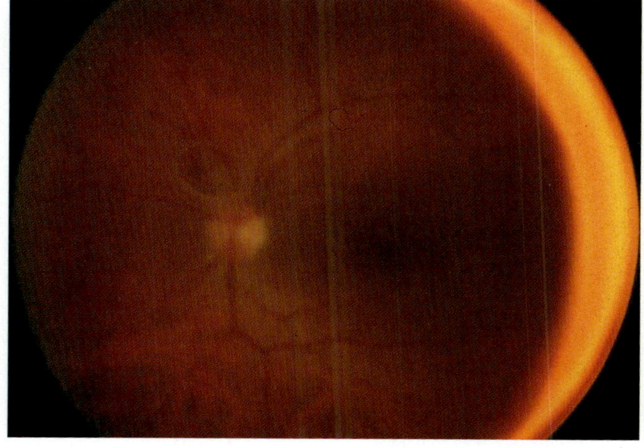

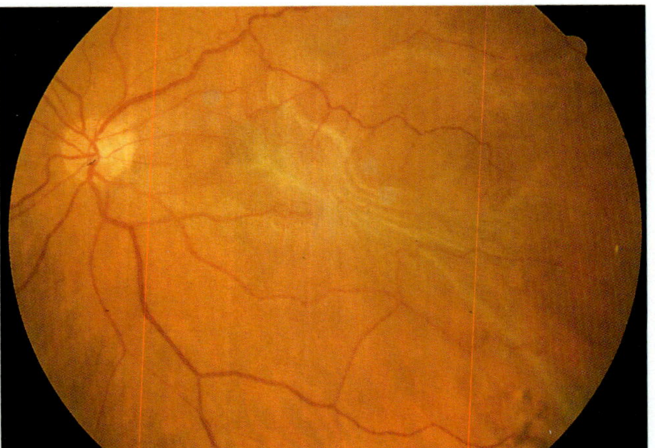

Figure 10.13 Epiretinal membrane at the posterior pole. The figure shows a dense, slightly undulated membrane with streaky condensations towards the temporal periphery, distortion of retinal vessels along the inferotemporal arcade and incipient traction retinal detachment. Vitreoretinal membranes develop at the interface between the vitreous and the retina. Hyalocytes and the retinal pigment epithelium, which can migrate to the inner retinal surface, contribute to the formation of epiretinal membranes. Traction develops owing to contractile properties of cellular components of the membranes (myofibroblasts). The membranes themselves can cause visual impairment. The major complication, however, is the progression to retinal detachment by contraction of the membranes. Even at early stages with very thin membranes, the patient may notice distortion while central vision is still fairly good. There is no conservative treatment available. The condition has a tendency to progress, for that reason, surgical removal should be considered. Recurrences are possible.

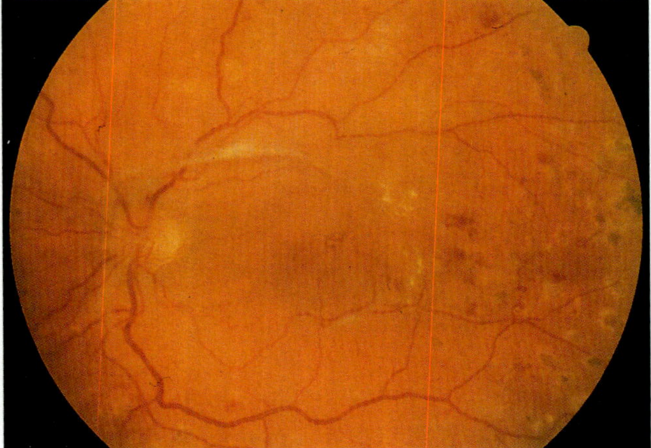

Figure 10.14 Vitreous membrane in proliferative diabetic retinopathy. Superior to the optic disc is an arc shaped vitreous membrane, which is attached to the retina temporal to the macula. A contraction of this vitreous membrane associated with traction and, in the later course, retinal detachment is possible (compare with figure 10.13). In the temporal mid-periphery are grey lesions that result from laser coagulation. This procedure was carried out as treatment of the proliferative retinopathy. Progression of pre-existing membranes can be induced by laser treatment.

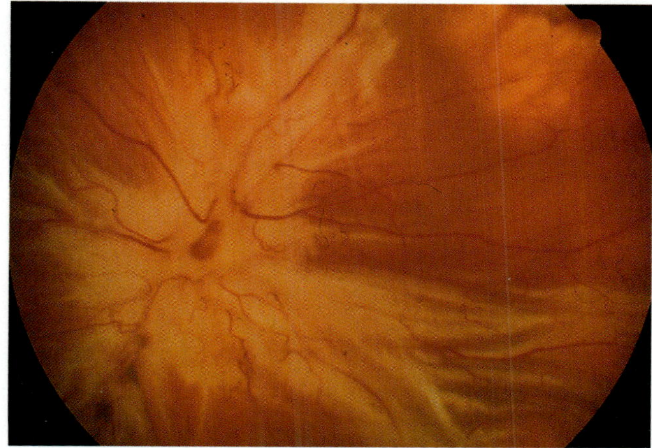

Figure 10.15   Proliferative vitreo-retinopathy (PVR). The figure shows a detached retina with rigid folds, which developed after contraction of an overlying vitreous membrane. Following rhegmatogenous retinal detachment, detachment surgery or trauma, formation of tractive epiretinal membranes and shrinkage of the vitreous body can occur. Cells from the retinal pigment epithelium contribute to the development of PVR. They can migrate to the inner retinal surface with or without pre-existing retinal breaks (compare with figure 10.13). Preretinal and subretinal membranes give rise to rigid retinal folds. Surgical management comprises combined vitreoretinal procedures.

Figure 10.16 Juvenile retino-schisis. The figure shows a central retinoschisis with a wheel-like appearance. The disorder is hereditary and progressive. The macular changes lead to progressive loss of vision. Peripheral changes with vitreous membranes (compare with figure 10.17) are common. In cases with atypical fundus picture, electroretinography can contribute to the diagnosis, showing a characteristic reduction of the b-wave amplitude.

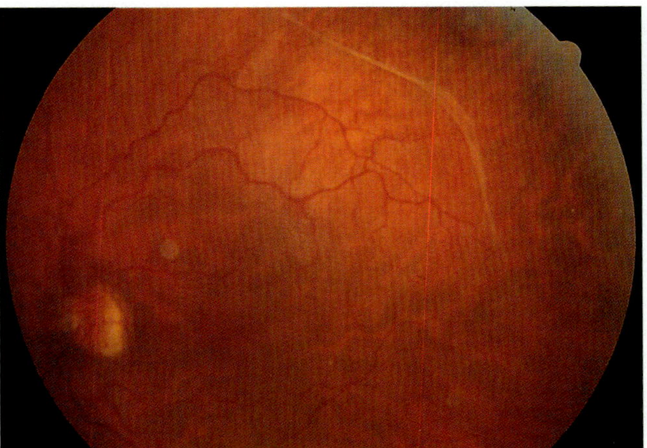

Figure 10.17 Juvenile retino-schisis. The figure shows a fine avascular preretinal membrane in the superotemporal periphery. The macular changes are less pronounced than in figure 10.16. For course and prognosis see figure 10.16.

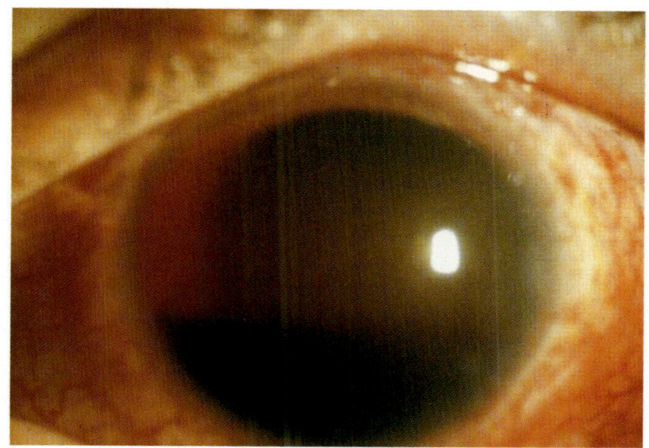

Figure 10.18   Vitreous hemorrhage extending into the anterior chamber in proliferative diabetic retinopathy and aphakia. The figure shows an anterior chamber hemorrhage with a horizontal level and an opacity in the vitreous cavity. Vitreous hemorrhages can have various causes. Aside from trauma, which can usually be ruled out by medical history, the most common underlying pathologies are retinal breaks, disorders associated with vascular proliferations (e.g. diabetes mellitus, vascular occlusions), as well as proliferating subretinal vessels and vascular anomalies. A vitreous hemorrhage obscures the view of the fundus. Clinical examination is based on ultrasosonography and visual field testing. The tendency to spontaneous resorption varies, depending on the kind and localization of the vitreous hemorrhage. If spontaneous resorption does not occur, a vitrectomy should be carried out after 6 months at the latest – and usually earlier in the young diabetic patient.

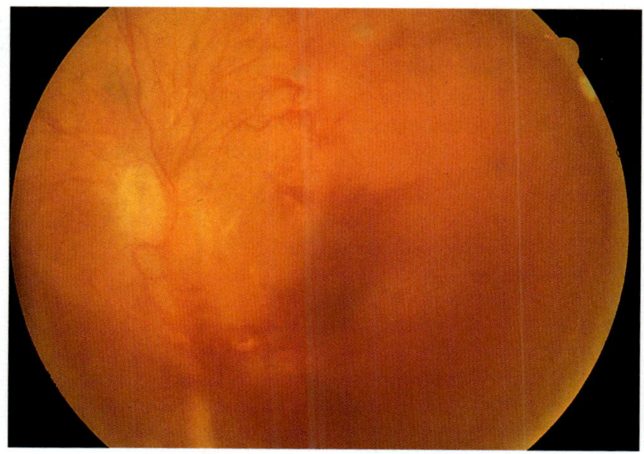

Figure 10.19   Vitreous hemorrhage in diabetic retinopathy. In this case, the vitreous hemorrhage is restricted to the posterior portion of the vitreous body. Fundoscopic examination is possible. Hemorrhages in the posterior vitreous have a tendency to spontaneous resorption. Following resolution of the opacities, the underlying retinal changes can be treated (e.g. laser treatment).

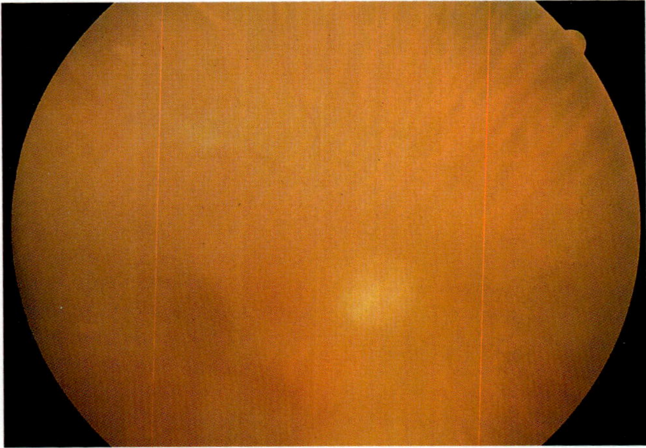

Figure 10.20   Vitreous hemorrhage in uveitis. The figure shows a severly blurred fundus picture. The optic disc appears pale and there is vascular sheathing. The vitreous is frequently involved in uveitis. The resorption of the opacities within the avascular vitreous is slow. Treatment is to be aimed at the underlying pathology (compare with chapter 7). Removal of the vitreous (vitrectomy) can be considered for functional improvement as well as treatment of uveitis.

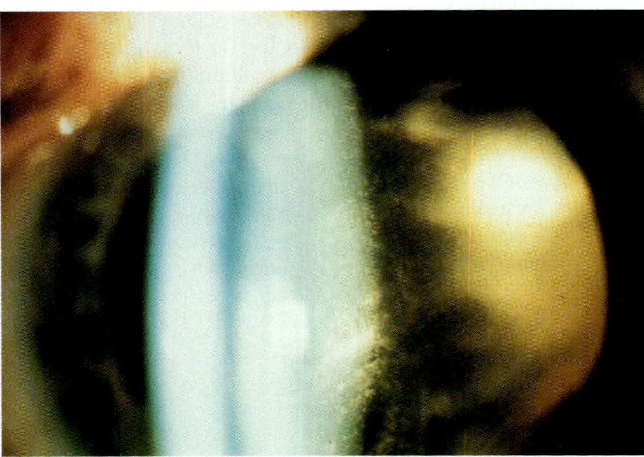

Figure 10.21   Vitreous abscess following a dog-bite injury. The figure shows dense yellowish opacities in the central vitreous. Bacterial vitreous abscesses occur following trauma, rarely after intraocular surgery, and may also be endogenous. Conservative treatment is usually not successful. An immediate surgical removal of the vitreous (vitrectomy) is required in order to avoid secondary retinal changes. Intensive systemic treatment aimed at the causative organism recovered from the eye should be conducted subsequently.

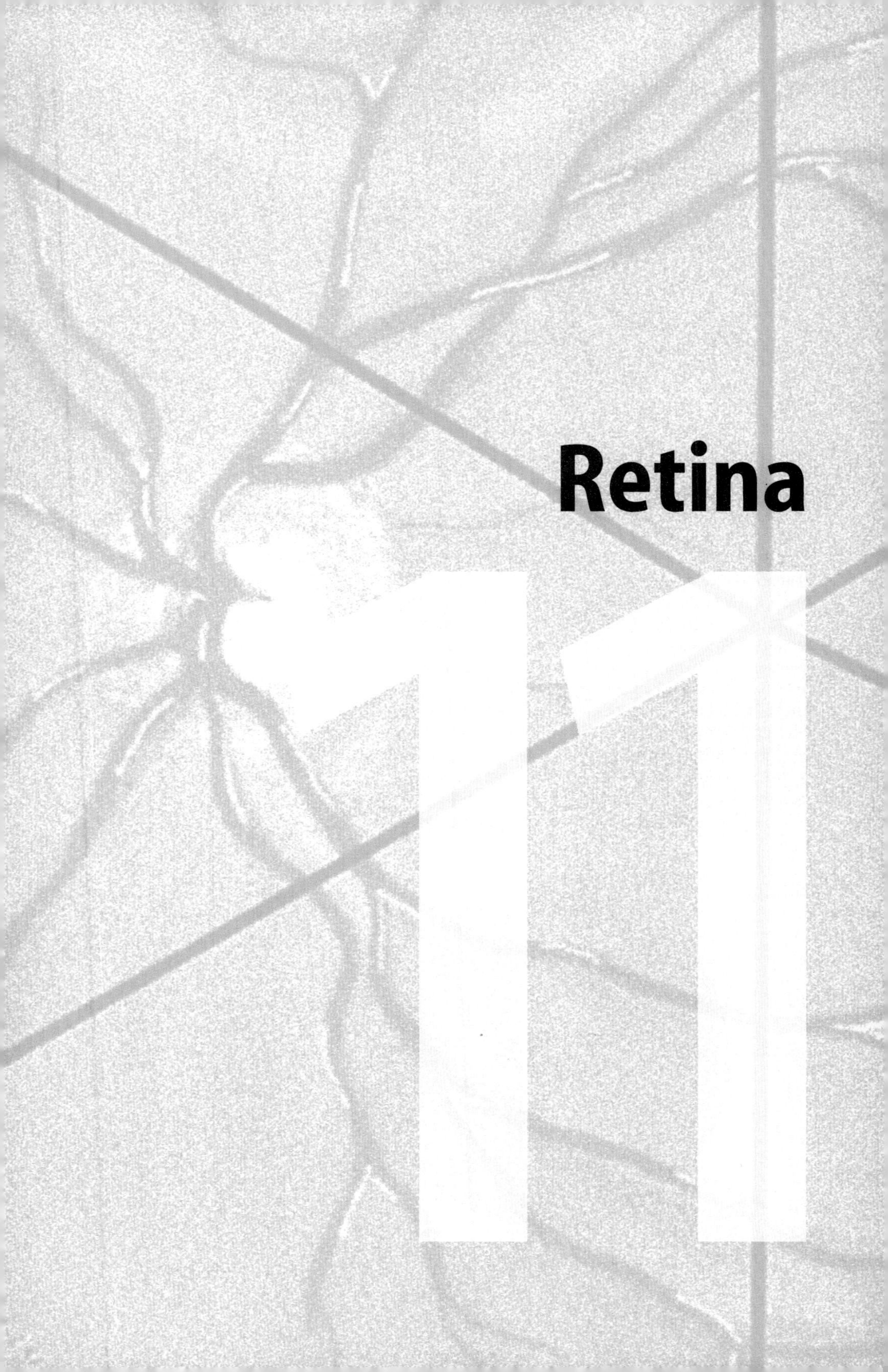

Retina

11

11.1 Applied anatomy and physiology

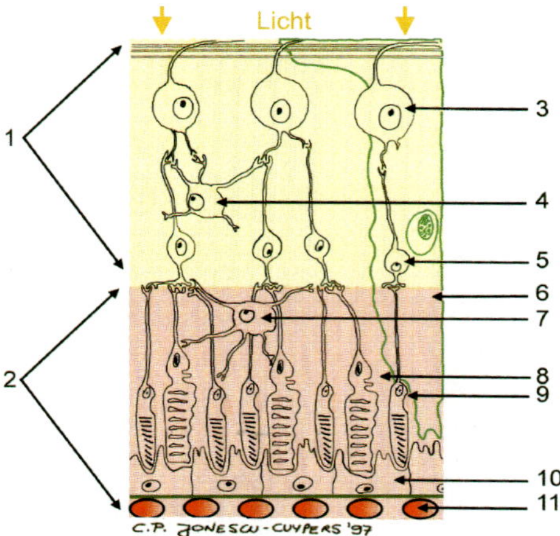

Figure 11.1 Schematic diagram of the retina with pigment epithelium, Bruch´s membrane and choriocapillaris. In the sensory retina, the light stimulus is conveyed by three neurons [(photoreceptores (8, 9) bipolar cells (5), ganglion cells (3)] into the optic nerve. Lateral interactions are established through amacrine and horizontal cells (4, 7). Müller cells and their processes serve as supportive tissue (glia). The photoreceptors comprise rods (scotopic vision) and cones (photopic and colour vision). Their outer segments contain the visual pigments (rhodopsin in rods and different opsins in cones). The absorption of light energy leads to a change in configuration of the prosthetic group (11 cis retinal -> all trans retinal). This reaction causes an excitation or inhibition of connected bipolar and ganglion cells via modulation of the transmembrane potential. In the fovea, exclusively cones are found (density: 150.000 per squaremillimeter). Three different types of cones are known to mediate color vision. The pigment epithelium (19) plays an important role in photoreceptor metabolism, including degradation of metabolic substances. The blood supply of the photoreceptors is effected through the choriocapillaris (11), while the inner layers of the retina are supplied through the central retinal artery (1,2 mark the areas of distribution). There is no anastomosis between these two vascular systems.

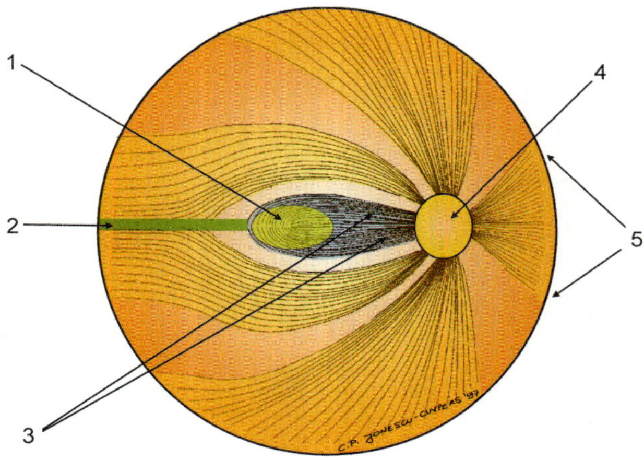

Figure 11.2 Nerve fiber pattern. From the macula (1) the neural axons (papillomacular bundle, 3) lead to the temporal margin of the optic disc (4). Temporal pallor of the optic disc is therefore associated with an impairment of central vision. The nasal axons (5) lead to the nasal margin of the disc. The axons from the upper and lower temporal quadrants lead in an arciform manner to the upper and lower margin of the disc. A raphe divides the areas from which the axons originate. The figure explains the relationship between visual field defects and axonal defects resulting from glaucomatous cupping.

Figure 11.3 Schematic diagram of the retina in the posterior pole. The foveola is marked by an excavation of the retina. It contains only cones, which are densely arranged. In the foveal margin, ganglion cells are clustered (6-8 layers) (2), constituting a slight elevation, which is visible upon ophthalmoscopic examination. This area is avascular, blood supply is effected through the chorocapillaris (see ophthalmoscopic picture in central artery occlusion). The content of melanin of the pigment epithelium is considerably higher in the central region.

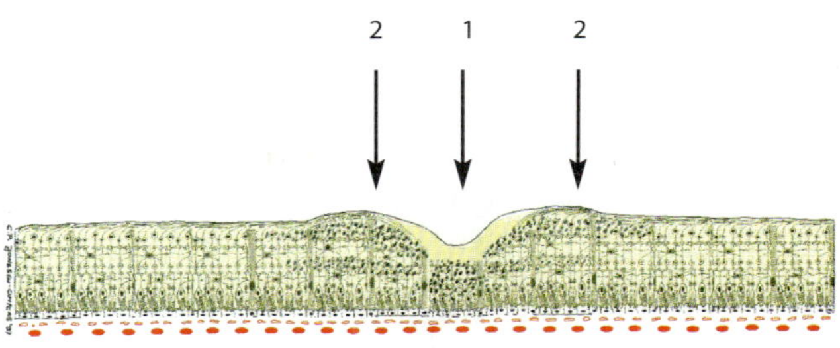

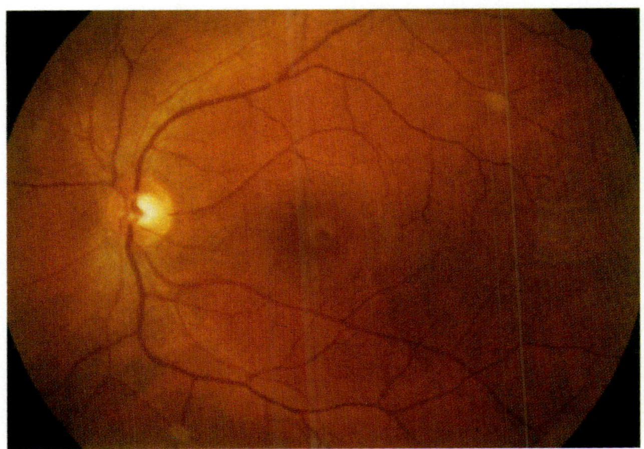

Figure 11.4 Normal fundus. The sensory retina is transparent. The red color of the normal fundus results from the choriocapillaris and the overlying pigment epithelium. Within retinal breaks, the red color is even more intense, making the diagnosis of retinal breaks is possible. If the retina becomes visible (edema, necrosis), this is always considered a pathologic condition. The excavation of the foveola is emphasized by the foveal margin, which results from clustering of ganglion cells. An area of approx. 0.5 mm is avascular. The central retinal artery and vein divide into four major vessels. A cilioretinal artery emerging from the choroidal vasculature is often present.

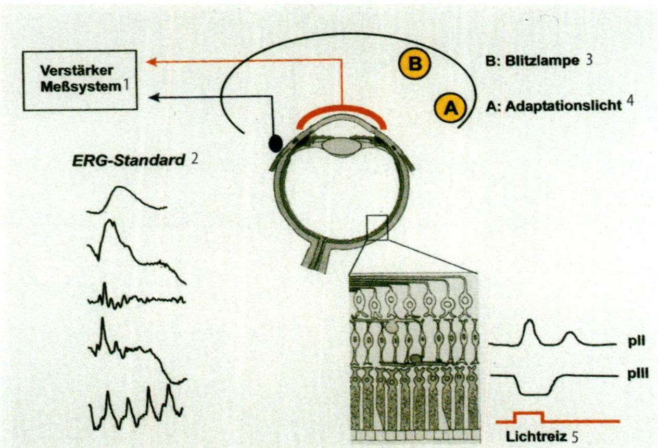

Figure 11.5   Electroretinogram. The absorption of light quanta leads to a hyperpolarization of the transmembrane potential in the photoreceptors (pIII). Changes in the phasic transmembrane potential of the inner retina are mediated via synaptic connections. The integrated light-elicited neuronal activity can be recorded with electrodes, which are placed on the corneal surface, via the ERG. Depending on the intensity of the stimulus and the stage of light adaption, standardized responses can be obtained, which comprise an early negative wave (a-wave, receptor activity) and a late positive wave (b-wave, postsynaptic activity). Standardized ERG *(from top to bottom)*: rod response, combined rod and cone response, oscillatory potentials, cone response and flicker-ERG. The localization and type of pathologic process can be inferred from pathologic changes in the ERG, allowing for an early diagnosis even before clinical detection.
Footnote: [1] amplifier/acquisition system; [2] standard ERG; [3] flash light source; [4] background light source; [5] light stimulus.

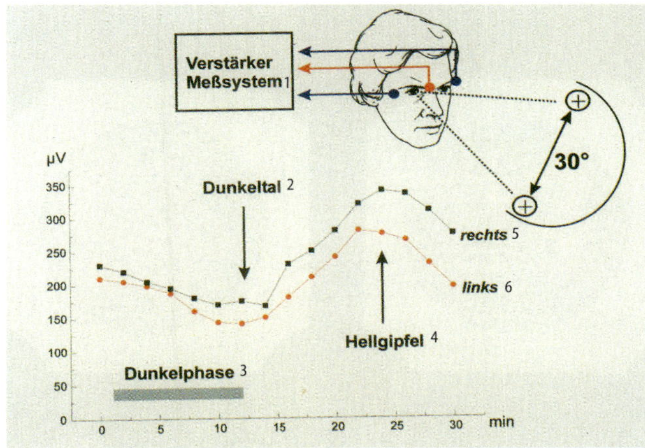

Figure 11.6 Electro-oculogram (EOG). The electric potential between the two poles retina and cornea can be measured during horizontal eye movements with surface electrodes that are placed at the lateral canthus on both eyes. In darkness, the measured potential is low (dark trough) ,while it rises in bright light (light peak). The ratio between light peak and dark trough provides information on the function of the pigment epithelium and the photoreceptors. The EOG is particularly applied in disorders of the retinal pigment epithelium, making an early diagnosis possible. *Footnote:* [1] amplifier / acquisition system; [2] dark trough; [3] dark adaption: [4] light peak; [5] right; [6] left.

Figure 11.7 Amsler grid. Minimal changes within the central visual field can be assessed with an Amsler grid. Macular alterations are symptomatic as scotomas or distortion of lines. This test is simple, can be performed by the patient himself and allows for an early detection of beginning or progressive macular alterations. For visual acuity testing see chapter 15.

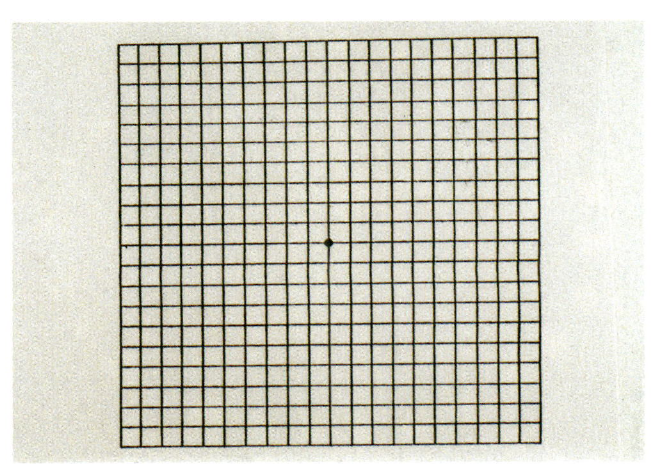

11.2 Diagnostic procedures and techniques

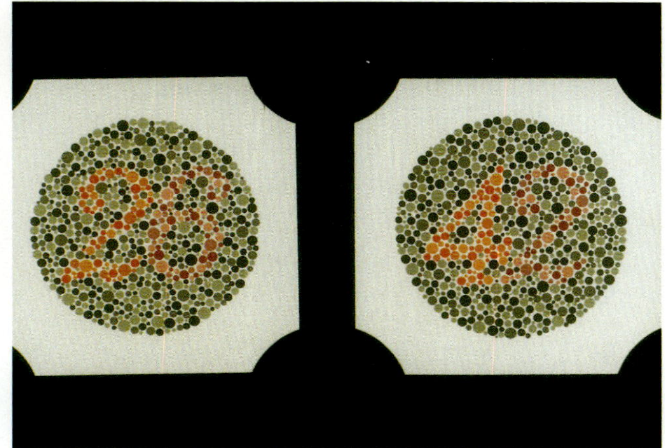

Figure 11.8 Color vision testing, pseudoisochromatic plates. Color vision testing offers a means of assessing color vision deficiencies. It allows a differentiation between congenital and acquired conditions, within the acquired conditions between retinal alterations and those of the optic nerve. Easy-to-use clinical tests are the pseudoisochramtic color plates and the Farnsworth-Munsell (Hue28) color arrangement test. Pseudoisochromatic color plates consist of an array of color spots, which are placed in between a camouflage pattern of confusion colors and grey spots. In different color deficiencies, different readings of the plates result. Various patterns are used in order to identify different forms of color vision defects.

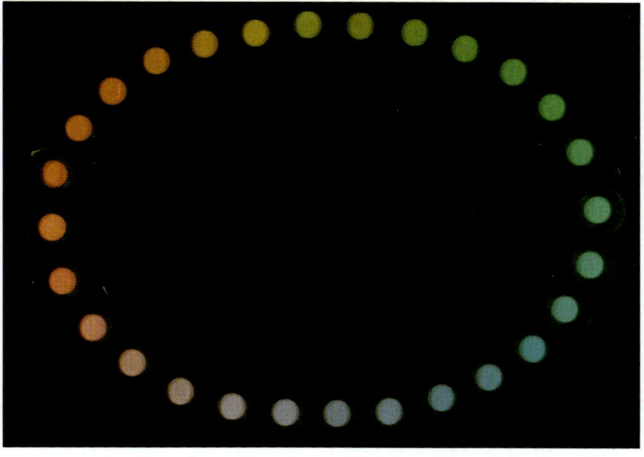

Figure 11.9 Farnsworth-Munsell Hue28 color arrangement test. The test consists of a set of colored round caps, which have to be arranged according to similarity. Different arrangements result, depending on the form of color defect (see 11.10).

Figure 11.10 Protanomaly. Color confusions in the Farnswort 28 Hue test with congenital red deficiency.

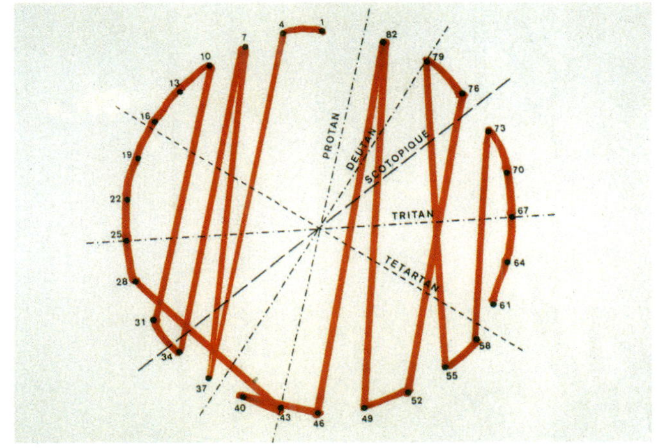

Figure 11.11 Nagel anomaloscope. In the Nagel anomaloscope, white light is divided into spectral colors. The patient is asked to match the brightness and color of a presented spectral yellow to a red/green mixture. The mixture ratio of red and green points to the subject´s red/green color deficiency.

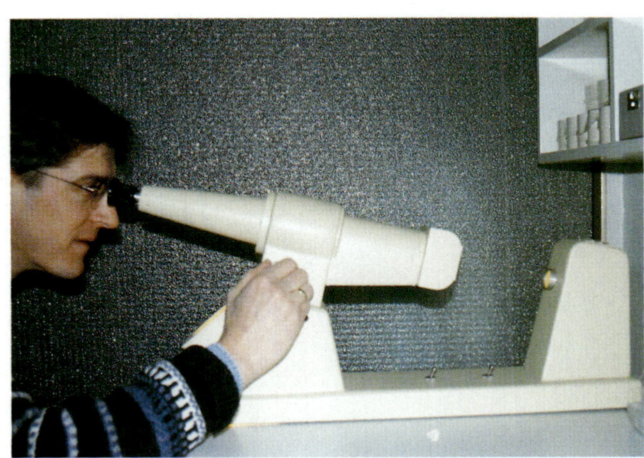

Figure 11.12 Visual sensitivity testing with the Goldmann-Weekers adaptometer. After bright-adaption, the time course of dark adaption is followed by exposure to visual test-types with changing background illumination.

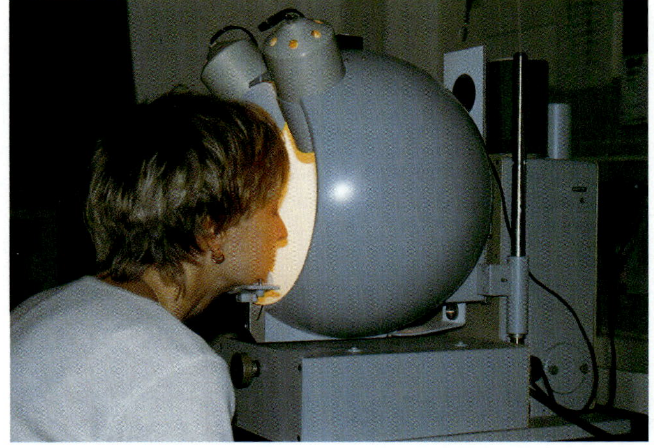

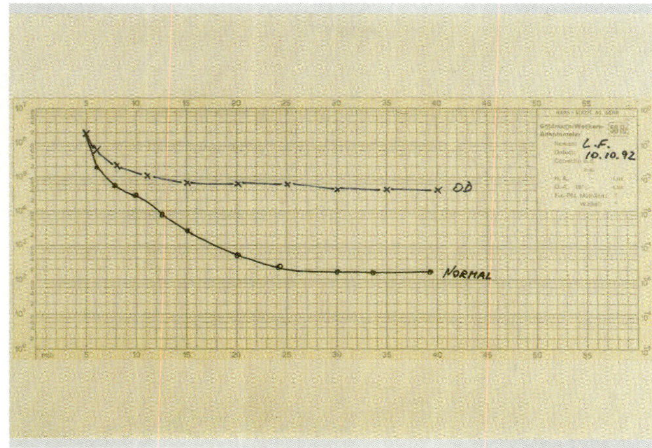

Figure 11.13 Time course of dark-adaption. The registration typically shows a biphasic curve with an initial phase of rapid increase in retinal sensitivity (cone adaption) follwed by a slow phase (rod adaption). A shift in the dark-adaption threshold is characteristic of night blindness.

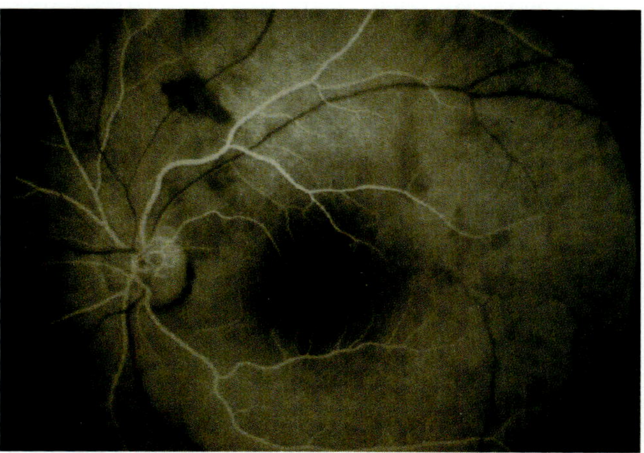

Figure 11.14 Fluorescein angiography. Fluorescein angiography is an important technique for detection of pathologic changes in the retina, the pigment epithelium, Bruch´s membrane and the choroid. The pigment epithelium and the endothelium of the retinal vessels are normally impermeable for fluorescein. A leakage of the pigment epithelium or the retinal vessels is considered a pathologic finding. Marked hyper- and hypofluorescence reveal corresponding pathologic processes (alterations in retinal vasculature, defects in pigment epithelium, neovascularizations arising from the choriocapillaris, occlusions of vessels, edemas). The frame shows an early phase of a normal fluorescein angiogram with dye-filling of the arterioles.

Figure 11.15 Late phase of fluorescein angiogram. The arterioles are less dye-filled, an increasing venous filling is noted. The macular region appears darker than the surrounding fundus (darker pigmentation of the pigment epithelium in this area).

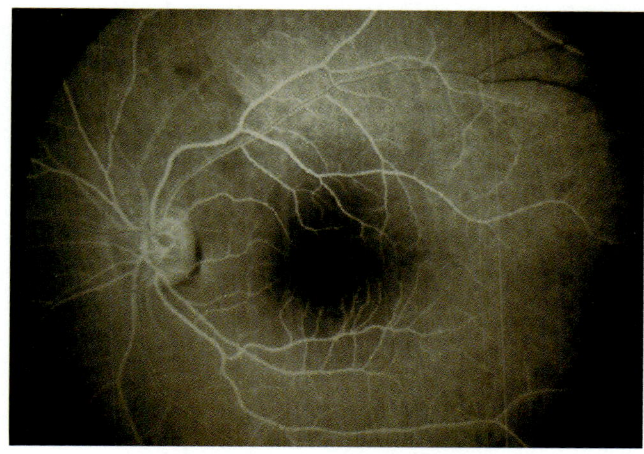

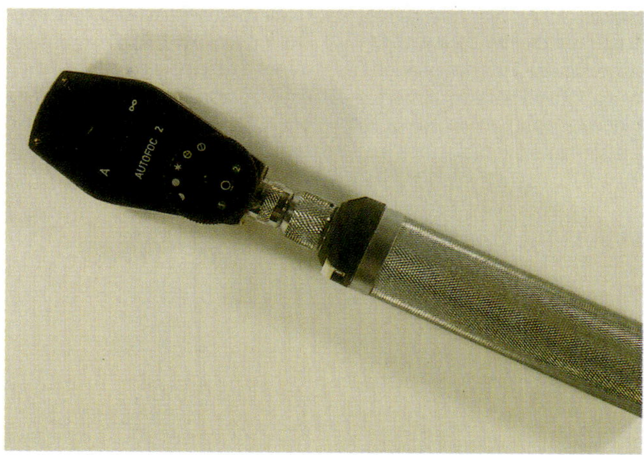

Figure 11.16 Ophthalmoscopy, true image, monocular and binocular. A true image of the fundus can be viewed through a monocular direct ophthalmoscope or in a binocular and stereoscopic fashion with the slit-lamp biomicroscope in conjunction with a Goldmann contact lens (see chapter 10). Direct ophthalmoscopy provides an examination of small portions of the retina at a time, it is not suitable for a quick overview. The advantage of the Goldmann three-mirror contact lens, apart from binocularity, is the visualization of the periphery (see chapter 10). The figure shows a direct ophthalmoscope, which is used for monocular ophthalmoscopy. Examination is performed through a dilated or undilated pupil at a very short distance from the examiner´s to the subject´s eye.

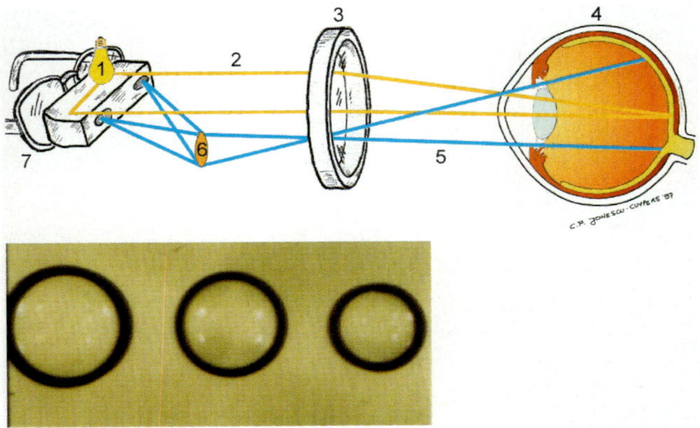

Figure 11.17 Binocular stereoscopic ophthalmoscopy with inverted image. The examination can be performed with an indirect binocular ophthalmoscope or with the slit-lamp biomicroscope in conjunction with a hand-held lens. The indirect ophthalmoscope allows a quick examination of the entire fundus including the periphery. Slit-lamp biomicroscopy in conjunction with various lenses allows for different enlargements, providing better possibilities of an exact stereoscopic examination of the midperiphery.

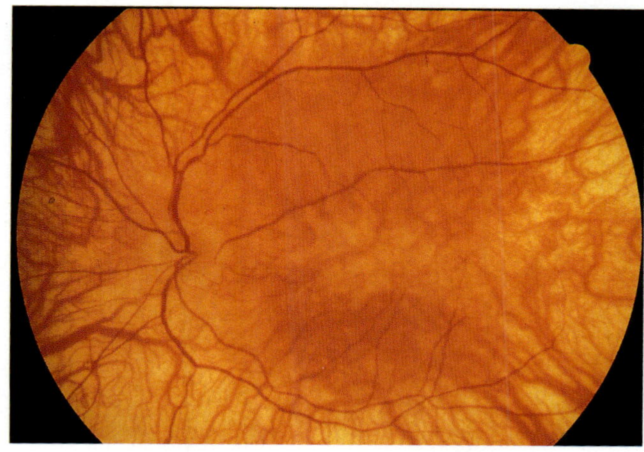

Figure 11.18 Albinism. Albinism is a disorder of the melanin synthesis, specifically of the thyrosine metabolism. In ocular albinism, the anterior segments (see chapter 7) and the fundus are abnormal. Normally, the pigment epithelium covers the choroid. In albinism, the choroidal vasculature is visible due to a decrease or loss in the amount of melanin. The clinical picture includes foveal hypoplasia, reduced visual acuity and an abnormal optic chiasm (see chapter 7).

Figure 11.19 Congenital hypertrophy of the retinal pigment epithelium (CHRPE). The figure shows a solitary, sharply demarcated, deeply pigmented flat lesion. CHRPE consist of inclusions of enlarged melanin granules in the retinal pigment epithelium. The lesions show no tendency to enlargement or malignancy. The sharp demarcation, the dark color and the flatness are features that help with the differential diagnosis.

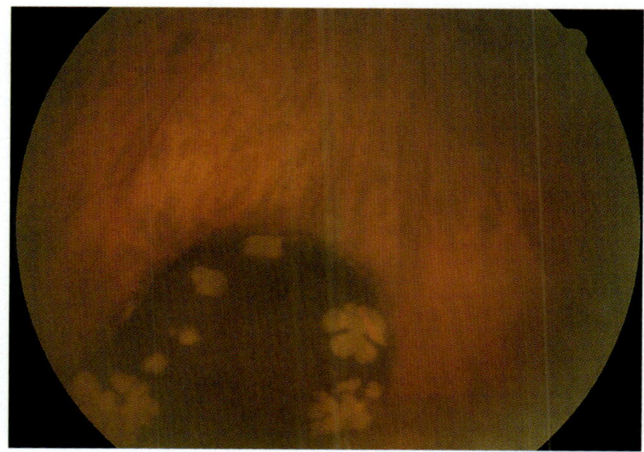

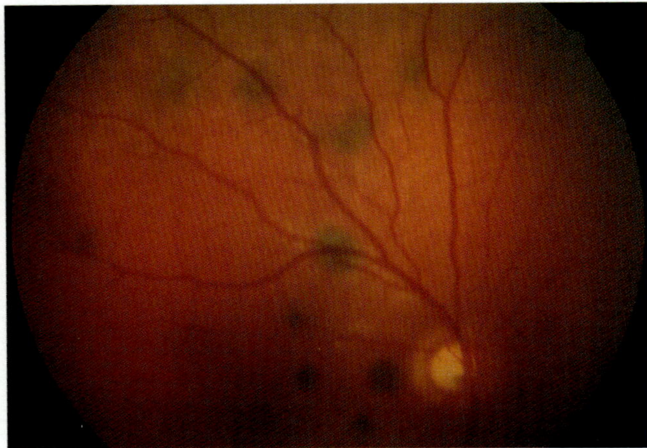

Figure 11.20 Congenital grouped hypertrophy of the retinal pigment epithelium ("bear tracks"). It is a variant of congenital hypertrophy of the pigment epithelium, in which multifocal small lesions are found.

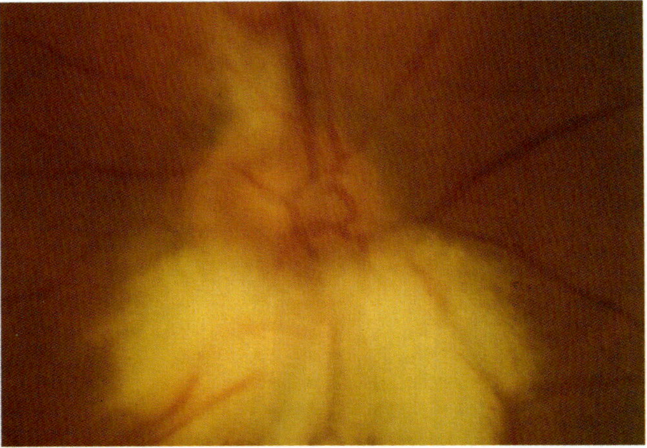

Figure 11.21 Myelinated nerve fibers. Myelination of the optic nerve is normally present only posterior to the lamina cribrosa. Myelinated nerve fibers, which are located mostly around the optic disc and sometimes peripherally, are an insignificant finding. They do not cause dysfunction, but have to be differentiated from inflammatory or occlusive disease. A characteristic feature is their fibrous structure, which is revealed by blue light, as well as the feathery margins.

Figure 11.22 Falciform retinal detachment, congenital retinal fold. Falciform retinal detachment mostly extends from the papilla to the ora. The figure shows the characteristic surrounding pigment and the vessels within the fold. Tractions often include the macula, resulting in severe vision loss. This condition is found in combination with persistent hyperplastic primary vitreous (see chapter 10).

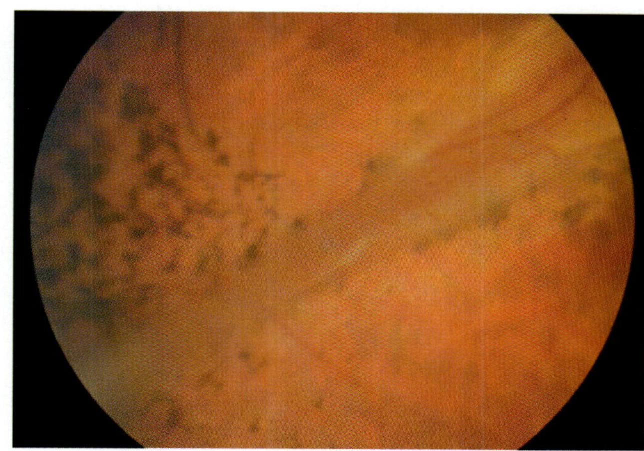

11.4 Vascular disorders

General: Arterial hypertension can lead to a variety of fundus changes, depending on the course (acute, chronic) as well as the ratio between systolic and diastolic pressure. Vascular changes almost always occur in prolonged hypertension, parenchymatous changes are found in advanced stages or acute rises in systemic blood pressure.

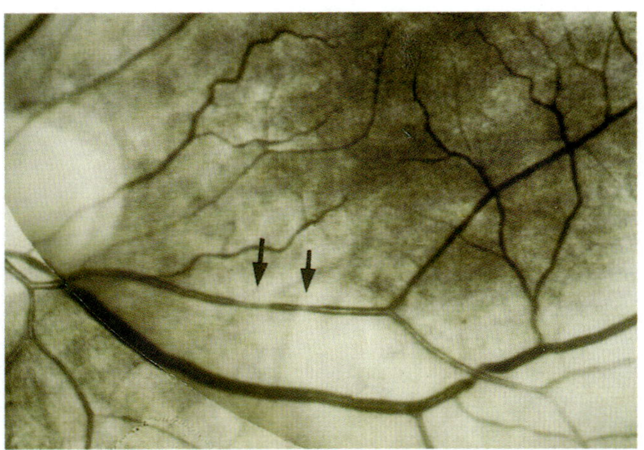

Figure 11.23   Hypertensive arteriolopathy with high diastolic pressure. The figure shows a focal narrowing of the temporal inferior arteriole *(arrows)*. Prolonged hypertension causes changes in the lumen of the arterioles. The resulting narrowing can be generalized (sometimes hard to diagnose) or focally emphasized. Assessing the vessel lumen by the the ratio between arteriole and vein, which is normally 2:3, may prove unreliable. Focal narrowing is easier to detect. In prolonged arterial hypertension, a compression of the vein in arteriolo-venous crossings occurs.

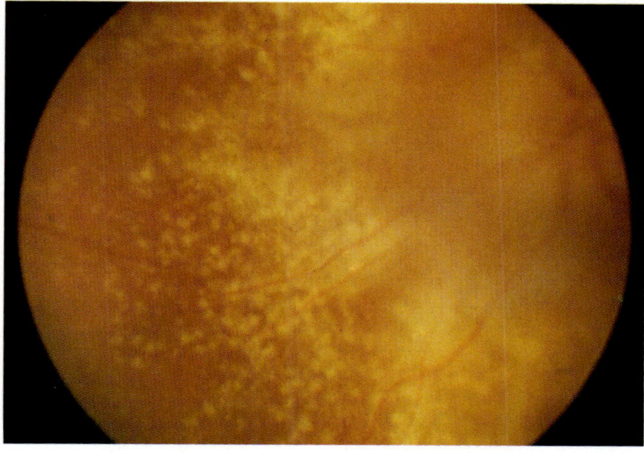

Figure 11.24 Hypertensive retinopathy, parenchymatous changes. In prolonged, severe hypertension but also in acute hypertension, parenchymatous changes in the fundus are described. A fibrinoid necrosis of the vessel walls causes a breakdown of the blood-retinal barrier, leading to hemorrhages in the nerve fiber layer, occlusion of superficial capillaries by cotton-wool spots, which are located in the nerve fiber layer, deep intraretinal edema and exudation. In advanced stages (figure shows stage IV), the arterioles are significantly narrowed, disc edema may be present in addition.

Figure 11.25 Hypertensive retinopathy, acute onset, stage of remission. In acute, but reversible rises in systemic blood pressure, the parenchymatous changes are reversible as well. After resorption of the deep edema, fine white exudates in the posterior pole remain, forming a "macular star". The exudate collects in the outer plexiform layer. The changes are reversible and usually of no visual consequence.

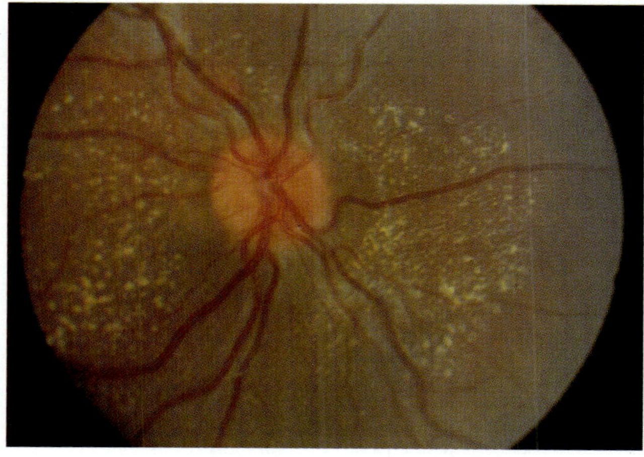

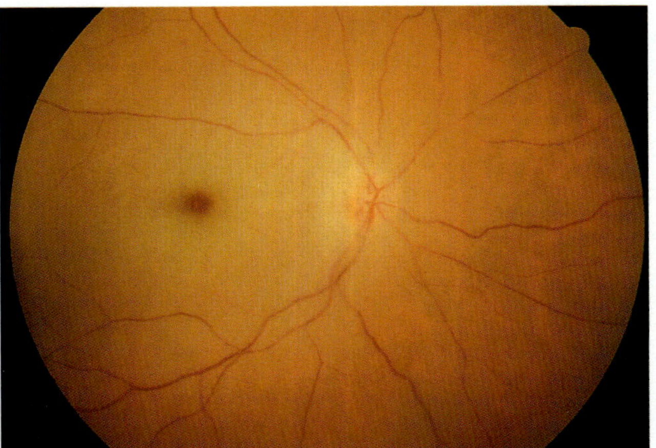

Figure 11.26 Central retinal artery occlusion (CRAO). CRAO leads to a mostly irreversible severe loss of vision. The onset is sudden and painless, there is failure in direct pupillary light response. Funduscopically, a pale edema of the retina with a charcteristic cherry-red spot in the fovea can be observed. This pathognomonic finding is explained by the fact that the fovea is exclusively perfused by the choroid, while the inner retinal cell layers of the surrounding macula are perfused by the central retinal artery. The case history and the clinical picture give the diagnosis. Causes for CRAO may be: genuine embolization (less common), a combination of atheromatous changes in the vessel wall and a drop in blood pressure, reduced blood flow in the proximal vessels. Genuine emboli (among others cholesterol) may arise from proximal arteries (carotid). If an immediate restoration of blood flow cannot be achieved, a necrosis of the inner retinal layers develops, sparing the periphery, which is supplied by the choroid. Treatment is usually unsuccessful, due to the patients seeking medical attention after several hours at the earliest. By that time, the permanent cell loss in the inner retinal layers is already advanced. With time, the normal fundus color is restored, the arteries remain narrowed (late diagnosis). In some cases, rubeosis may develop as a late complication. In every CRAO, as well as episodes of transient vision loss, carotid testing must be conducted.

Figure 11.27 Embolus with partial occlusion of a vessel. The figure shows a yellowish area in the optic disc at the bifurcation of the inferior artery. The branches of the superior artery show significant narrowing. The embolus has obviously only caused a partial occlusion of the vessel.

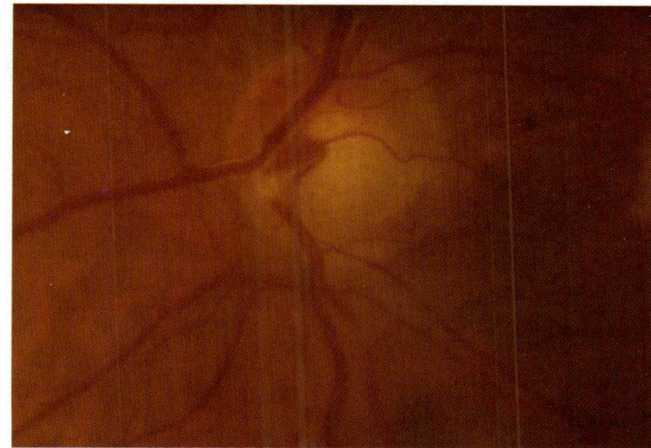

Figure 11.28 Branch retinal artery occlusion (BRAO), caused by multiple emboli. Sometimes the emboli may be carried into the periphery by the blood flow. The nonperfused retinal area shows whitening and is sharply defined against areas with intact blood supply. The emboli, which are mostly lodged at bifurcations, may disappear spontaneously.

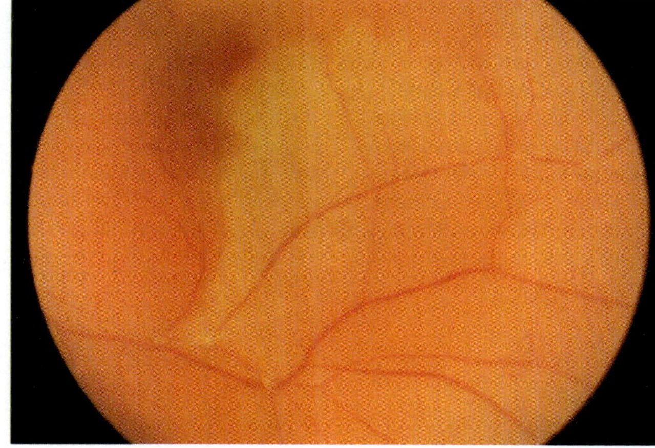

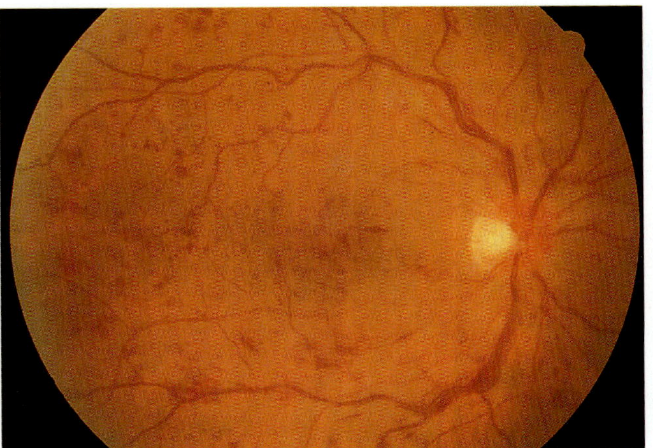

Figure 11.29 Central retinal vein occlusion (CRVO), partial, nonischemic form. The figure shows dilated, tortuous, dark-colored retinal veins. Intraretinal hemorrhages are scattered across the entire fundus. In this incomplete form of CRVO, retinal ischemia does not develop (detection by fluorescein angiography). Visual acuity is usually good, but may be lowered by a grey-whitish macular edema. The nonischemic form of CRVO may progress to the ischemic form (follow-up required). The prognosis of partial CRVO is good. If areas of capillary nonperfusion are identified by fluoresein angiography, laser photocoagulation of the affected areas is indicated. The most important component of the work-up is the evaluation for systemic causes, among which are cardiovascular disease, diabetes mellitus, hyperviscosity syndromes and blood dyscrasias. There is an association between CRVO and chronic open-angle glaucoma.

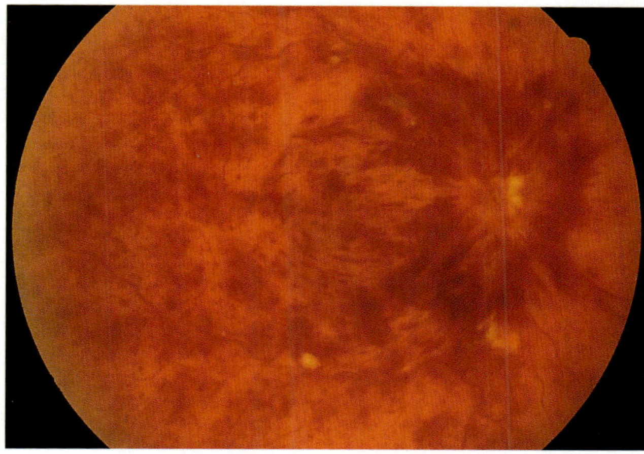

Figure 11.30 Central retinal vein occlusion (CRVO), ischemic form. The figure shows the complete picture of central retinal vein occlusion with disc edema, extensive peripapillary hemorrhages, slight elevation of the optic disc and intraretinal hemorrhages scattered across the entire fundus. In this variety of CRVO, an ischemic component is present. Secondary macular changes, including macular holes with irreversible vision loss, may occur. Unlike the nonischemic form of CRVO, older patients are mostly affected. The prognosis is relatively poor. The formation of collateral vessels may improve the prognosis. Therapy includes i.v. infusions and laser coagulation in the later course. The same systemic causes as in the nonischemic form of CRVO must be ruled out. The most severe complication is a neovascularization of the iris leading to neovascular glaucoma (see chapter 9). Panretinal photocoagulation cannot restore visual acuity, but it reduces the risk of neovascular glaucoma.

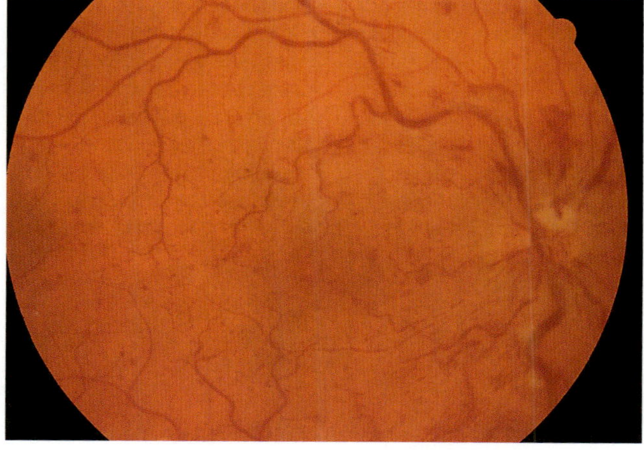

Figure 11.31 Venous stasis retinopathy. Carotid artery occlusive disease can show venous congestion in the fundus. Unlike CRVO, the veins are more tortuous, hemorrhages are less and located in the periphery. Carotid artery occlusive disease may cause severe pain (ischemic pain), despite low intraocular pressure.

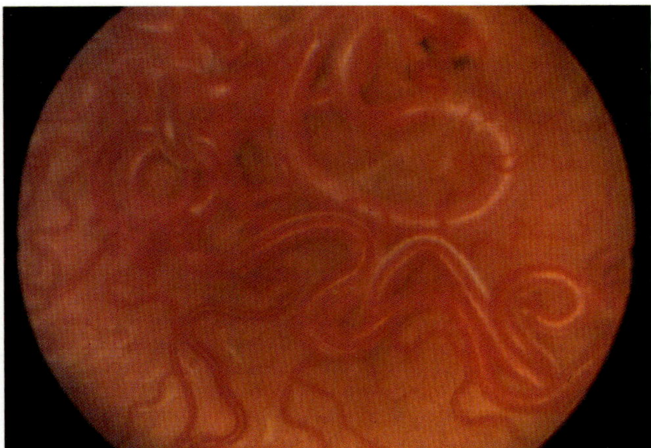

Figure 11.32 Racemose angioma. Unilateral anomaly characterized by excessively dilated and tortuous arteries and veins as well as arteriovenous shunts. An association with cerebral vascular malformations may be found in some cases (Wyburn-Mason syndrome). Central vision is usually decreased. The condition is non-progressive. There is no possible treatment. Cerebral lesions must be ruled out.

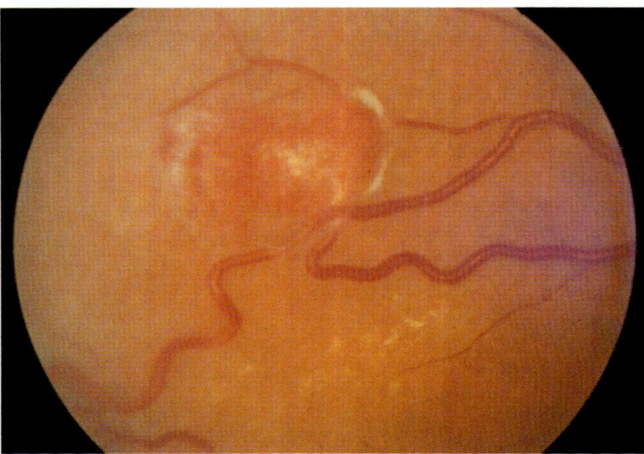

Figure 11.33 Capillary hemangioma of the retina, von Hippel-Lindau tumor, von Hippel-Lindau syndrome. The figure shows a reddish tumor with dilated and tortuous feeding and draining vessels. The picture is pathognomonic. The tumor consits of endothelial cells. Exudative changes (nasal and temporal margins of the tumor) are sometimes present. Hemorrhages, transsudates and retinal detachments may occur in addition. Treatment options, depending on the size and localization of the lesion, are laser photocoagulation, cryotherapy and surgical resection. In untreated lesions, the condition is complicated by retinal detachment, neovascularization and glaucoma. The tumor may occur solely in the eye or in asssociation with other hemangiomas (cerebral). An appropriate work-up has to be conducted. Family examination may be considered.

Figure 11.34 Capillary hemangioma, status post cryotherapy. The figure shows the remaining tumor with less filled feeding and draining vessels. A vitreous traction is present towards the tumor. The surrounding area shows a scar resulting from cryotherapy (lacking choroid). Treatment was done in order to reduce vitreous traction.

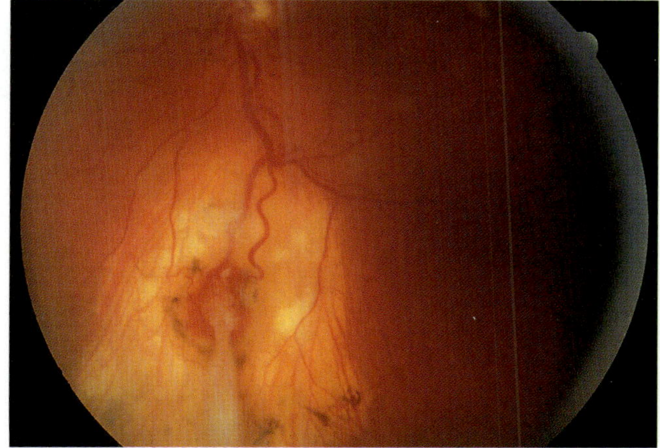

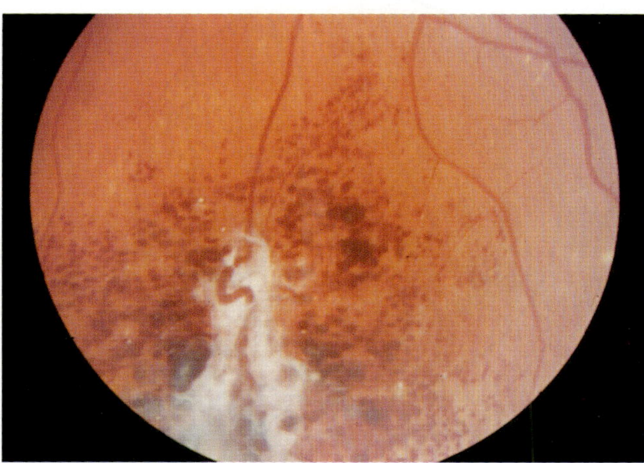

Figure 11.35 Coats´disease. The clinical picture includes retinal vascular anomalies with severe exudation and retinal detachment. The disorder is primarily defined by the presence of teleangiectasia, aneurysms and shunts. The breakdown of the blood-retinal barrier leads to hemorrhage and exudation. Subretinal cholesterol deposits are found. The condition mostly occurs in young males, but might also be found in older patients. The disorder is progressive and leads to vision loss, if not treated. Treatment is usually surgical (vitrectomy). The entity should always be suspected in young patients presenting with a combination of vascular anomalies, exudation and retinal detachment, without any underlying systemic disease like diabetes mellitus.

11.6 Neovascularizations

General: Neovascularizations can occur in the course of various disorders. The cause for vascular proliferation is mostly ischemia or inflammation. The release of angiogenic factors, which target the endothelial cells, is triggered. The newly grown vessels are permeable, hemorrhages and exudations occur. The resulting fundus changes include vasoproliferation, fibrovascular membranes, hemorrhages and exudates. Various disorders therefore lead to similar clinical manifestations.

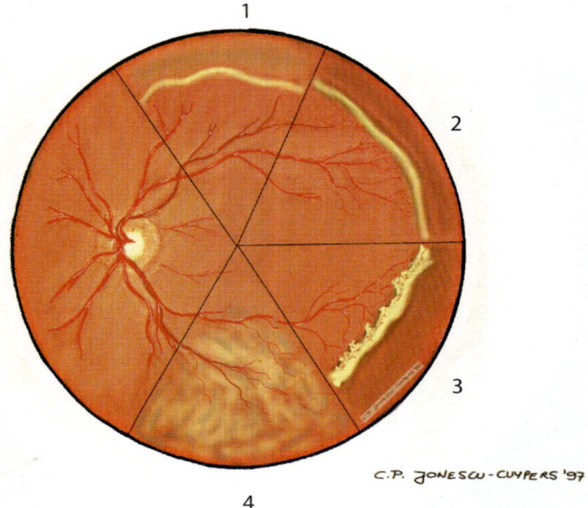

Figure 11.36   Retinopathy of prematurity (ROP), scheme of the disease stages. The precondition for the development of ROP is an incomplete vascularization of the peripheral retina, mainly the temporal periphery, and the fact that oxygen causes a vasoconstriction or even vaso-obliteration. The result is a progressive vasoproliferation, which has been classified into stages. The vasoproliferations occur on the margin of normally vascularized to the avascular retina. Classifcation: *Stage 1:* Demarcation line between peripheral avascular and posterior vascular retina; *Stage 2:* Elevated ridge on the demarcation line with vasoproliferations and beginning shunts; *Stage 3:* Progressive vasoproliferation, formation of shunts, beginning vitreoretinal traction (sector 1-3). Spontaneous regression is possible. With progressive vitreoretinal traction, a retinal detachment develops (*Stage 4;* sector 4), ending in the formation of a dense retrolental cicatricial tissue and blindness. In advanced stages, the clinical presentation with leucocoria has to be differentiated from persistent hyperplastic primary vitreous (see chapter 10) and retinoblastoma. The retrolental membrane in ROP is vascularized. Treatment consists of laser- and cryotherapy of the peripheral avascular retina in stage 3 and scleral buckling in circumscribed retinal detachment.

General: The following changes occur in diabetic retinopathy: hemorrhages, microaneurysms, cotton-wool spots, hard exudates, macular edema, intra- and extraretinal proliferations and vitreous traction. The underlying cause is a thickening of the basal membrane and a loss of endothelial cells due to hyperglycemia.

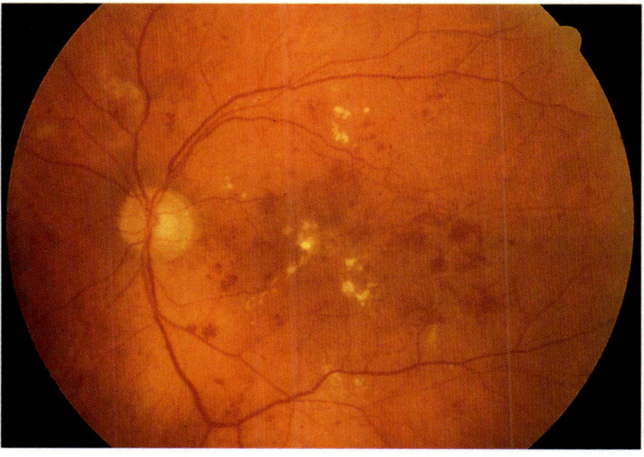

Figure 11.37 Nonproliferative diabetic retinopathy. The figure shows a combination of cotton-wool spots, exudates, fine-spot hemorrharges and microaneurysms. There are no proliferative changes. In progressive disease (follow-up) laser photocoagulation therapy is performed to debride ischemic regions. Before initiation of treatment, the changes should be evaluated by fluorescein angiography. Microaneurysms, which cannot be seen funduscopically, can be detected with fluorescein angiography.

11.6 Neovascularizations

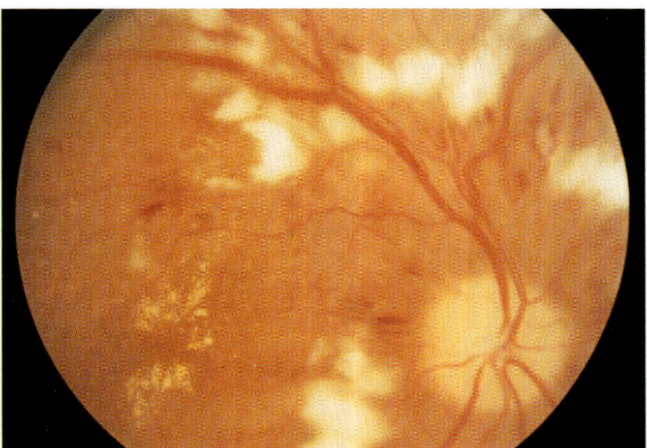

Figure 11.38 Nonproliferative diabetic retinopathy, advanced stage. In advanced nonproliferative retinopathy, an abnormal permeability of the retinal vessels leads to macular edema, accounting for vision loss and deposition of lipids, particularly in the regions with marked vasculopathy. Treatment of the vasular abnormalities and lipid deposits with laser photocoagulation gives a good prognosis.

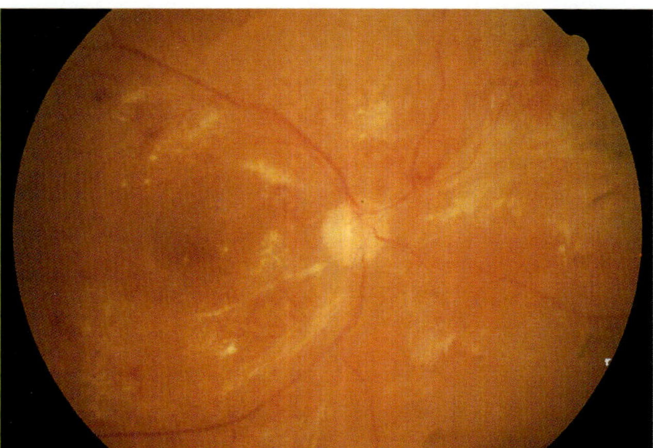

Figure 11.39 Proliferative retinopathy. In addition to the changes in nonproliferative retinopathy, in proliferative retinopathy vasoproliferations occur, forming fibrovascular vitreous membranes. Ischemic retinal areas (visualized by fluorescein angiography) are thought to trigger the vessel growth. Therapy: panretinal laser photocoagulation.

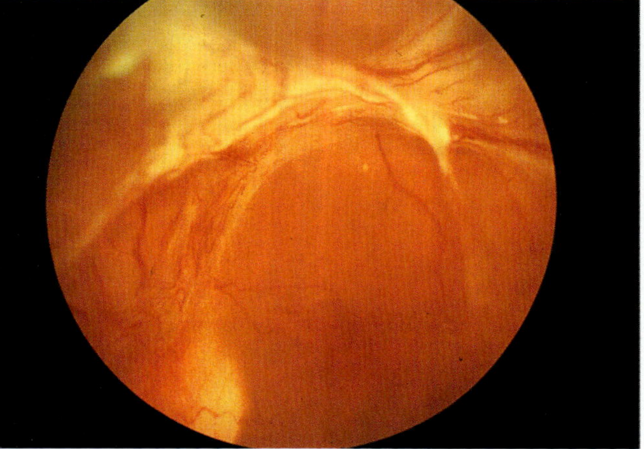

Figure 11.40 Proliferative diabetic retinopathy with vitreous membranes. The figure shows neovascularizations which form an elevated vitreous membrane. Tractions from these fibrovascular membranes causes retinal detachment. Therapy: panretinal laser photocoagulation.

Figure 11.41 Diabetic retinopathy, status post panretinal laser photocoagulation.

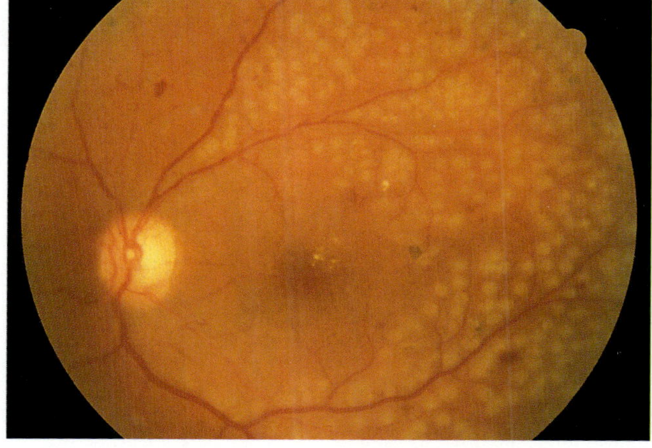

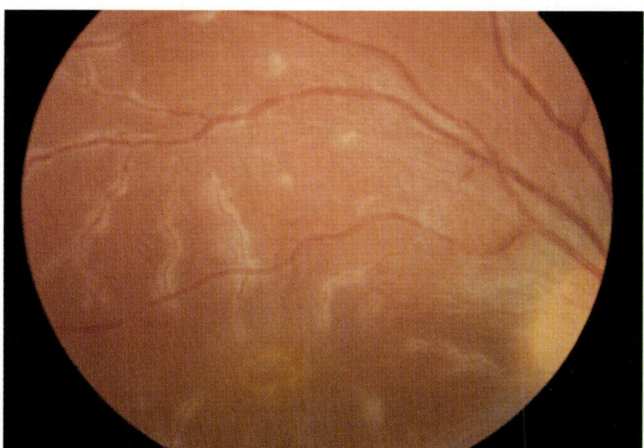

Figure 11.42 Eales´disease (retinal perivasculitis, vasculitis). The figure shows white-greyish sheathing of arterioles and venules. The vascular disorder predominantly occurs in young men and is mostly bilateral. The peripheral venules are more often affected than the arterioles. In advanced stages, obliterations develop, leading to neovascularizations, recurrent vitreous hemorrhages and sometimes macular edema. Patients have no complaints in the early stages of the disease. Vitreous hemorrhages and macular edema account for severe vision loss. The cause for the condition remains unknown. Laser photocoagulation therapy is indicated in order to prevent vasoproliferation. Systemic disease has to be ruled out.

11.6 Neovascularizations

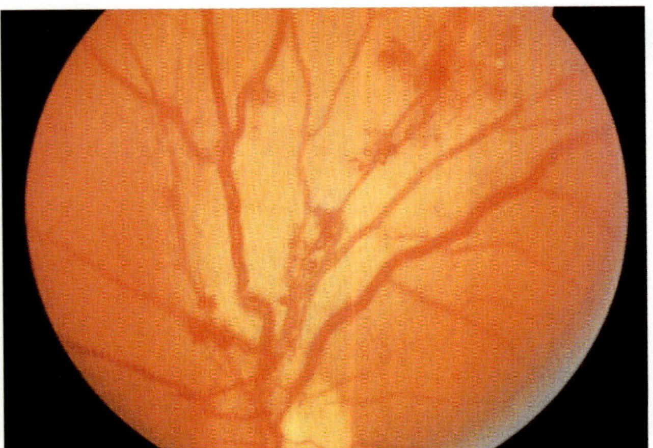

Figure 11.43 Retinal periphlebitis, vasoproliferations.

General: Infectious processes in the fundus often involve the retina along with the choroid. A differentiation between a primary affection of the retina (retinochoroiditis) and a primary affection of the choroid (chorioretinitis) is not always possible (see chapter 7). Viral inflammations are restricted to the retina.

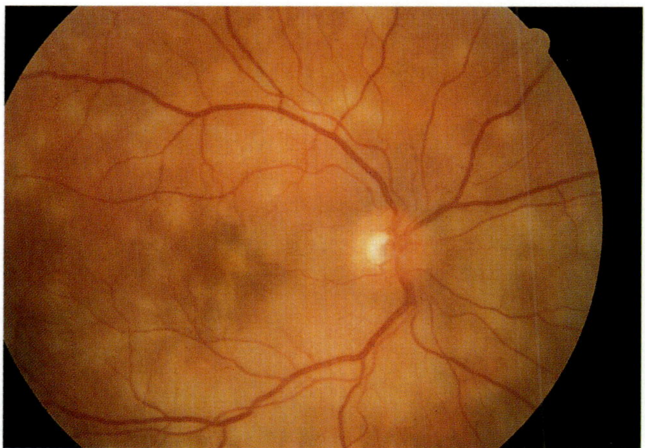

Figure 11.44 Acute multifocal posterior placoid pigment epitheliopathy (AMPPPE). The condition represents a disorder of the pigment epithelium of unknown cause. Viral infections and immunologic factors are presumed to cause the disorder. The clinical picture is characterized by flat, grey-white lesions, which are irregularly scattered across the posterior pole. The fluorescence angiographic finding is pathognomonic (see 11.45). In the further course, the edema resolves, leaving discrete pigment epithelial alterations. Despite the striking initial finding, the prognosis is good and vision is fully recovered in most cases. There is no valid therapeutic concept. The clinical presentation can be confused with multifocal choroiditis.

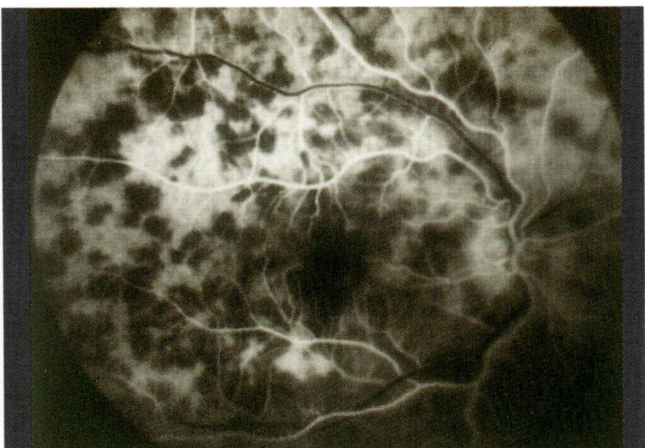

Figure 11.45 Acute multifocal posterior placoid pigment epitheliopathy (AMPPPE), fluorescein angiogram. The lesions show hypofluorescence during the early phase. This fact has led to the assumption, that AMPPPE is associated with a perfusion defect of the choriocapillaris.

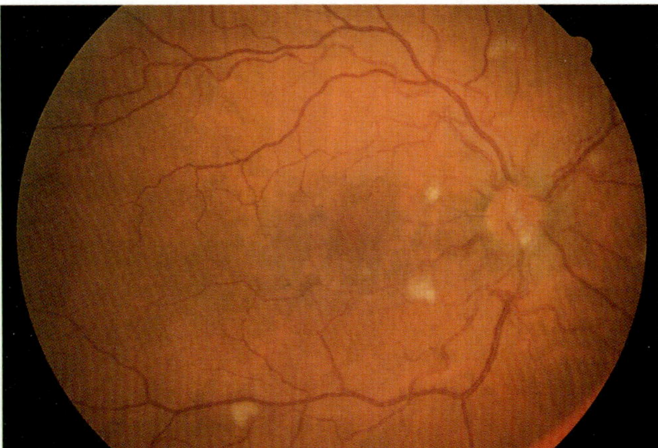

Figure 11.46 Cytomegalovirus (CMV) retinitis, early stage. This condition mostly occurs in patients with aquired immunodeficiency (AIDS) and drug induced immunodeficiency. In early stages, circumscribed grey lesions (cotton-wool spots) and hemorrhages are found. This clinical presentation may be confused with collagen-vascular disease. The case history should consider the question of possible HIV infection.

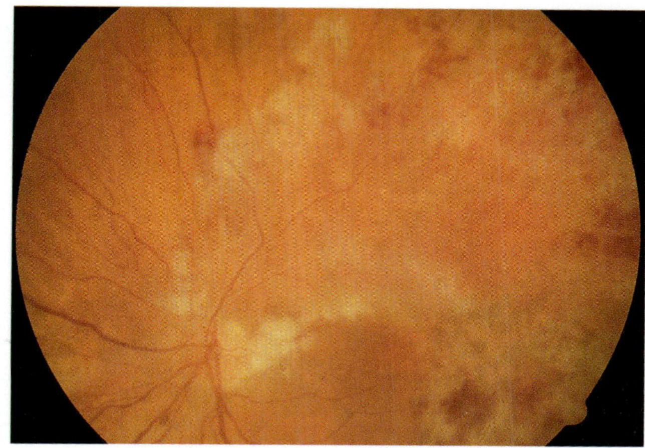

Figure 11.47 CMV retinitis, advanced stage. The invasion of the retina is directed from the posterior pole towards the periphery, causing an almost complete destruction. The figure shows an area of visible choroid in the temporal upper quadrant where no retinal vessels are present. This area is delimited towards the intact retina by edematous zones and hemorrhages. This clinical finding indicates active disease. Without therapy, the condition results in blindness within a short period of time. Treatment with virustatic drugs may stop the progression. Discontinuation of therapy is not possible. At present, "pellets" loaded with virustatic drugs are successfully implanted into the vitreous cavity.

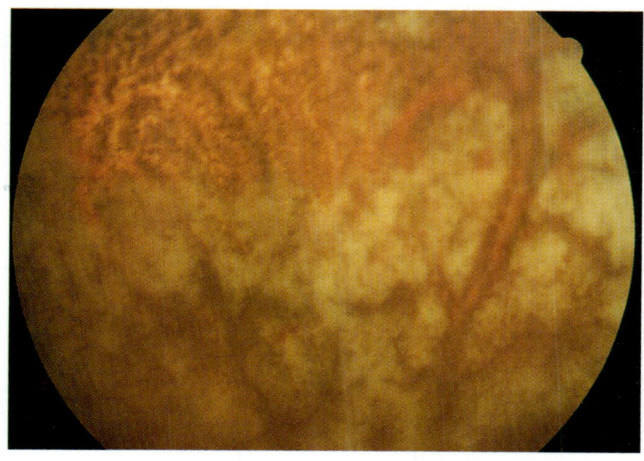

Figure 11.48 CMV retinitis, end stage. The figure shows a status post retinal necrosis. *In the upper half* granular pigmentations can be seen, *in the lower half* areas of grey, necrotic retina prevail. Retinal vessels cannot be detected.

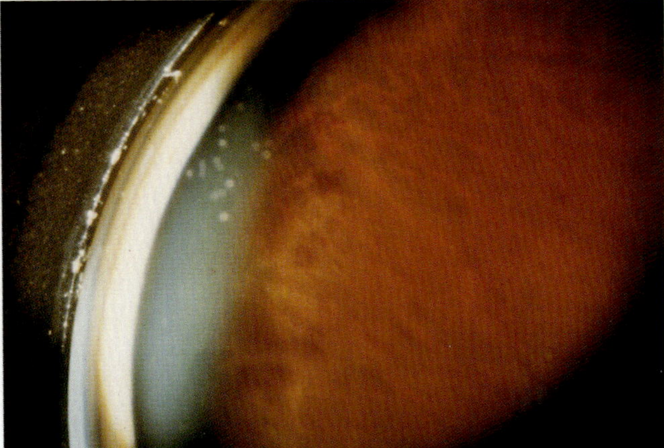

Figure 11.49 Herpes retinitis. Herpes retinitis, as well as CMV retinitis, leads to a selective destruction of the retina. Unlike CMV retinitis, the process commences in the periphery (figure shows view through a Goldmann contact lens). Therapy consists of virustatic drugs, which can stop the progression. Permanent therapy is not necessary.

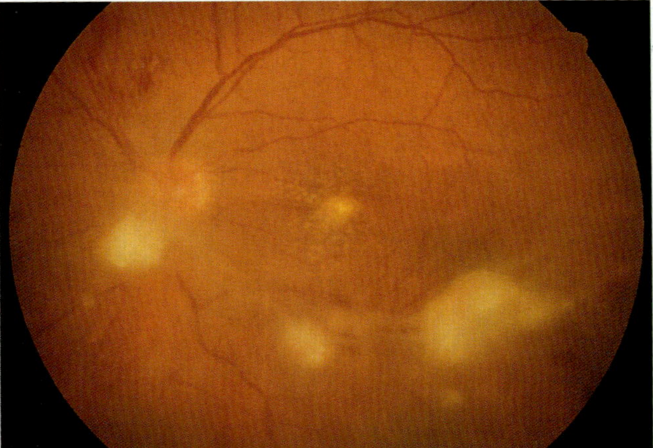

Figure 11.50 Candida mycosis / chorioretinitis with involvement of the vitreous. Endogenous candida mycosis typically occurs in patients receiving intensive long-term therapy with antibiotics, corticosteroids and immunosuppressive agents. The initial focus often is an intravenous catheter. The condition represents a chorioretinitis, fundoscopic findings are large, white, poorly demarcated lesions, which have invaded the vitreous. The tentative diagnosis is based on the clinical picture and the case history. It can be confirmed upon detection of germs after vitrectomy. Without therapy, the condition leads to blindness. Systemic antifungals in combination with vitrectomy can lead to recovery.

Figure 11.51   Subretinal granuloma in toxocara infection. Toxocara larva can invade the eye and cause a massive granulomatous reaction. A concomitant retinal detachment often resolves. In end stage disease, an elevated nodulous scar is found, which can be confused with a tumor.

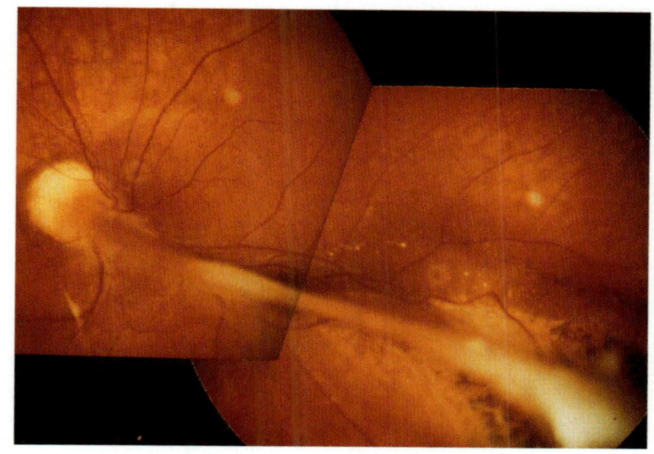

11.8 Macular disorders and degenerations

General: Macular disorders are located in the various layers of the retina, the pigment epithelium, Bruch´s membrane and the choriocapillaris. Edemas, serous detachments, hemorrhages, neovascularizations, ingrowth of fibrovascular tissue and scarring are described. Early symptoms can be visual disturbances including photopsia, distortion of lines, micropsia and macropsia. Later on, the process leads to an impairment of visual acuity.

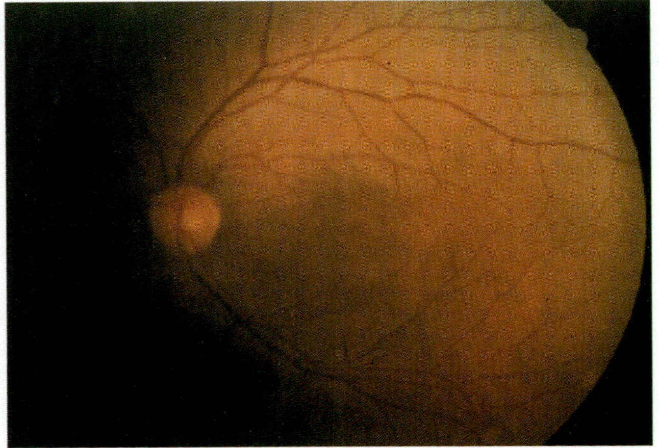

Figure 11.52   Serous detachment of the retina (central serous chorioretinopathy). The clinical picture includes a shallow, often hardly visible detachment of the retina with ill-defined borders. There is an accumulation of fluid in the subretinal space. The patient notices a deterioration of vision, macropsia and a relative scotoma. Fluorescein angiography classically reveals a small fluorescent spot, which progressively increases in size. In this so-called "leak" the fluorescein dye transits from the choriocapillaris via a small defect in the pigment epithelium to the subretinal space. The cause of the disorder remains unclear, spontaneous resolution is often seen. Laser photocoagulation can be considered in recurrent disease.

Figure 11.53   Fluorescein angiogram in central serous chorioretinopathy. The frame shows the typical fluorescent spot defining the defect in the pigment epithelium through which the fluid transits.

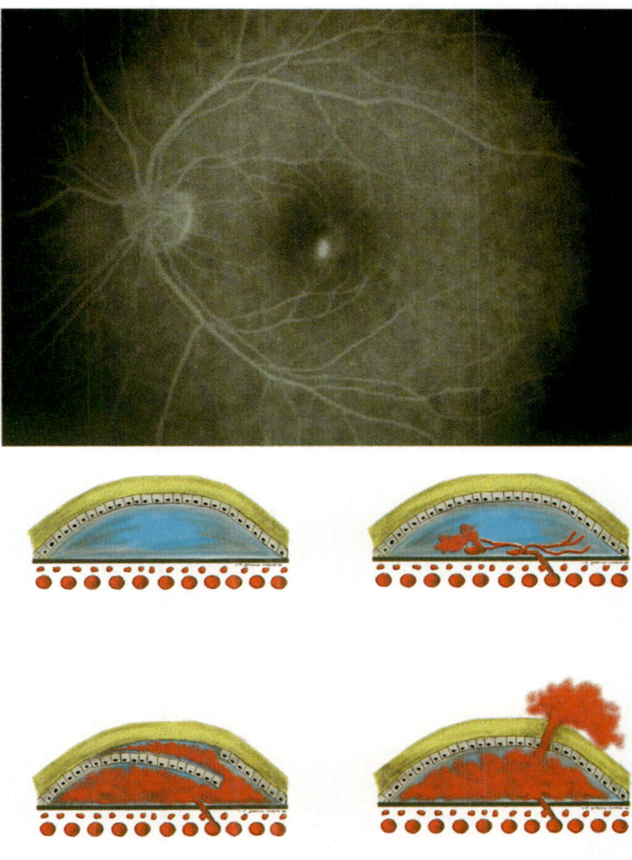

Figure 11.54   Pigment epithelial detachment / schematic diagram of the development of macular degeneration. In pigment epithelial detachment, fluid is located underneath the pigment epithelium *(top left)*. Compared with central serous retinopathy, the elevated area is better visible, has a domed configuration and is well demarcated. A concomitant serous detachment of the retina may develop. Pigment epithelial detachment occurs in the exudative form of age-related macular degeneration and may be associated with choroidal neovascularization, i.e. vessels expand into the subretinal space *(top right, bottom left)*. Hemorrhages may originate from these vessels *(bottom right)*.

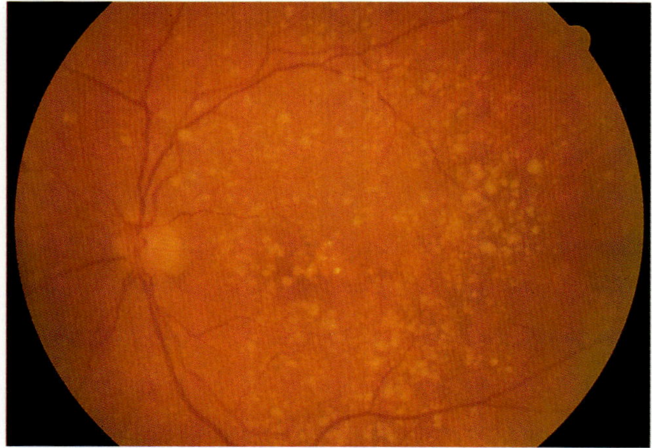

Figure 11.55 Age-related macular degeneration, hard drusen. In this form of macular degeneration, hyalin material is deposited in a nodular shape underneath the pigment epithelium. The clinical picture is characterized by white spots, which are evenly scattered across the posterior pole. This impressing clinical finding may be harmless. The visual acuity is usually not significantly impaired. The condition may remain unchanged for a long period of time. Therapy is not available and not required.

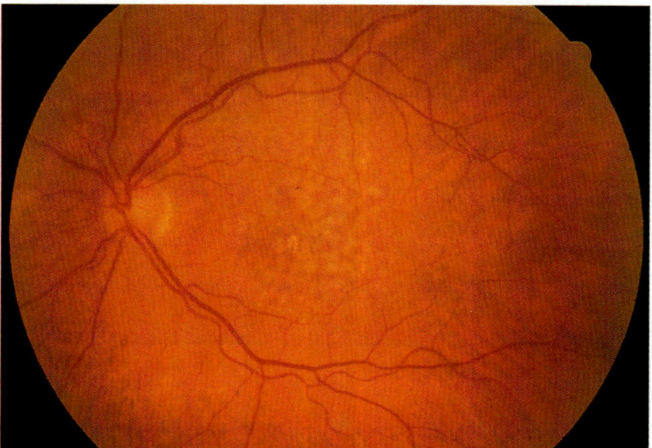

Figure 11.56 Age-related macular degeneration, soft drusen. Soft drusen is a different form of deposition of material within the pigment epithelium and Bruch´s membrane. The figure shows that this type of drusen is larger in comparison with hard drusen, sometimes confluent and with indistinct margins. With this appearance of drusen, which may change in size and become confluent, a tendency to deterioration and development of neovascular membranes (compare with 11.57) is observed. Vision testing, which can be performed by the patient himself (Amsler grid), is essential for the early detection of deterioration.

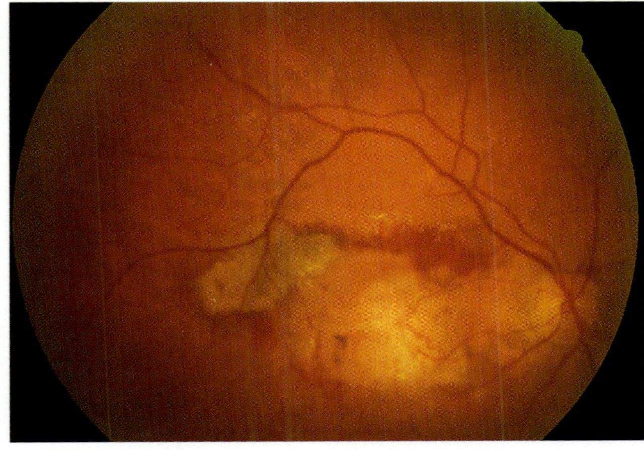

Figure 11.57 Age-related macular degeneration, choroidal neovascularization. The figure shows a yellow-orange lesion in the macula on the basis of edema and fibrotic changes. Temporally above, there is an area of greyish color indicating a choroidal neovascularization and in between this area and the papilla there is an arc shaped intraretinal hemorrhage. Choroidal neovascularizations are the most dreaded complication in degenerative alterations of the macula. They develop from a defect in Bruch´s membrane, which may have various causes, followed by the formation of neovascular membranes expanding from the choriocapillaris to underneath the pigment epithelium (compare with 11.54). Clinically, a shallow elevation of grey color indicates this process. The combination with exudate and blood leads to the typical picture of "disciform macular degeneration".

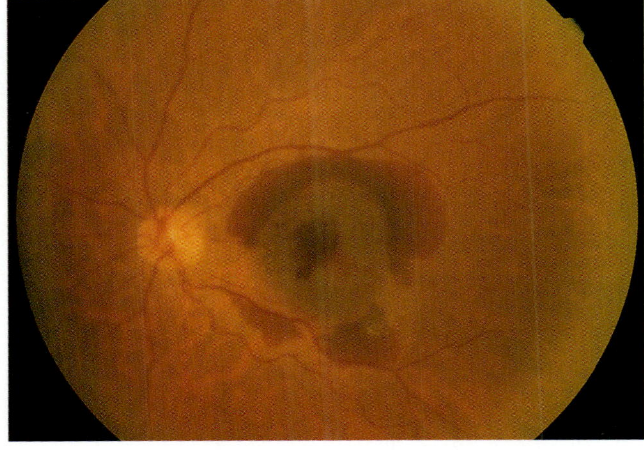

Figure 11.58 Choroidal neovacularization with intraretinal hemorrhage at the margin. The figure shows the typical finding of a choroidal neovascularization underneath the pigment epithelium with cinically notable greyish color. These pathologic vessels can be the origin of hemorrhages into the retina, seen here as marginal hemorrhages.

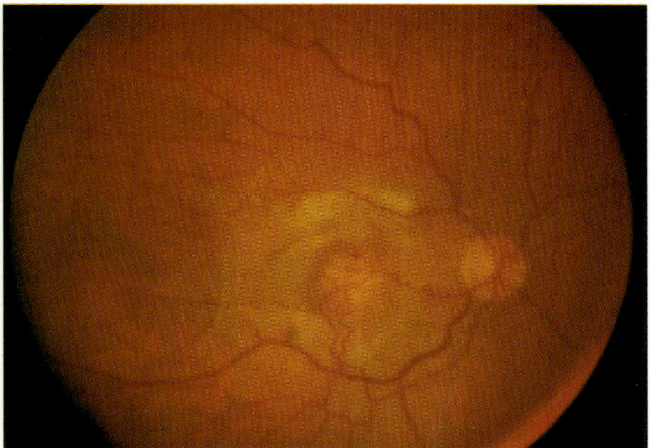

Figure 11.59 Macular degeneration, anastomosis of choroidal and retinal vasculature. The figure shows a disc-shaped macular degeneration with exudate and a central indrawing. In the central fibrotic area, an anastomosis of the choriocapillaris and retinal vessels has formed.

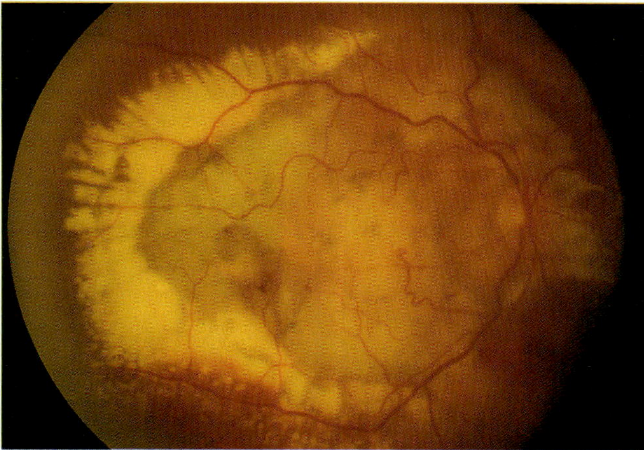

Figure 11.60 Disciform macular degeneration. The figure shows the complete picture of a so called "wet", disciform macular degeneration. In the central area is an elevation of greyish color (edema). Above, below and temporally it is limited by regions of yellowish exudate. On the lower margin and underneath the optic disc, intra-retinal hemorrhages are found. In the surroundings of neovascularizations, which always show a pathologic permeability of the vessel walls, a combination of edema, fatty changes and hemor-rhages typically appears. The clinical picture may change, a resorption of blood, exudate and edema is possible, thus resulting in a fibrose scar, which makes an improvement of central vision unachieveable.

Figure 11.61 Macular degeneration, "dry" form. The figure shows an atrophy of the pigment epithelium and a partial atrophy of the choricapillaris in the macula. The retinal vessels are preserved and the large choroidal vessels are bared. Edema, exudate and blood are not present. This finding is named "dry" form. Usually, an impairment of vision is found, of which the extent cannot be judged based on the clinical appearance. Magnifying devices may be applied in order to improve vision.

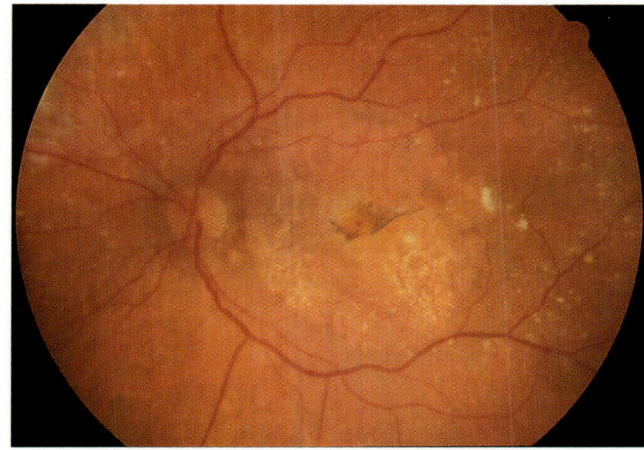

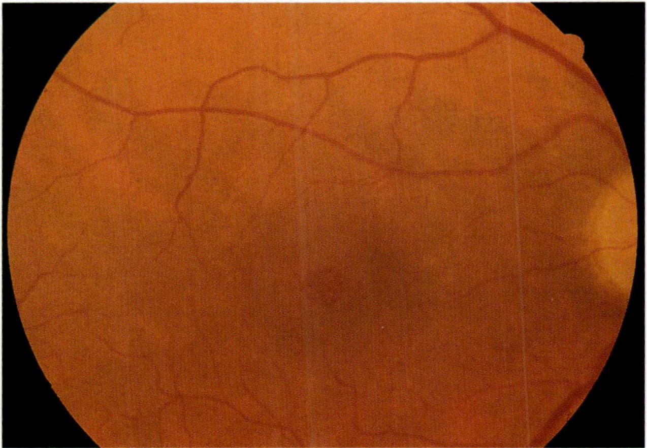

Figure 11.62 Macular hole. Macular holes may develop following macular edema on the basis of various underlying disorders (uveitis, complicated surgery, trauma). The figure shows a round, sharply defined lesion in the foveal area, which appears like a hole with a blurred, slightly elevated surrounding cuff. This finding may be easy to typify, but a clinical differentiation between a lamellar or pseudo hole and a full-thickness hole is difficult. Full thickness holes lead to a significant visual loss. Idiopathic macular holes are thought to be related to vitreoretinal tractions in the fovea. Surgical treatment consists of vitrectomy and application of substances that lead to closure of the foramen.

11.9 Hereditary degenerations

General: Hereditary degenerations may occur solely in the eye or in association with systemic disorders. They combine changes in the pigment epithelium with degeneration of photoreceptors. The resulting pigmentations are various and have characteristic appearances in the particular disorders. Due to alterations in the pigment epithelium the choroid may be bared, the optic disc is usually pale.

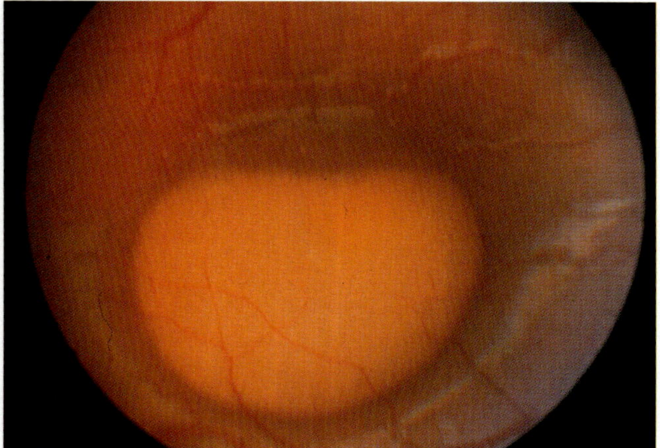

Figure 11.63   Vitelliform macular dystrophy. The figure shows a round yellow lesion in the macular region, which, due to its shape and color, is referred to as an "egg-yolk" lesion. The onset of this hereditary disorder is during childhood. The macular alterations may vary, with disruption of the cystic lesion and resorption of the yellow material, leading to the picture of a "dry" maculopathy. It is remarkable that the visual acuity is usually normal at early stages and may then decrease. Occasionally, multiple vitelliform lesions can be observerd within the posterior pole. Electrophysiology is an important diagnostic tool. In vitelliform dystrophy, the electroretinogram is usually normal, the electro-oculogram, however, is highly abnormal. This finding reflects the disturbance of the pigment epithelium. In the later course, multiple changes, leading to different forms of macular degeneration, may occur.

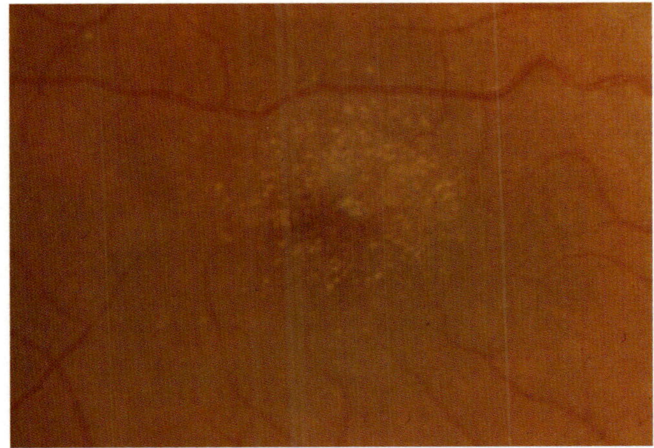

Figure 11.64 Stargardt's disease, juvenile macular degeneration (fundus flavimaculatus). Hereditary disorder that occurs bilaterally during childhood and leads to severe deterioration of central vision. Clinical findings in advanced stages include white-yellowish flecks within the posterior pole associated with pigment epithelial abnormalities. The macula may appear metallic, described as "beaten bronze". The most prominent feature is the vision loss, while the visual field, ERG and EOG remain normal. Fundus flavimaculatus (compare with 11.65) and Stargardt juvenile macular degeneration are thought to be variations of a single disorder.

Figure 11.65 Fundus flavimaculatus. The figure shows white-yellowish flecks scattered in the periphery, which are ill-defined and "fishtail"-shaped. These lesions are composed of lipofuscin. They may be present in combination with alterations within the posterior pole. The ERG and EOG can be slightly pathologic. An EOG reduction reflects the alteration of the pigment epithelium. Differential diagnoses are retinitis punctata albescens and fundus albipunctatus.

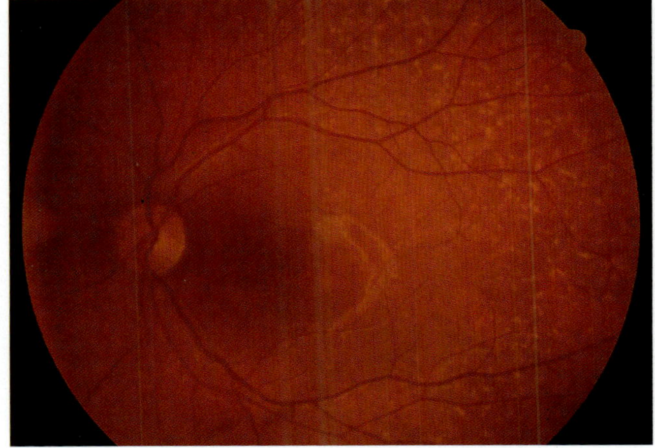

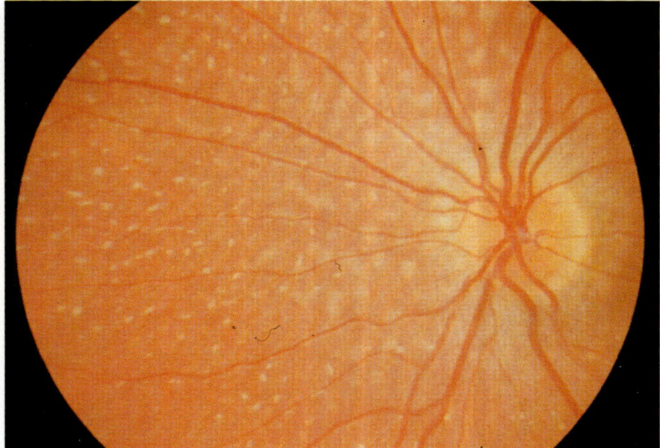

Figure 11.66 Retinitis punctata albescens. The figure shows small white-yellowish lesions scattered across the entire fundus. The disorder leads to progressive visual field defects, the ERG is pathologic. Fundus albipunctatus, a condition with normal visual field and ERG, may be considered as differential diagnosis.

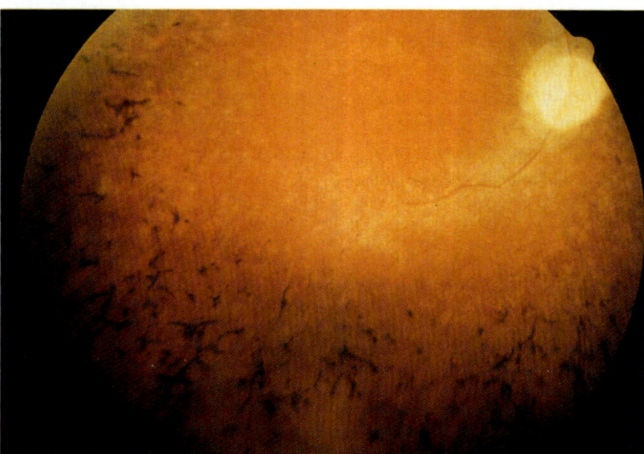

Figure 11.67 Retinitis pigmentosa. The figure shows the typical fundus picture with so-called "bone-spicule" pigmentations, bared choroid (rarefaction of the pigment epithelium), narrowed vessels and optic atrophy. In early stages, the patient complains of night blindness. As the disease progresses, the viusal field narrows. Therapy is not available. Besides visual field testing, the electro-retinogram is an important diagnostic tool, revealing patho-logic findings even in early stages.

Figure 11.68 Sectoral retinitis pigmentosa. The retinitis pigmentosa may be restricted to only one sector of the eye. This condition is usually stable, the pathologic changes, including visual field and ERG, are found in the affected area only. Follow-up is important and cases with progression to the complete picture of retinitis pigmentosa have been described.

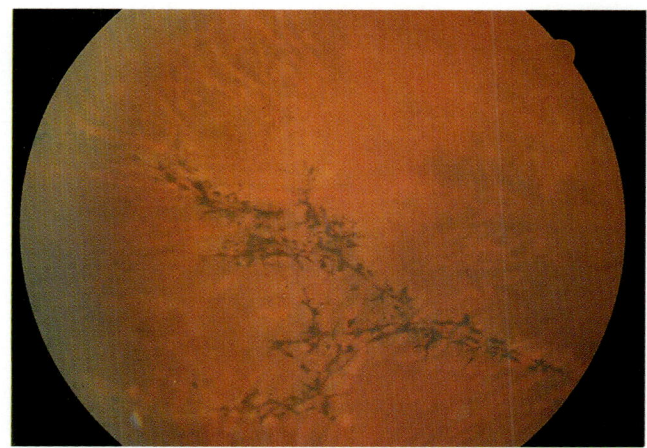

Figure 11.69 Pattern dystrophy. The fundoscopic picture shows a slightly abnormal pigmentation in the posterior pole. Changes in the pigment epithelium occur, leading to an impairment of central vision. The diagnosis is made by electropysiological testing (pathologic EOG) and fluorescein angiography (see 11.70).

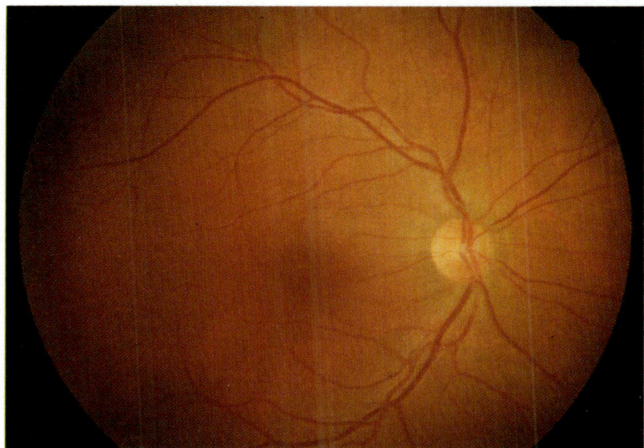

Figure 11.70 Pattern dystrophy, fluorescein angiogram. After injection of the fluorescein dye, the circumscribed pigment epithelial defects are revealed. The combination of reduced central vision, typical fluorescein angiogram and pathologic EOG implies the diagnosis.

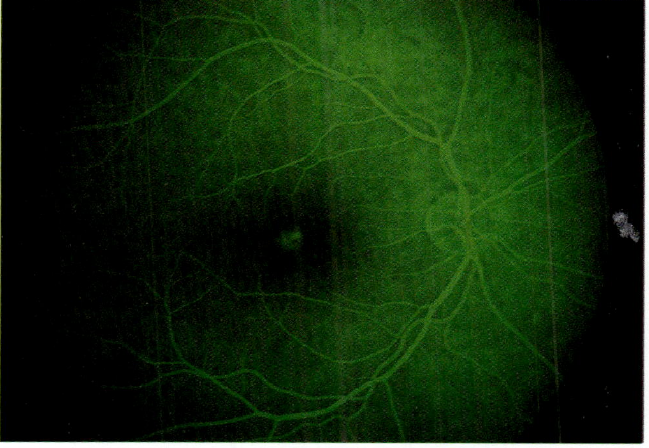

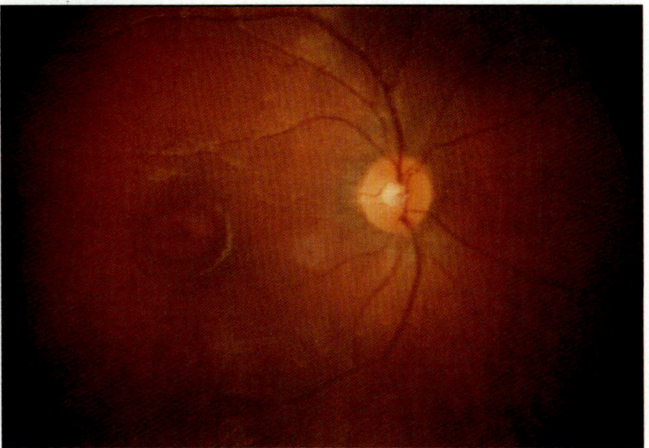

Figure 11.71 Cone dystrophy. The clinical picture of cone dystrophy is characterized by changes in the posterior pole that occur in a so-called "bulls eye" pattern. The origin is an annular atrophy surrounding the darker central area. Cone dystrophy leads to a reduction of central vision together with an impairment of color vision. The ERG is pathologic. The disorder might be found in combination with rod dystrophy. The funduscopic picture resembles that of chloroquine maculopathy.

General: When atypical pigmentations of the fundus are present, a combination with systemic disorders has to be ruled out. Metabolic, neurologic as well as renal disorders must be considered and respective tests carried out.

Figure 11.72 Refsum syndrome (Heredopathia atactica polyneuritiformis). The typical fundoscopic appearance is of fine-grain pigmentation ("salt-and-pepper"). The changes may be subtle. Symptoms are nightblindness and visual field defects. The association with polyneuropathy, changes in cerebrospinal fluid and cerebral alterations implies the presence of Refsum syndrome. A hereditary enzyme deficiency in the fatty acid metabolism underlies the disorder.

Figure 11.73 Usher syndrome. The figure shows minimal changes in the pigment epithelium, narrowed arterioles and a pale optic disc. The Usher syndrome includes congenital deafness. The combination of deafness and pigmentary alterations in the fundus demands a meticulous clinical examination, for many syndromes include this combination of symptoms.

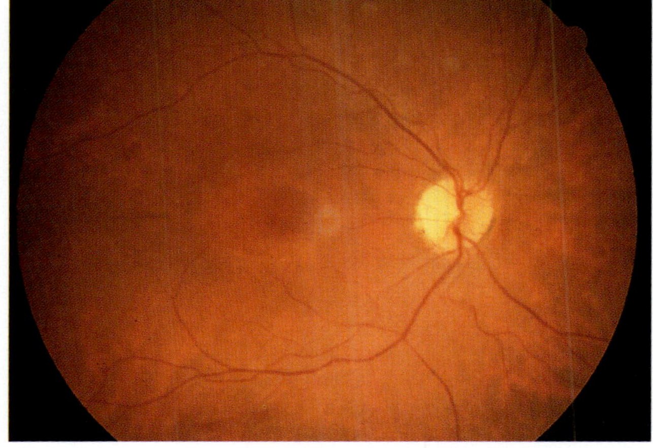

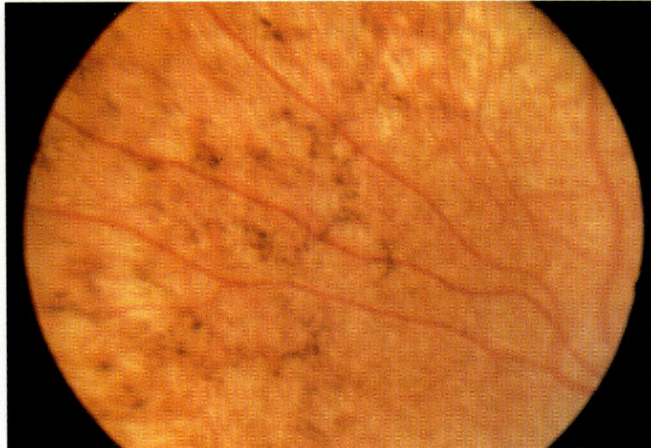

Figure 11.74 Cystinosis. Cystinosis is caused by a disturbance in the cysteine metabolism. Fundus pigmentations might be the earliest symptom of the disease and therefore are of high diagnostic importance. The peripheral retina is affected at first, macular changes lead to vision loss. For anterior segment in cystinosis see chapter 4.

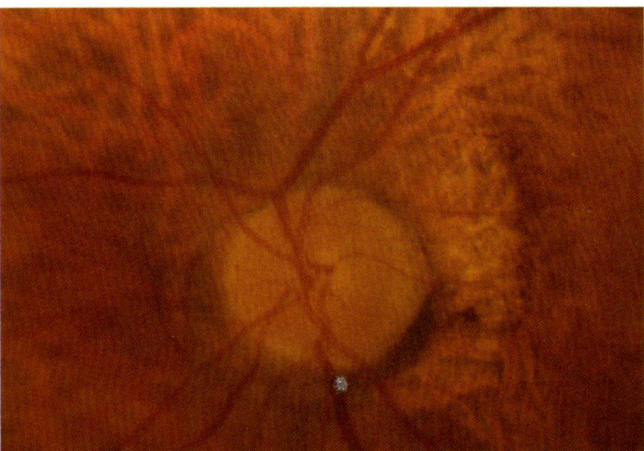

Figure 11.75 Nephronophthisis. Nephronophthisis is a renal disorder characterized by thickening of the basal membrane and cystic changes in the tubular system. The fundus picture includes pigmentations of various kinds. They may resemble the picture of retinitis pigmentosa or appear as an attenuation of the pigment epithelium and the choriocapillaris. In later stages, the retinal vessels narrow, irrespective of the renal hypertension. The visual field shows progressive deterioration. The funduscopic changes may be early symptoms and are therefore of high diagnostic importance.

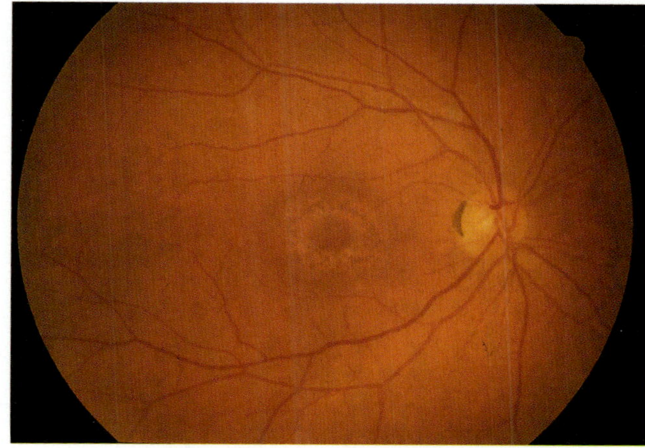

Figure 11.76 Chloroquine retinopathy. After long-term therapy with high doses of chloroquine, irreversible retinal changes occur. The fundus picture shows a typical ring of depigmentation surrounding more normal foveal pigment ("bull´s eye"). Besides this characteristic finding, narrowed vessels and an irregular pigment clumping in the periphery are seen. Visual field testing reveals paracentral scotomas, the EOG is abnormal. Binding of chloroquine to melanin is thought to be the toxic mechanism. Established visual abnormalities are irreversible, hence an early diagnosis should be achieved. In order to detect early and reversible abnormalities a comparison with an EOG taken before initiation of therapy is important. In contrast to the toxic retinal changes, the corneal abnormalities (see chapter 4) are reversible.

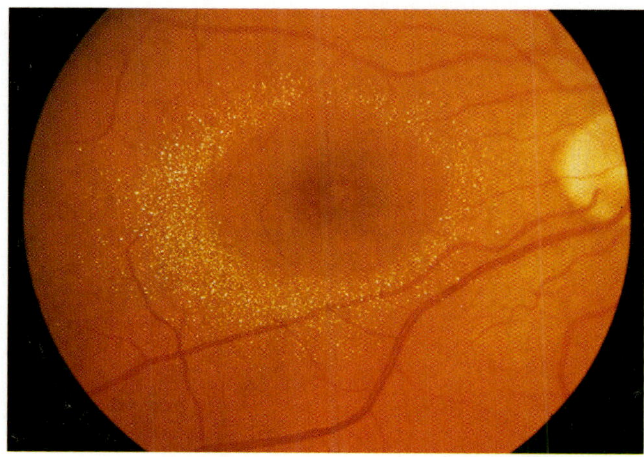

Figure 11.77 Canthaxanthin inclusion. Following ingestion of the carotenoid canthaxanthin retinal inclusions are described, typically seen as a ring of fine gold- colored pinpoint particles in the posterior pole. The finding is pathognomonic, a confusion with other clinical pictures is impossible. There is no visual impairment. The inclusions are reversible within years after cessation of drug usage.

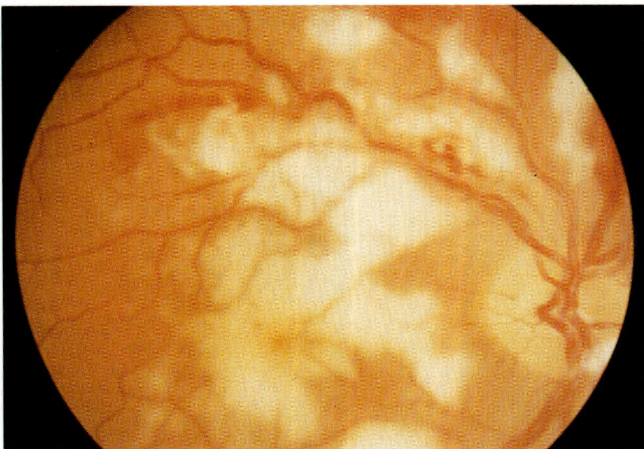

Figure 11.78 Retina in acute pancreas necrosis. The figure shows multiple confluent white-greyish lesions, which resemble cotton-wool-spots. Vascular occlusions in the choriocapillaris are the cause.

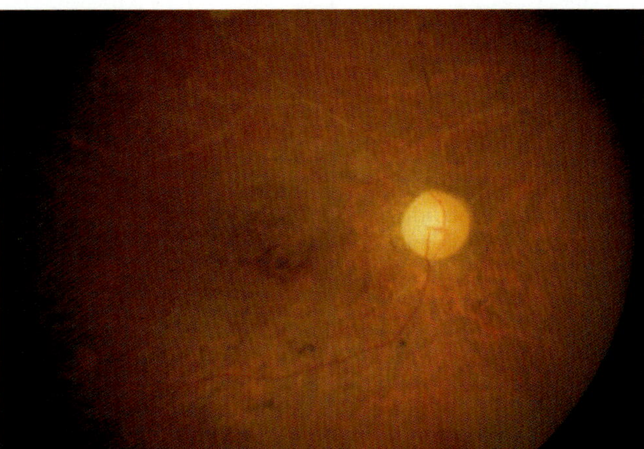

Figure 11.79 Behçet-syndrome/vascular changes. The figure shows an extremely narrowed, partly obliterated arterial vascular tree and a pale optic disc. Apart from the changes in the anterior segment, the retinal manifestations nearly always occur in longstanding disease, being the cause for severe vision loss.

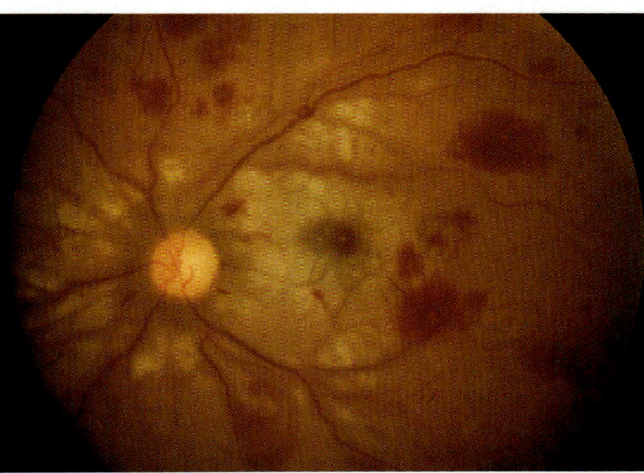

Figure 11.80 Moschcowitz syndrome (thrombotic thrombocytopenic purpura, TTP). The prominent findings are thrombocytopenia, abnormalities of erythrocytes, hemolysis, polychromasia and severe ischemia of various organs. The illustration shows extensive white-greyish lesions as a result of ischemia in choriocapillaris and retina.

Figure 11.81   Lupus erythematosus. The figure shows multiple
cotton-wool-spots and fine
hemorrhages in the posterior pole
as well as severe vascular obstruction. The retinal changes are manifestations of the obliterative
microangiopathic disease.
Collagen disease must always be
considered when this fundus
picture is present.

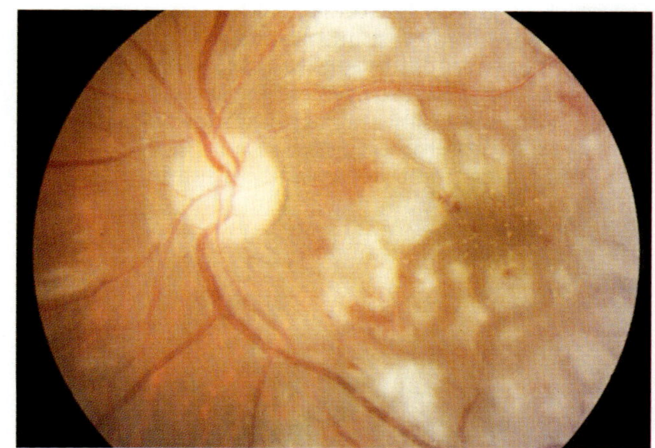

11.13 Peripheral retinal degeneration

General: In the peripheral retina, which is defined as the region expanding from a little anterior to the ocular equator to the ora serrata, significant thinning and degenerative changes occur. The combination of vitreoretinal tractions with certain degenerations predisposes to the formation of holes, which may cause retinal detachment. The knowledge of the various forms of peripheral degeneration and their judgement with reference to the formation of retinal tears is therefore important.

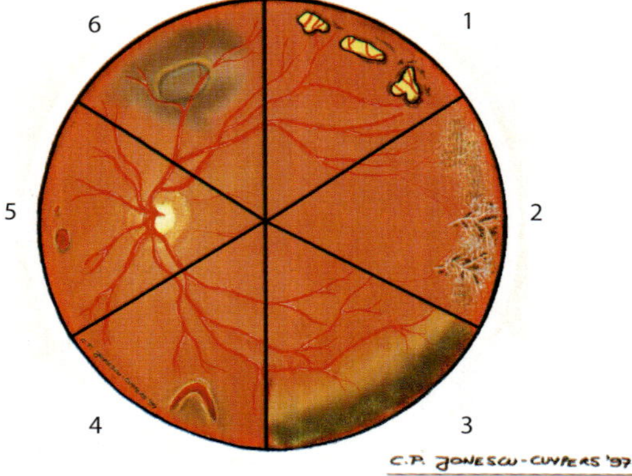

Figure 11.82   Schematic diagram of the various characteristic forms of peripheral degeneration:

1. Paving stone degeneration: localized thinning of the choriocapillaris, scarred retina and choroid, no risk of retinal detachment. Harmless finding.
2. Lattice degeneration: Thinned retina, obliterated vessels, vitreoretinal attachment at the margin of the lesion. High risk of retinal detachment. Prophylactic treatment with laser coagulation has to be considered.
3. Peripheral oral pigmentation: No clinical significance, no need for follow-up.
4. Horseshoe tear: Configuration of the tear indicates vitreoretinal traction. High risk of retinal detachment. Requires treatment with laser coagulation, cryoretinopexy or surgery (see 11.84).
5. Round holes: Atrophic lesions, no vitreoretinal traction, prophylactic laser coagulation is recommended.
6. Retinoschisis: Can be followed conservatively.

Figure 11.83   Horseshoe tear along the edge of an equatorial degeneration with associated retinal detachment. The figure shows a large horseshoe tear, a flap of retina is still hinged. The finding implies the development from vitreoretinal traction. Centrally to the tear, the retina appears grey and wrinkled indicating a beginning retinal detachment. For surgical therapy see retinal detachment.

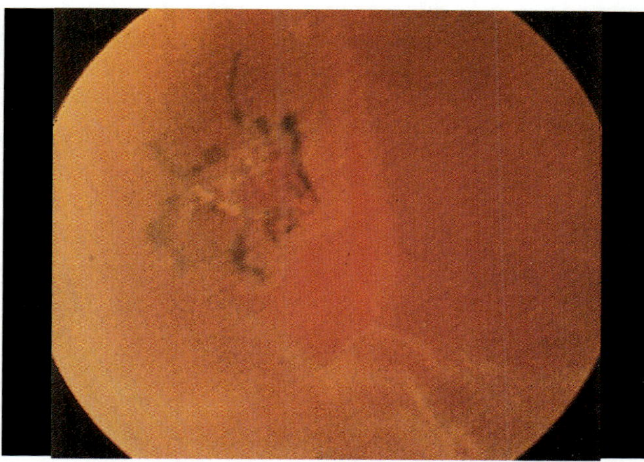

Figure 11.84   Peripheral retinoschisis. Retinoschisis is a degenerative change, which is most commonly located in the inferotemporal quadrant. The figure shows a transparent, even schisis cavity. The condition is usually stable and treatment is not necessary. The distinction between retinoschisis and retinal detachment is very important. The outer layer of a retinoschisis has a beaten metal appearance, the affected region produces an absolute scotoma

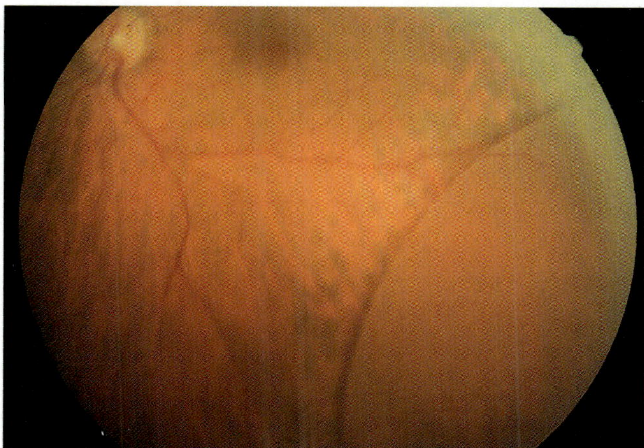

11.14 Retinal detachment

General: Retinal detachment is a separation of the sensory retina from the pigment epithelium. The causes are various: retinal breaks with or without vitreous traction (the resulting detachment is named rhegmatogenous), tractions of the vitreous, shrinking preretinal membranes and exudation (nonrhegmatogenous).

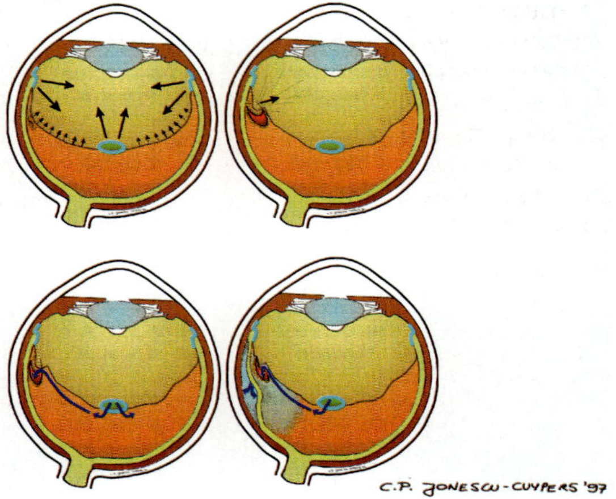

Figure 11.85   Schematic diagram of the development of a retinal detachment from a retinal break and vitreous traction. The drawing shows that liquified vitreous gains access through the retinal break to the subretinal potential space causing the detachment. *Top left* posterior vitreous detachment, vitreous traction; *top right* formation of a break in preexisting degenerations; *bottom left* liquified vitreous transits through the break; *bottom right* formation of a retinal detachment.

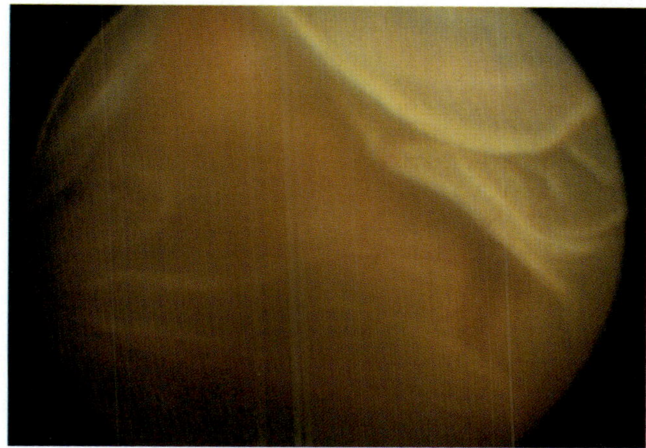

Figure 11.86 Bullous retinal detachment. The figure shows the typical appearance of detached retina with grey color and folds. The separation of sensory retina from the pigment epithelium and the choriocapillaris leads to edema, loss of transparency and corrugation, which appears as sand dune-like. Every retinal detachment leads to damage of the photoreceptors, which develops very quickly in the macula. The classical symptom of a retinal detachment is the appearance of a curtain-like shadow, which expands more or less rapidly. Patients with predisposing conditions should be apprised of this phenomenon. The treatment of a retinal detachment is surgical (see figure 11.88 and 11.89). If the retina cannot be permanently reapposed, blindness results.

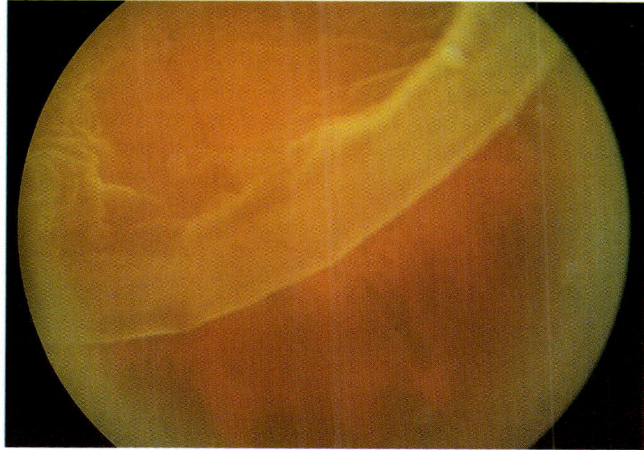

Figure 11.87 Folded retina in oral dialysis. On the basis of pre-existing degenerations or following blunt trauma, a large avulsion of the retina in the periphery can occur. The retina may then fold over its interior surface. The figure shows a giant tear, the retinal vessels can be discerned only up to the folded retina, more peripherally the choroid is visible and retinal vessels are missing. The surgical management may consist of scleral buckling (circumferential buckle).

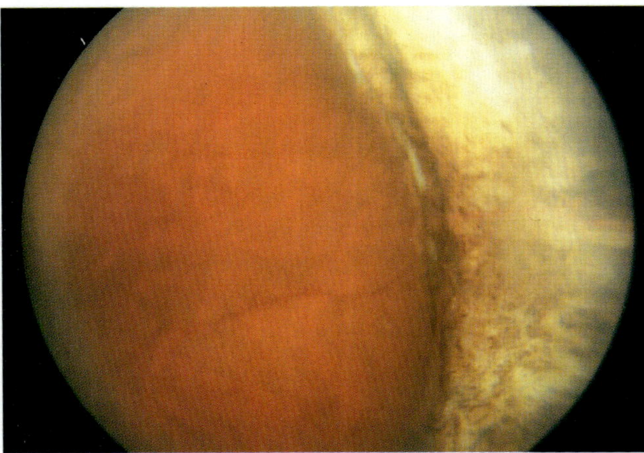

Figure 11.88   Status post encircling band in retinal detachment. The figure shows a peripherally located circumferential bulge, which is caused by a band encircling the globe. The encircling element is used to compensate vitreous traction. The white color of the retina results from laser photocoagulation.

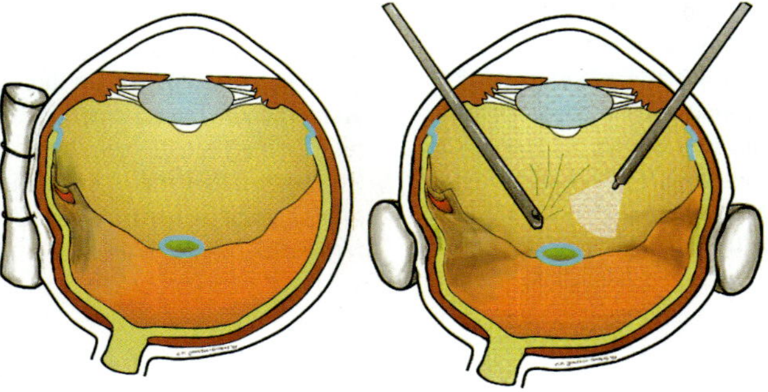

Figure 11.89   Schematic diagram of different surgical approaches in the management of a retinal detachment. Depending on the underlying cause of a retinal detachment, isolated measures on the retina, the vitreous or a combination of both can be taken. Retinal breaks without signs of traction and without detachment can be treated with laser coagulation or cryopexy. In cases with defined localization of the breaks, closure can be achieved by scleral buckling. A vitrectomy is additionally required when the vitreous is markedly changed or in complicated retinal detachments (traction detachment, unclear localization of breaks).

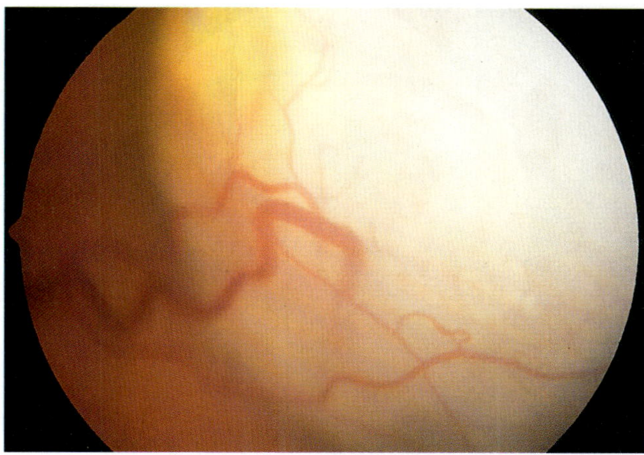

Figure 11.90 Retinoblastoma. Retinoblastoma is the most common intraocular tumor in childhood. Funduscopic examination reveals a single or multiple white-greyish tumors. The tumor is highly malignant, it responds to therapy, but has to be treated agressively. Growth can be endophytic (into the vitreous cavity, figure 11.92) or exophytic (combination with exudative retinal detachment and invasion of the optic nerve). A concomitant retinal detachment may complicate the diagnosis. A typical finding in advanced retinoblastoma is leucocoria (white pupillary reflex). The condition must be differentiated from persistent hyperplastic primary vitreous (see chapter 10). Diffuse infiltrating growth may lead to hypopyon. Retinoblastoma can be hereditary (early onset, bilateral, multiple tumors) or sporadic (later onset). Therapeutic management varies, depending on the size and extent of the tumor. Photocoagulation, cryotherapy and external beam radiation are used as well as enucleation in advanced stages, if needed, in combination with chemotherapy. The prognosis for life is good, as long as metastasis or invasion of the optic nerve has not ocurred. Recurrent tumors have been described, giving the need for frequent follow-up examinations.

Figure 11.91 Retinoblastoma, leucocoria. Whenever leucocoria, strabism or glaucoma are found in an infant, retinoblastoma must be ruled out. A white pupillary reflex can be noticed early when the tumor is located in the posterior pole. With peripheral localization, this finding is present not until larger extents of the tumor.

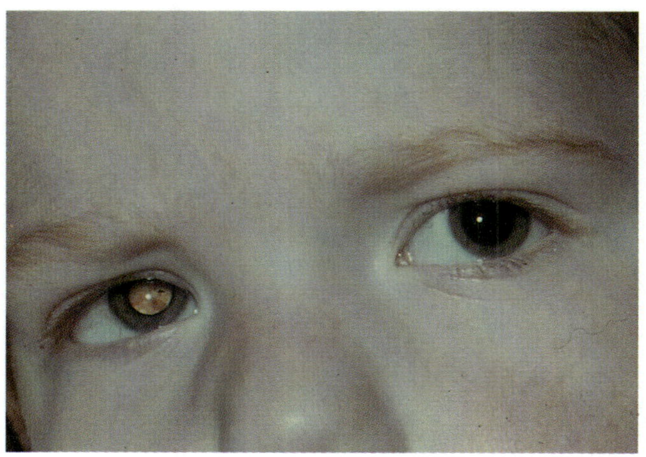

11.15 Tumors of the retina

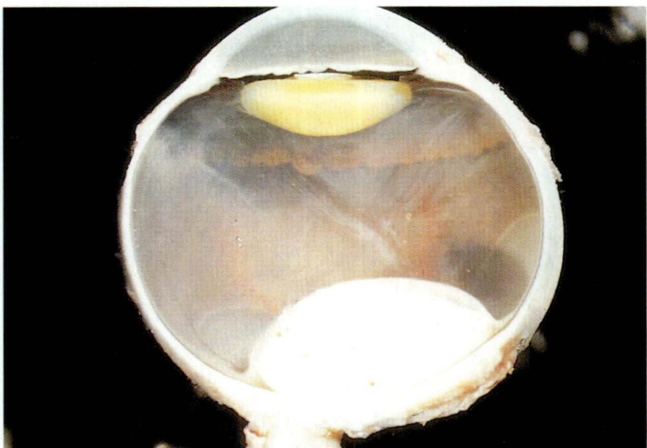

Figure 11.92 Macroscopic picture of a retinoblastoma in the posterior pole.
(Figures 11.90-11.92 Courtesy of Prof. Förster, University Eye Clinic Benjamin Franklin, Berlin)

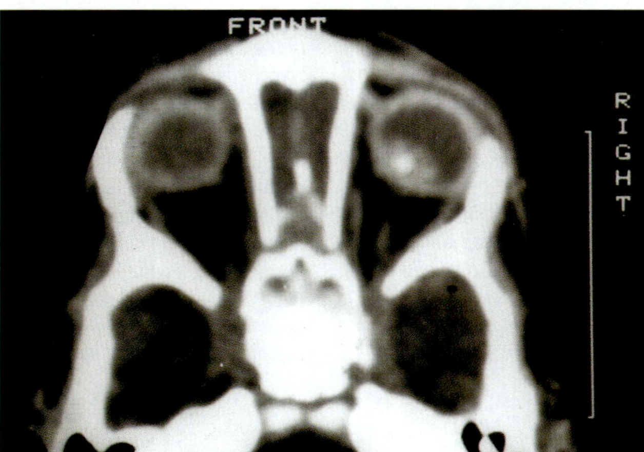

Figure 11.93 Retinoblastoma, CT-scan. When differentiation is difficult (concomitant retinal detachment), a CT-scan should be considered. The figure shows a tumor in the posterior pole of the right eye.

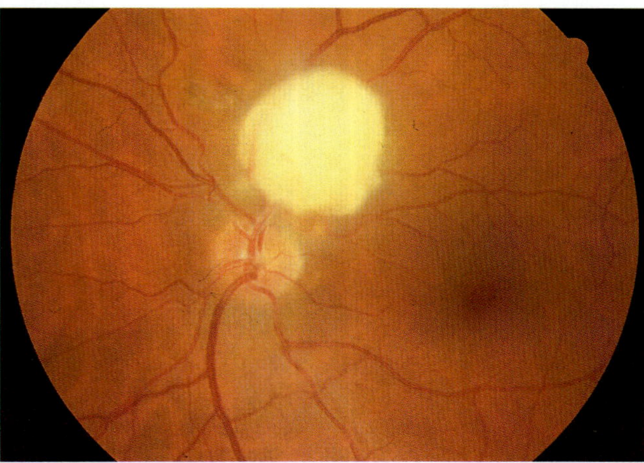

Figure 11.94 Tuberous sclerosis (astrocytic hamartoma). In tuberous sclerosis (Bourneville-Pringle-syndrome), the characteristic finding upon fundoscopical examination is a whitish, nummular, mulberry-like tumor in the posterior pole, located mostly near the optic disc. It may resemble retinoblastoma. The combination with the typical nodular skin lesions gives the diagnosis. The condition is usually stationary, treatment is not indicated.

Optic nerve

12

12.1 Anatomy and examination techniques

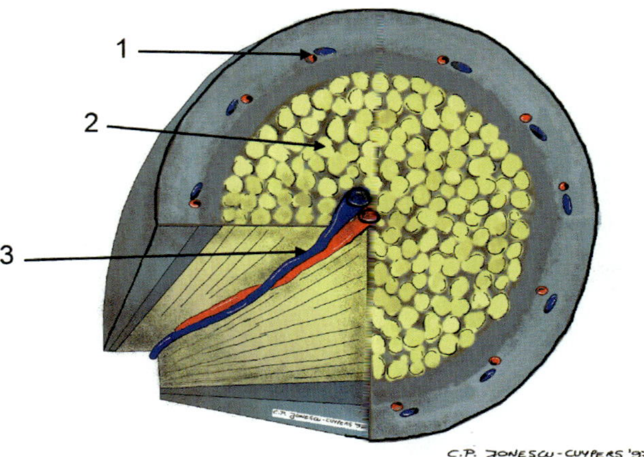

Figure 12.1 Structure of the retrobulbar optic nerve, schematic drawing. The optic nerve connects the retinal ganglion cell layer to the lateral geniculate body. It consists of approximately 800,000 to 1 million nerve fibers, wich are grouped in nerve fiber bundles (2). About 10-15 mm posterior to the globe the central retinal artery and vein enter the optic nerve (3). The optic nerve is sheathed by prolongations of the meninges, it is supplied by pial blood vessels (1). Since the meninges covering the optic nerve are continuous with those of the brain, the optic nerve comprises a subarachnoid space with connection to the cerebrospinal canal. An increased intracranial pressure is transmitted to the optic disc and leads to papilledema.

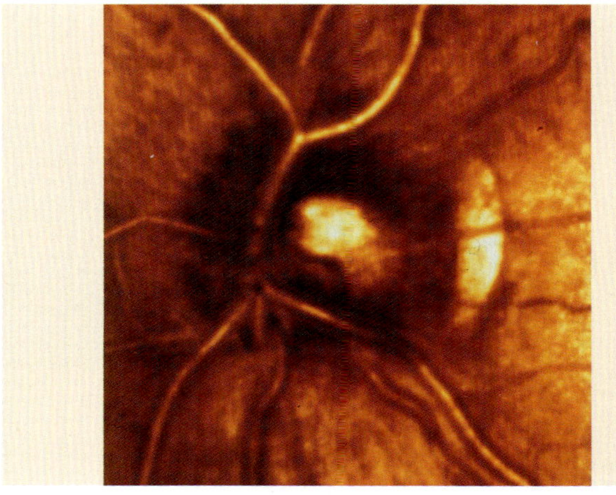

Figure 12.2 Depiction of the intraocular optic disc (papilla nervi optici) with laser-scanning tomography (Heidelberg retinal tomograph). In laser scanning tomography, confocal laser beams are used to obtain high resolution tomographic images, which allow for quantitative biomorphometry of the optic disc. The area of the disc and the cup, its depth and volume as well as the thickness of the peripapillary nerve fiber layer can be measured. This way, the morphologic changes with pathologic significance can be differentiated from the physiologic variability of the optic disc.

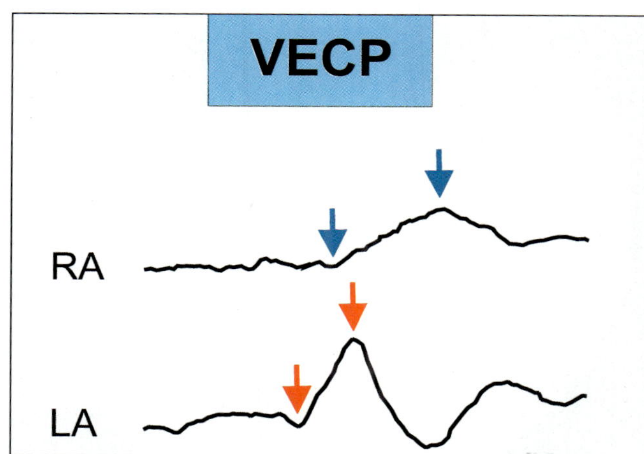

Figure 12.3 Visually evoked cortical potentials (VECP) with pathologic changes of the curve obtained from the right eye of a patient *(top, blue arrows)*, compared to a normal curve obtained from the left eye *(bottom, red arrows)*. The VECP is used to evaluate the quality of signal transmission in the optic nerve and the central visual pathways from the retina to the visual cortex. The potentials of the visual cortex are recorded with special electrodes placed on the occipital scalp. After electronic summation and averaging, a typical curve results with two peaks, one trough and a late potential. Differences from normal curves can affect both amplitude and latency. In inflammatory diseases of the optic nerve, the latency of the response in the VECP is increased. In the pattern or flash-VECP, disturbances in retinal function as well as optic nerve function are reflected by a change in amplitude.

12.2 Abnormalities of the optic disc

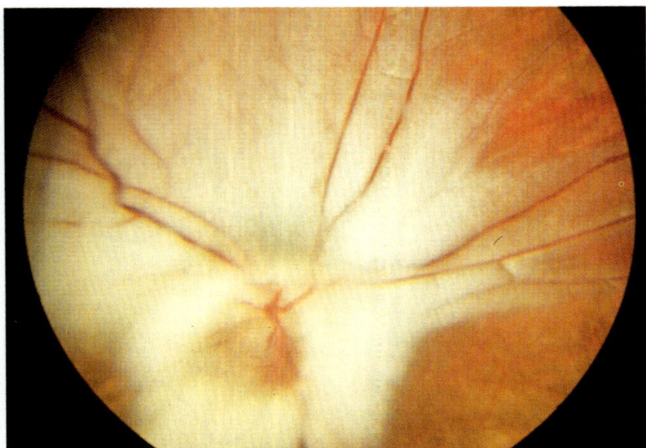

Figure 12.4 Myelinated nerve fibers in the retina. The fibers of the optic nerve are usually only myelinated in the retrobulbar portion. Myelination in the retinal nerve fiber layer appears as characteristic peripapillary white patches with feathery peripheral edges. Myelinated nerve fibers in the retina are a common finding in animals. In the human eye, they are considered a stationary, benign anomaly.

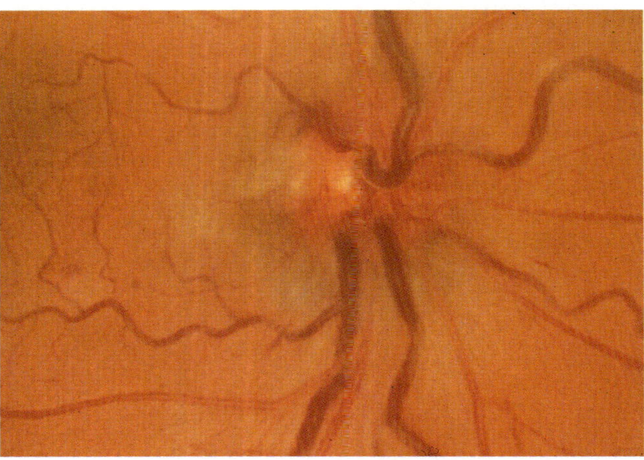

Figure 12.5 Micropapilla ("crowded disc","pseudoneuritis nervi optici"). The size of the optic disc in the human eye shows considerable variability. If the optic disc is very small, it may appear hyperemic and elevated and the disc margin may be blurred. This finding is frequently associated with venous engorgement in the posterior pole (chronic retinal venous stasis). This explains the terms "pseudoneuritis nervi optici" and "crowded disc". There is an increased risk of central retinal vein occlusion or buried drusen of the optic nerve head with corresponding visual field defects. The transition to optic nerve hypolasia with associated impairment of visual acuity and visual field is gradual.

Figure 12.6 "Tilted disc" syndrome. This congenital abnormality represents a combination of abortive optic disc coloboma and micropapilla. There is an incomplete inferotemporal coloboma of the disc, retina and choriod in combination with an abnormally small optic nerve head. The disc appears longer horizontally than vertically. Longitudinal, "glaucoma-like" visual field defects are often seen in this kind of abnormal optic disc.

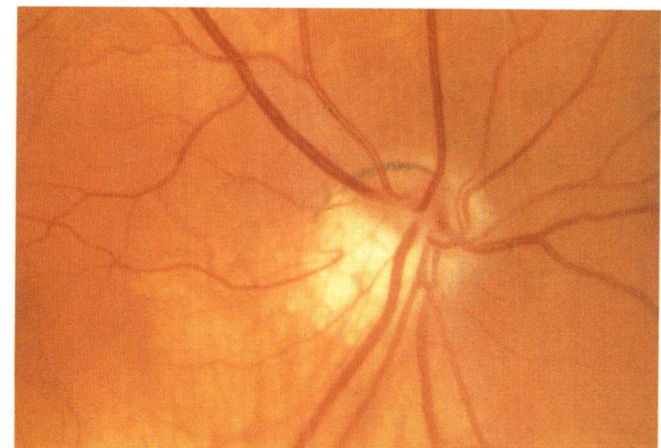

Figure 12.7 Visual field defects in "tilted disc" syndrome (shown in figure 12.6), grey-scale graphical depiction of the central 30 degree visual field tested with threshold perimetry *(left)* and cumulative defect curve *(right)*. Note the loss of the superonasal quadrant as well as a longitudinal scotoma in the temporal periphery starting from the blind spot.

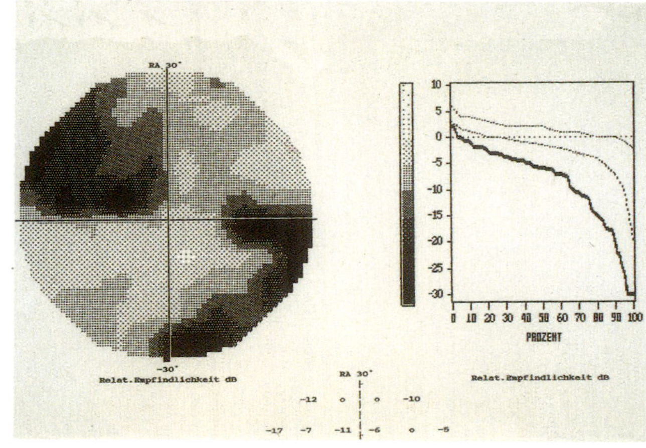

Figure 12.8 Macropapilla. A physiologically large optic disc with a large physiologic central cup is termed macropapilla. There are no intra- or peripapillary signs of pressure-induced, pathologic cupping. Biomorphometry with the scanning laser tomograph confirms the diagnosis of an abnormallyl large optic disc. The large central cup matches the size of the disc. There are no neuronal lesions, the visual field is normal.

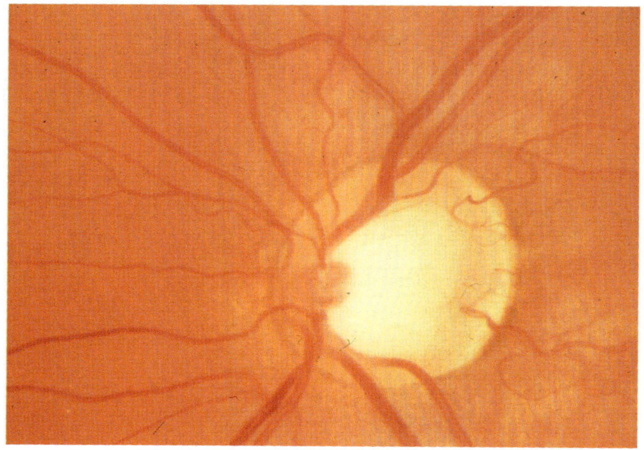

12.2 Abnormalities of the optic disc

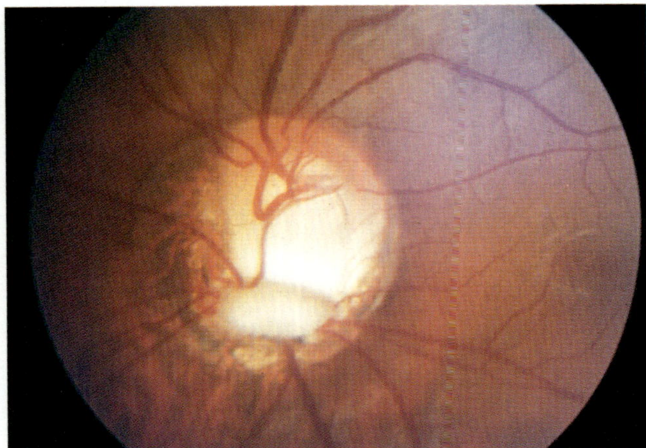

Figure 12.9 Optic disc coloboma with optic disc pit. Note the large optic disc with large central cup, abnormal vessels and a "pit" at the inferior pole with connection to the subretinal space. Visual field and central visual acuity are impaired.

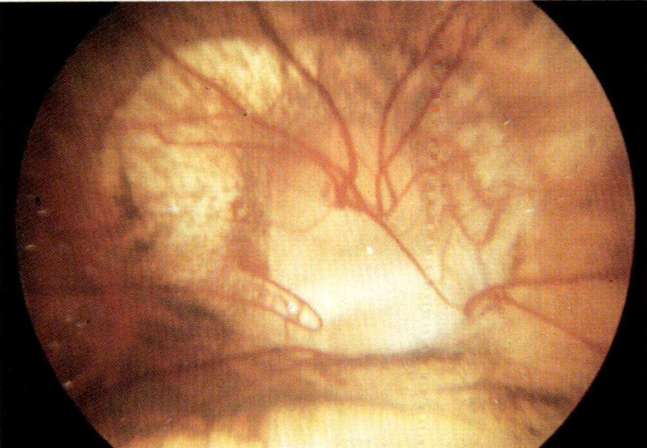

Figure 12.10 Peripapillary coloboma of the optic disc in combination with an inferior retinochoroidal coloboma. The colobomas of the central fundus result from faulty closure of the embryonic fissure of the optic stalk and cup, thus colobomas of the optic disc are commonly associated with inferior colobomas of the retina and choroid. In the present case there is an inferior peripapillary coloboma, separated by a broad pigmented band from an inferior retinochoroidal coloboma.

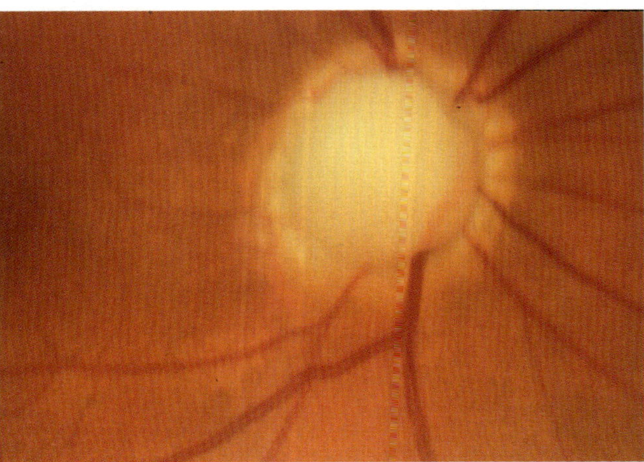

Figure 12.11 Coloboma of the optic disc. Note the abnormally enlarged disc with total, deep excavation and absent neuro-retinal rim. Visual field and acuity are greatly impaired. The presence of the condition since early childhood, the lack of progression (morphologic and functional) and normal intraocular pressure at repeated measures are features that help in making the diagnosis. Mophologically, only a small portion of the optic nerve neurons are present.

Figure 12.12 "Morning glory" syndrome of the optic disc. This condition corresponds to a total coloboma of the optic disc, the deep excavation is filled with retained glial tissue. A characteristic feature is the hyperplasia of the retinal pigment epithelium forming a dark ring around the disc. The emerging vessels are abnormal. Visual acuity is diminished to light perception or hand motion.

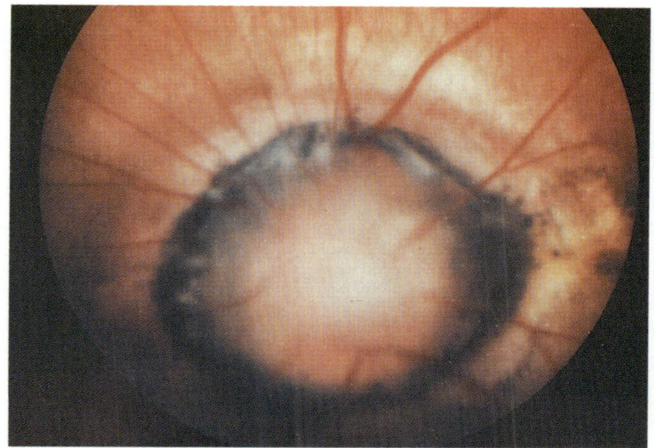

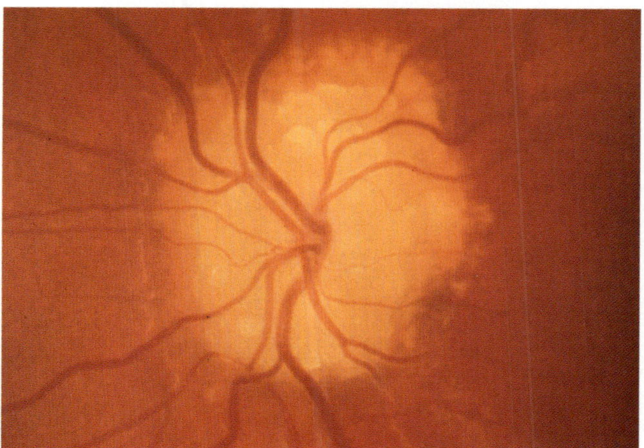

Figure 12.13 Drusen of the optic disc. Drusen are calcified, hyalin deposits located in between the nerve fibers of the optic disc. As in the present case, they can be found in the prelaminar portion of the optic nerve head, ophthalmoscopically appearing as superficial nodular lesions with blurred disc margin, elevated disc and retinal venous stasis. Superficial drusen are easily detectable upon ophthalmoscopy, buried drusen show fluorescence in blue light and can be easily evaluated with ultrasonography or computer tomography. Advanced stages of optic disc drusen are usually associated with visual field defects and decreased visual acuity, caused by a compressive effect on the axoplasmatic transport in the optic nerve neurons.

12.2 Abnormalities of the optic disc

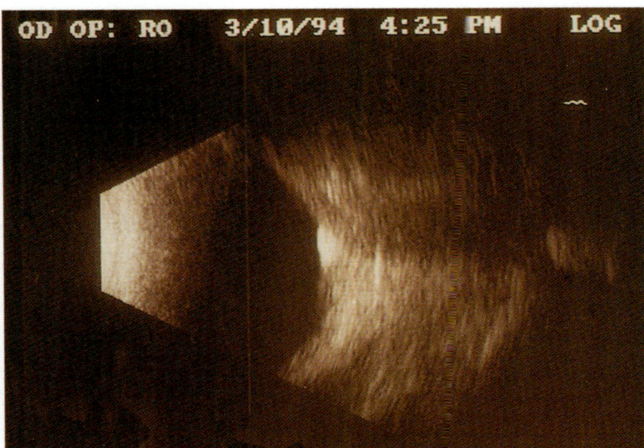

Figure 12.14 Optic disc drusen displayed in ultrasonographic B-scan. The white area at the posterior pole corresponds to an elevated optic disc with drusen, which alter the reflexivity of the ultrasound waves.

Figure 12.15   Papilledema of increased intracranial pressure. The optic disc is elevated, swollen, the disc margin is blurred, there is peripapillary edema of the nerve fiber layer as well as small epi-papillary and radial hemorrhages. Increased filling of the retinal veins indicates impediment of drainage.

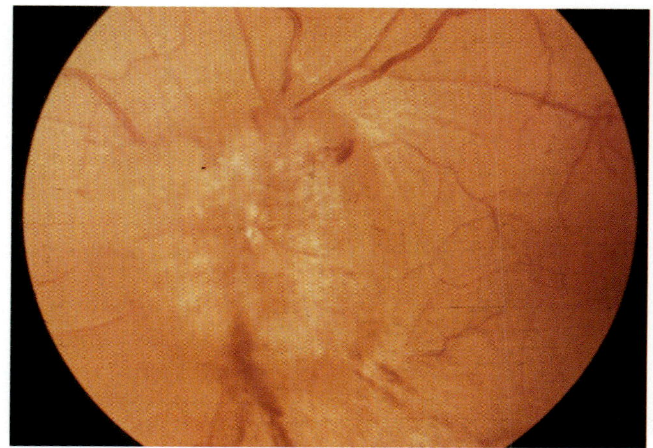

Figure 12.16   Chronic papilledema in intracranial mass. With long-standing papilledema, leakage of plasma into the nerve fiber layer occurs, resulting in a feathery opacification around the indistinct disc margin. Visual field testing reveals an enlargement of the blind spot, visual acuity is slightly diminished.

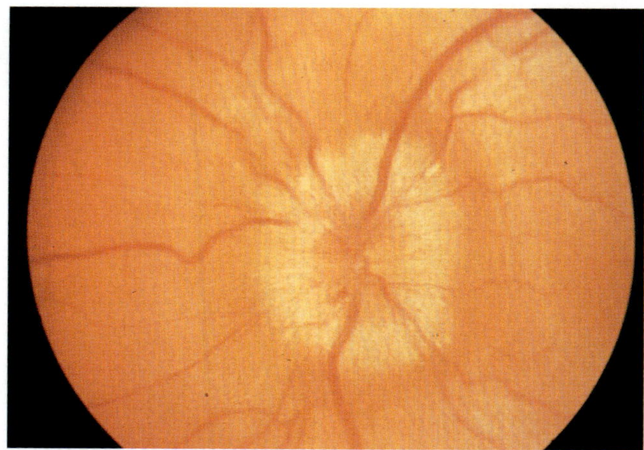

Figure 12.17   Optic disc swelling in chronic ocular hypotony ("e vacuo"). If the intraocular pressure is pathologically low, so-called chronic hypotony syndrome, swelling of the optic disc devlops as a result of the reversal of the pressure gradient between the subarachnoid space of the optic nerve and the inside of the eye. The characteristic ophthalmoscopic picture comprises swelling of the optic disc in the absence of hemorrhages or exudate, peri-papilary choroidal folds as well as folds in the inner limiting membrane in the papillomacular area.

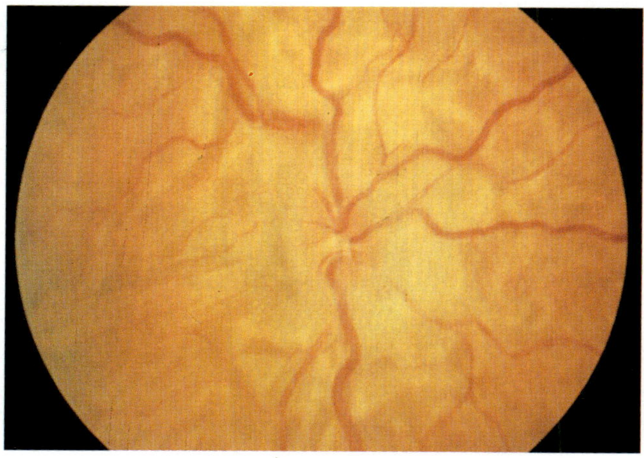

12.3 Optic disc swelling and papilledema

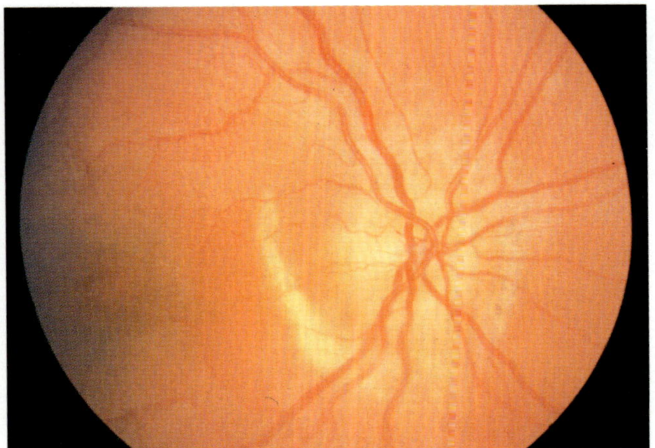

Figure 12.18 Minimal optic disc edema following blunt trauma with peripapillary choroidal rupture. Note the arcuate choroidal rupture between the optic disc and the macula with edema of the nerve fiber layer and the disc.

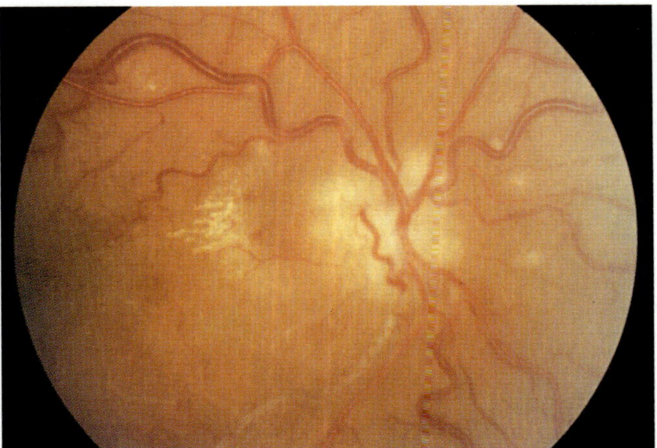

Figure 12.19 Optic disc swelling in optic nerve sheath meningioma. There is chronic papilledema with blurred disc margin, "hard" exudates and small hemorrhages in the papillomacular area ("hard" exudates = deposition of blood lipid in the nerve fiber layer). Note the venous congestion, which pathophysiologically accounts for the hemorrhages in the nerve fiber layer and the formation of hard exudates.

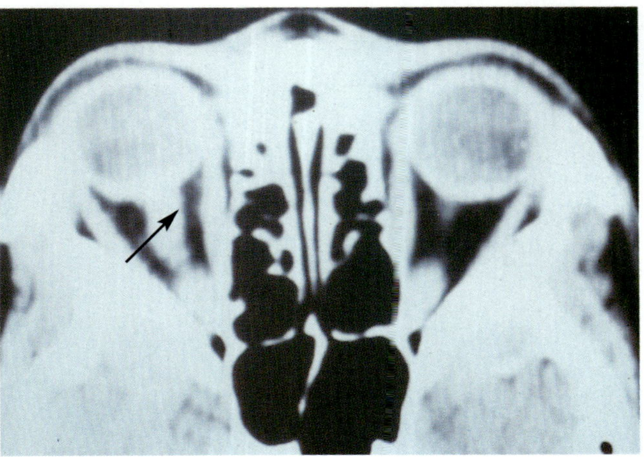

Figure 12.20 CT scan showing an optic nerve sheath menigioma in the left eye, which caused chronic swelling of the optic disc (shown in figure 12.19).

Figure 12.21 Hereditary optic atrophy. Note the pallor of the optic disc, most pronounced in its temporal portion with loss of visibility of the retinal nerve fiber layer above and below the disc. Normally, the retinal nerve fiber bundles are relatively thick at the superior and inferior poles of the optic disc, they appear as fine, white stripes emerging from the disc in an arcuate manner.

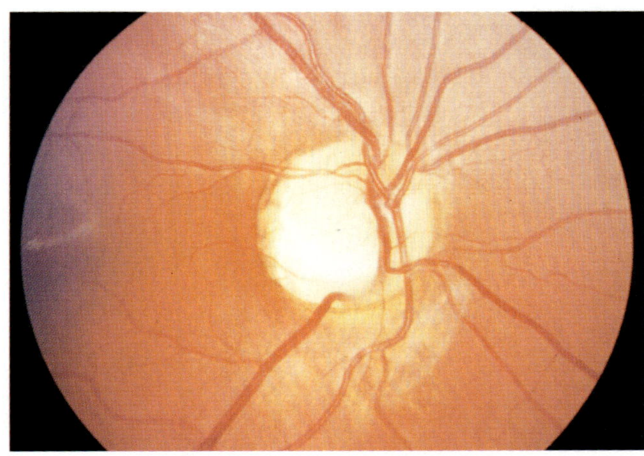

Figure 12.22 Toxic optic neuropathy secondary to thallium poisoning. Heavy metals, e.g. thallium, are toxic to the neurons of the optic nerve and lead to optic nerve atrophy within few weeks following exposure. Depending on the severity of poisoning, complete atrophy with white optic disc and blindness can result.

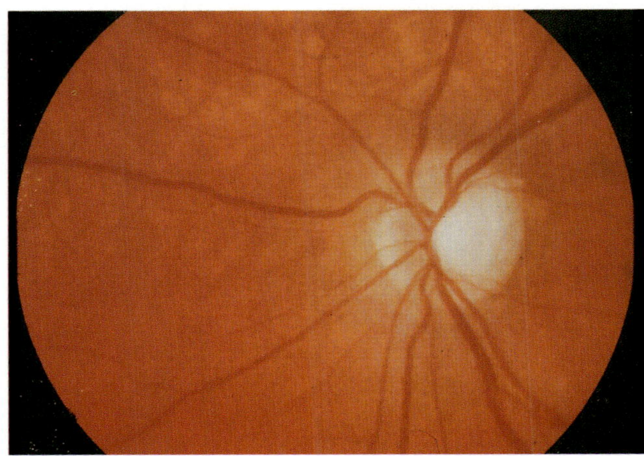

Figure 12.23 Peripapillary retinochoroidal atrophy in high myopia. Due to the stretching of the globe wall in high myopia, an atrophy of the retina and the choroid around the optic disc develops (conus). The myopic conus does not affect the disc itself, it appears healthy surrounded by the white, atrophic area. Only in very high myopia with extensive loss of retina and choroid a consecutive atrophy of the optic disc evolves.

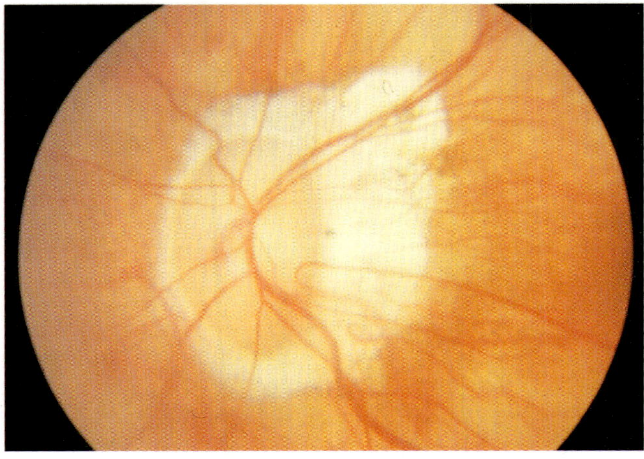

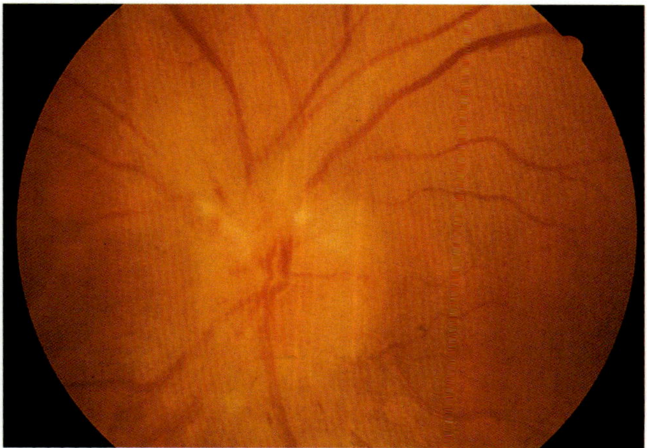

Figure 12.24 Acute papillitis. There is an inflammatory swelling of the optic nerve head with edema of the surrounding nerve fiber layer and splinter hemorrhages. The optic disc appears hyperemic and elevated. It is hard to differentiate an inflammatory swelling of the optic disc from papilledema of raised intracranial pressure upon ophthalmoscopy. Unlike papilledema, papillitis or an ischemic optic nerve swelling are associated with an acute loss of central vision.

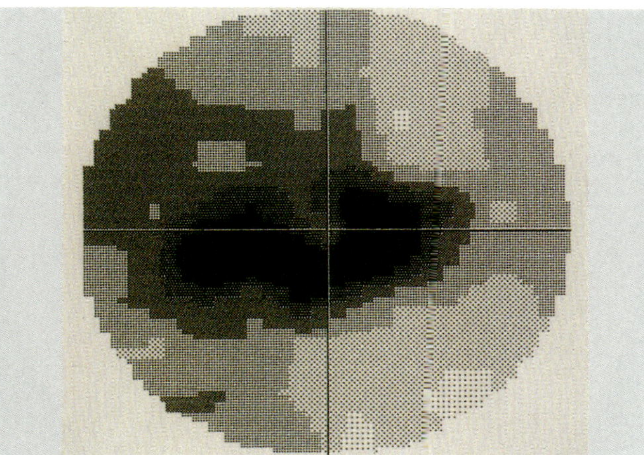

Figure 12.25 Central scotoma in optic neuritis with underlying multiple sclerosis. There is a large central scotoma with loss of fixation comprising approximately 15 degrees of the central visual field (grey scale printout of the central 30 degree visual field tested with automated, computer assisted perimetry).

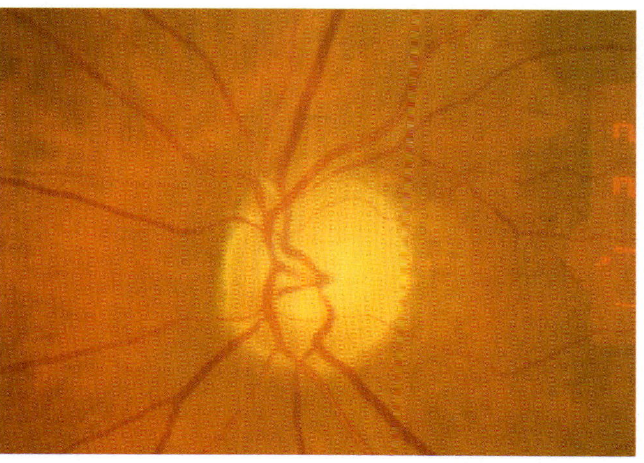

Figure 12.26 Postinflammatory, partial atrophy of the optic disc. The temporal portion of the disc is pale compared to the nasal portion. Note the loss of capillarization.

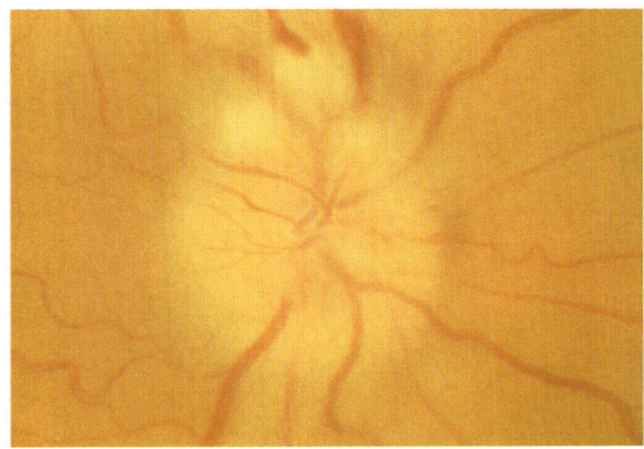

Figure 12.27 Ischemic optic neuropathy in arterial hypertension. The optic disc is diffusely swollen, the disc margin is blurred, capillarization is reduced, there are radial hemorrhages at the superior pole and edema of the retinal nerve fiber layer surrounding the hemorrhages. In contrast to papilledema from increased intracranial pressure or inflammations of the optic nerve head (e.g. in multiple sclerosis), the most prominent ophthalmoscopic finding in ischemic optic disc swelling is pale edema, which commonly extends to the peripapillary nerve fiber layer and is accompanied by radial hemorrhages.

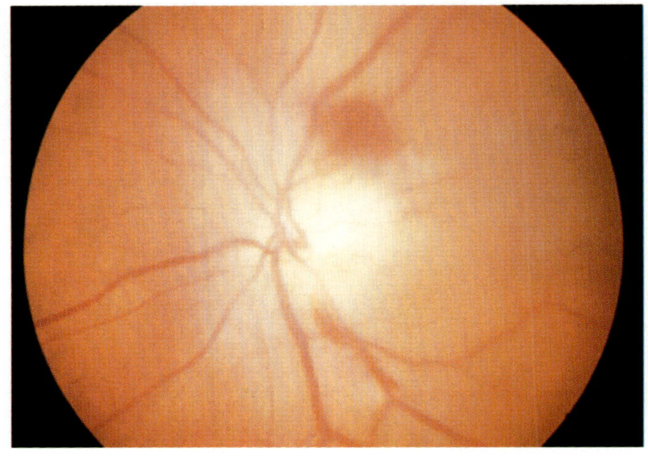

Figure 12.28 Acute anterior ischemic optic neuropathy (AION, "apoplexia papillae") in malignant hypertension. Note the pale swelling of the optic disc with peripapillary hemorrhages and edema of the peripapillary nerve fiber layer. Patients typically present with a sudden painless unilateral loss of vision.

12.6 Ischemic neuropathy

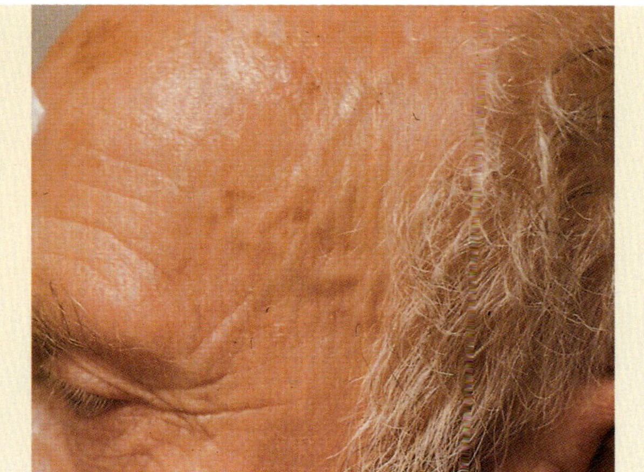

Figure 12.29 Thickened, tender, markedly pulsating temporal arteria in a patient with temporal arteritis (giant cell arteritis). The systemic inflammatory diease carries a high risk of acute loss of vision with involvement of the optic nerve head, as well cerebro-vascular accidents with high mortality. The patients present with severe headache, fatigue and malaise. A dramatically elevated erythrocyte sedimentation rate is considered pathognomonic.

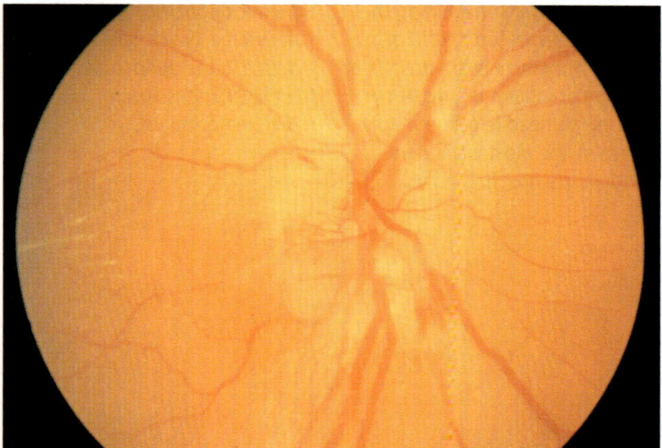

Figure 12.30 Ischemic optic disc swelling with hemorrhages and edema of the peripapillary nerve fiber layer, disc elevation and blurred disc margin in the patient shown in figure 12.29.

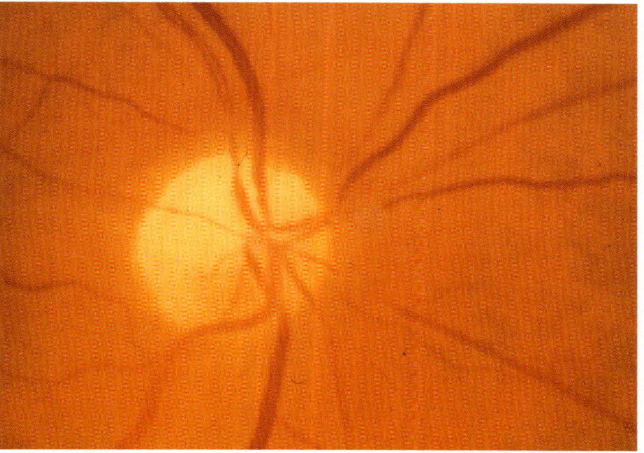

Figure 12.31 Partial optic nerve atrophy following acute ischemic optic neuropathy. Note the pallor of the superior pole of the disc with normal capillarization of the inferior pole a few weeks after the onset of an ischemic optic disc swelling. The nerve fiber bundles at the superior pole of the disc are atrophic, corresponding to a loss of the inferior half of the visual field. Note the irregularity of the retinal arteries with narrowing of the superior temporal artery at the optic disc margin.

Figure 12.32 Optic disc swelling in leukemia. In the course of the hematologic disease, acute ischemia of the optic nerve head occurred with disc edema, hemorrhages and ischemic edema of the surrounding nerve fiber layer. There is also venous congestion.

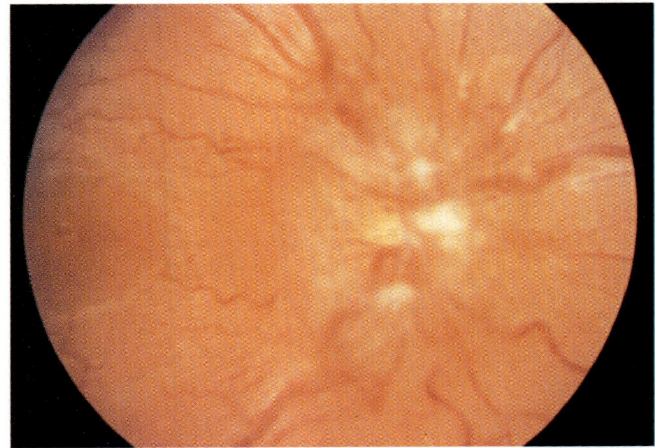

Figure 12.33 Optic disc edema associated with sarcoidosis. Note the mild disc edema with blurred disc margin and distinct capillary pattern (inflammatory involvement of optic disc and nerve in sarcoidosis).

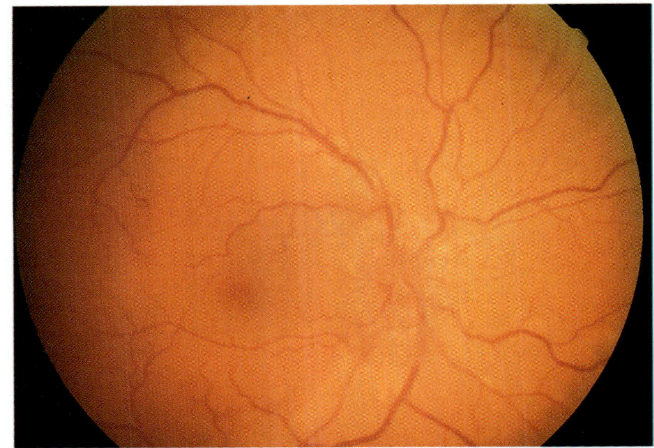

Figure 12.34 Central visual field of the right eye of the patient with sarcoidosis shown in figure 12.33. The granulomatous inflammation of the optic nerve caused destruction of the axial nerve fiber bundles, which correspond to the central visual field.

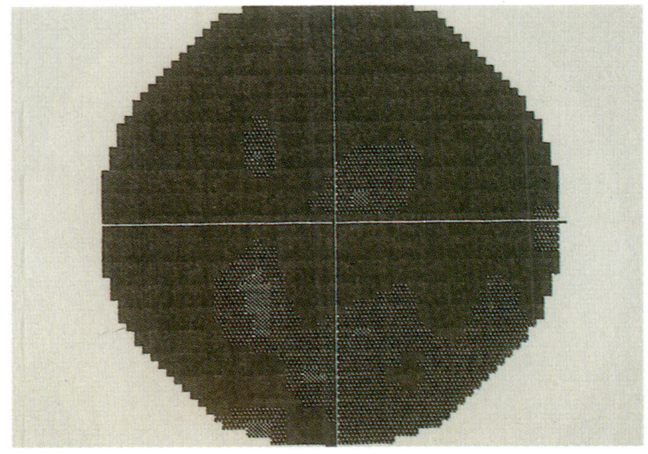

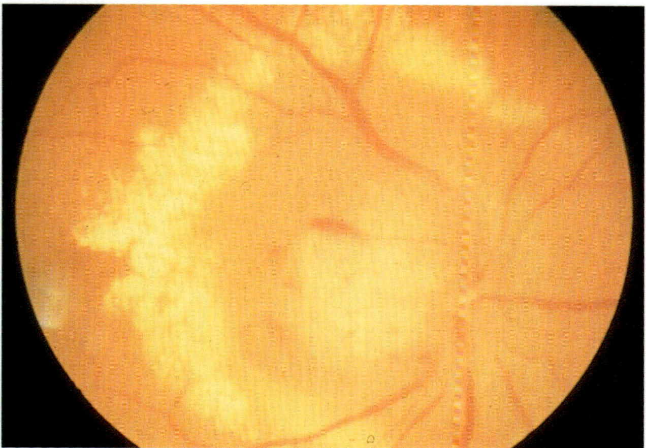

Figure 12.35   Metastasis to the optic disc from primary breast carcinoma. Note the ischemic disc edema with circular peripapillary hard exudates as residuals of chronic edema of the nerve fiber layer and leakage of blood components, resulting from breakdown of the blood-retinal barrier with tumorous invasion of the optic disc.

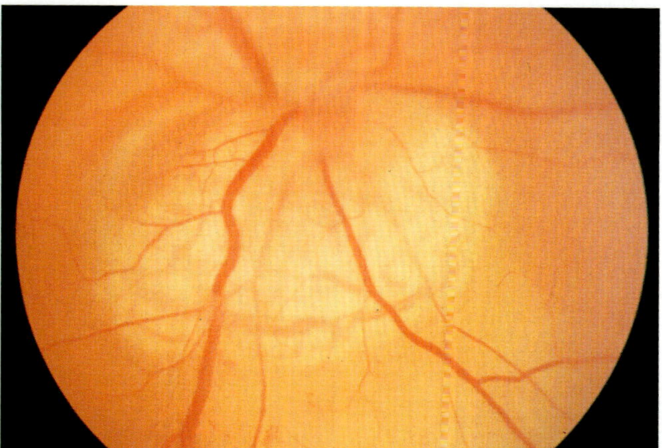

Figure 12.36   Metastasis to the optic disc from primary bronchial carcinoma. Note the elevated disc tumor, which is approximately 5 disc diameters in width, projecting downward.

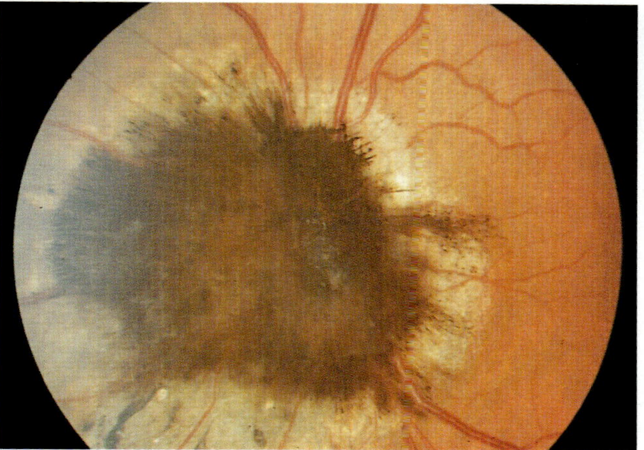

Figure 12.37   Melanoma of the optic disc. The structure and margin of the optic disc are obscured by darkly pigmented tissue, there is a surrounding ring of atrophic retina and choroid.

Figure 12.38 Fluorescein angiogram of the optic disc melanoma shown in figure 12.37. Note the hypofluorescence in the area corresponding to the darkly pigmented melanoma by virtue of blockage of the underlying choroidal vascular fluorescence, there is no capillary pattern or leakage identifiable within the tumor.

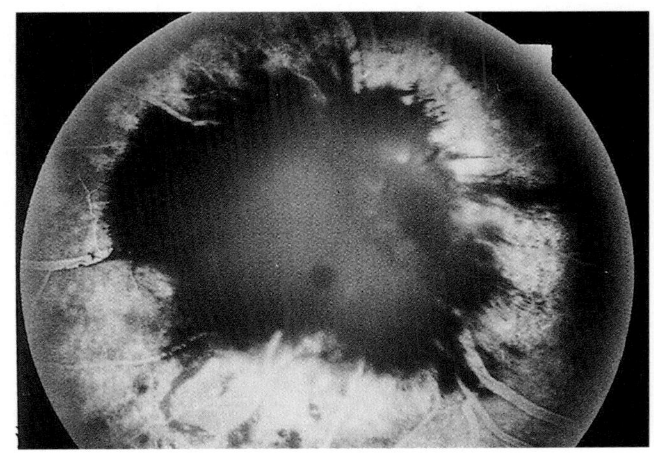

Visual pathways

13

13.1 Topographic anatomy

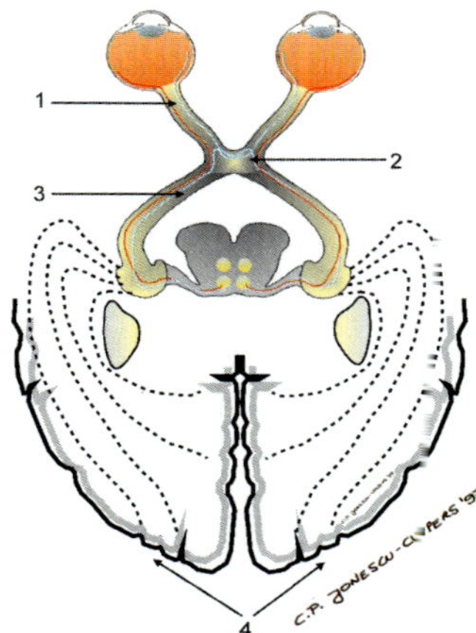

Figure 13.1   Visual pathways, schematic drawing: (1) optic nerve; (2) optic chiasm. In the optic chiasm, the axons from the medial halves of the retina cross to the contralateral optic tract, while the axons from the temporal retinal halves project to the ipsilateral optic tract. Only a fraction of the axons from the macular region crosses in the chiasm. The optic tract (3) terminates at the lateral geniculate body, which is connected to the quadrigeminal plate (tectum) for integration of eye movements. Between the lateral geniculate body and the visual cortex (4) extends the optic radiation.

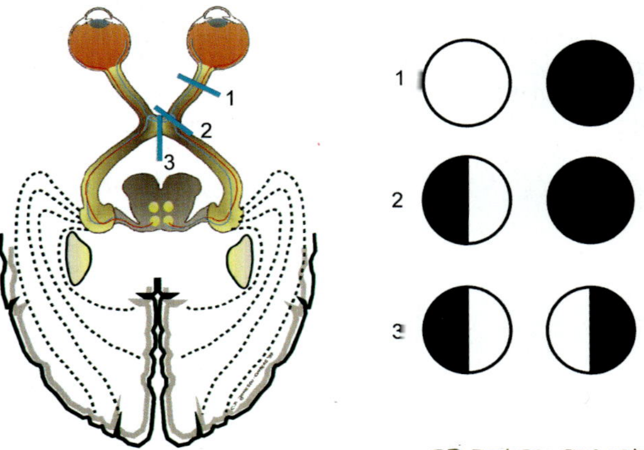

Figure 13.2   Visual field defects from prechiasmal lesions, schematic drawing. Total interruption of the optic nerve produces monolateral loss of vision (1). A lesion of the visual pathway in the anterior chiasm leads to hemianopic field defects in the contralateral eye and mostly to loss of vision in the ipsilateral eye. A disruption of neural conduction in the center of the chiasm mainly affects the crossing axons and produces bitemporal hemianopia (3).

Figure 13.3 Visual field defects from postchiasmal lesions, schematic drawing. On the *left side* the different interruptions of the postchiasmal visual pathways are marked, on the *right side* the resulting visual field defects are shown.

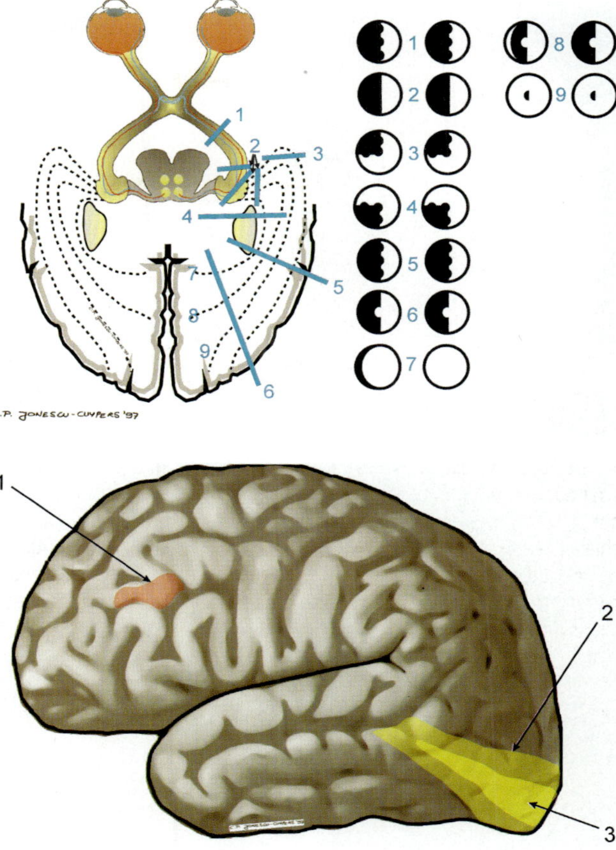

Figure 13.4 Schematic drawing of the visual cortical representation. The area 17 (3) corresponds to the primary visual cortex, it is located in the interhemispheral fissure (projected to the surface of the brain in the drawing). The visual field is represented in the primary cortex. Lesions in this area produce defects in the contralateral visual field. The area 18 (2, "area peristriata") is directly linked to area 17 (calcarine fissure). Lesions in the area 18 lead to visual agnosia, i.e. an object is clearly seen but cannot be recognized. The frontal eye field (1) is responsible for the coordination of horizontal eye movements. A lesion in this area leads to a loss of voluntary ocular movement.

13.2 Lesions of the optic nerve

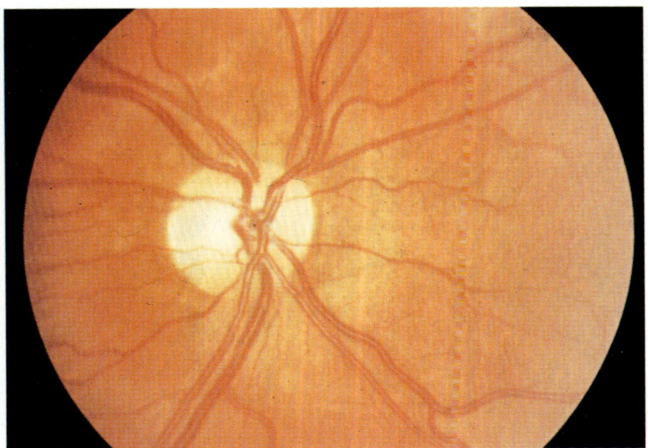

Figure 13.5   Pallor of the optic disc in descending atrophy of the optic nerve due to orbital vascular malformation. The orbital hemangioma causes chronic compressive neuropathy with descending optic atrophy.

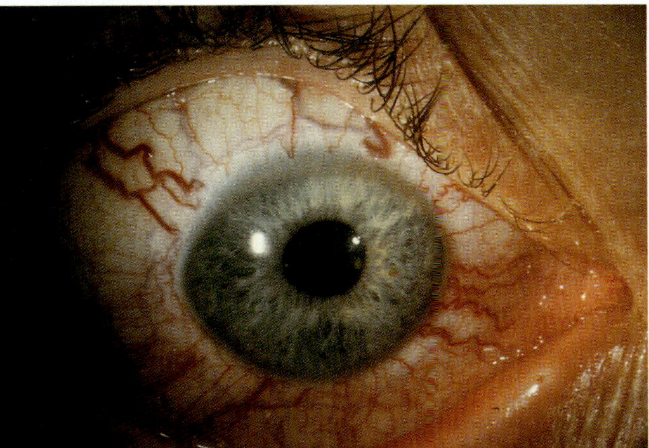

Figure 13.6   Massive episcleral venous congestion due to orbital vascular malformation (same eye as in figure 13.5).

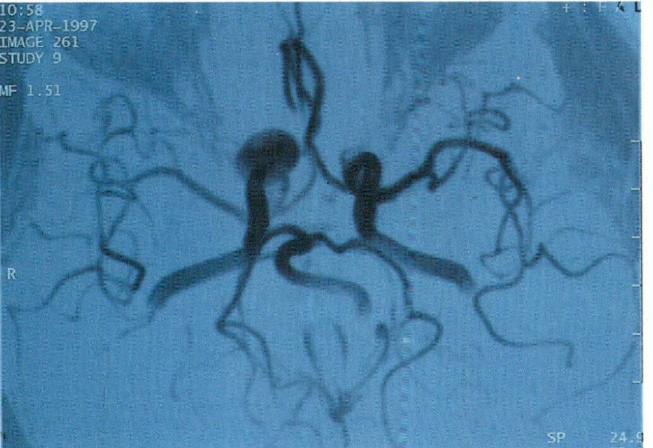

Figure 13.7   Intravenous digital subtraction angiogram showing two anerysms of the right internal carotid artery at the carotid siphon. Due to its particular hemodynamics, there is a predilection for the formation of aneurysms at the carotid siphon. As the optic nerve lies just above the siphon, aneurysms in this area produce a compressive neuropathy of the optic nerve in its intracranial portion between the optic canal of the orbit and the chiasm.

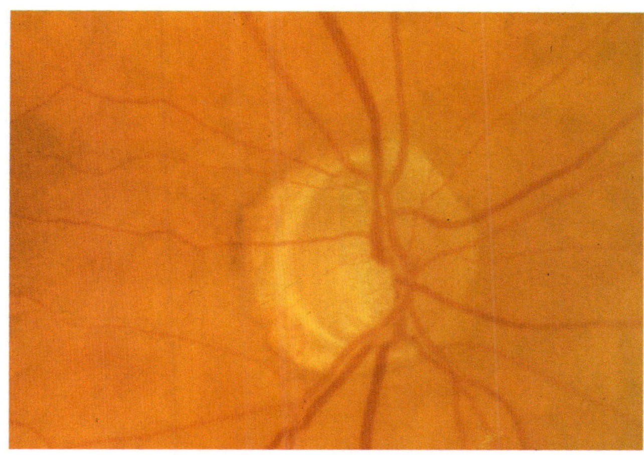

Figure 13.8 Pseudoglaucomatous cupping of the optic disc in the patient shown in figure 13.7. In the slow course of compressive neuropathy, an enlargement of the optic disc cup develops, which may resemble glaucomatous cupping. Damage to the optic nerve over a long period of time frequently produces so-called pseudoglaucomatous cupping. Note that the optic disc shown here has almost complete cupping, the fenestrated lamina cribrosa is visible in the vertical axis of the deep excavation.

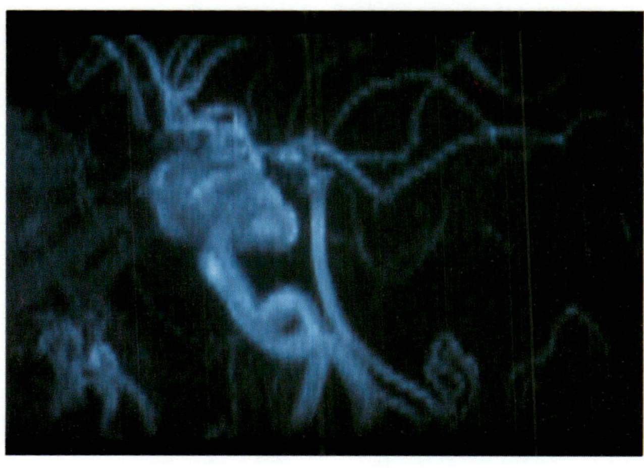

Figure 13.9 Angiogram showing an intracranial arterial aneurysm with calcification of its walls, which leads to chronic irritation and atrophy of the optic nerve.

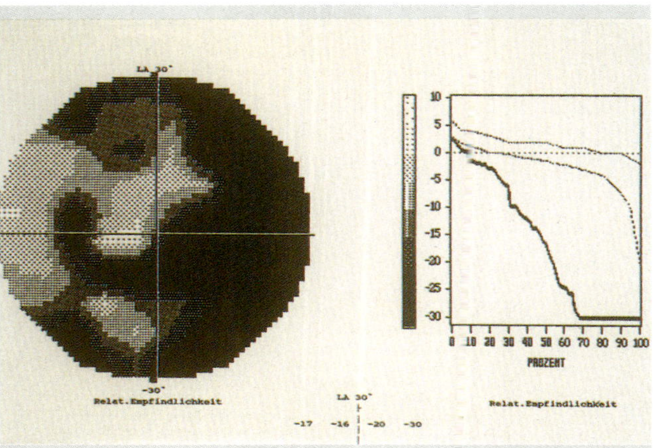

Figure 13.10   Central visual field of the affected eye of the patient shown in figure 13.9. On the *left side* is the grey scale printout showing advanced field defects, on the *right side* the cumulative defect curve is shown.

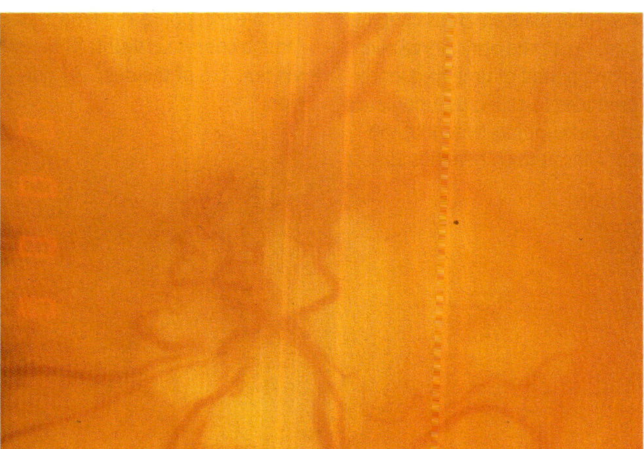

Figure 13.11   Optic disc swelling and massive epipapillary vascular congestion in optic nerve sheath menigioma. The obstruction of venous drainage in the posterior pole is the most prominent feature of the opthalmoscopic picture. The disc margin is blurred, the disc is pale, aptrophic.

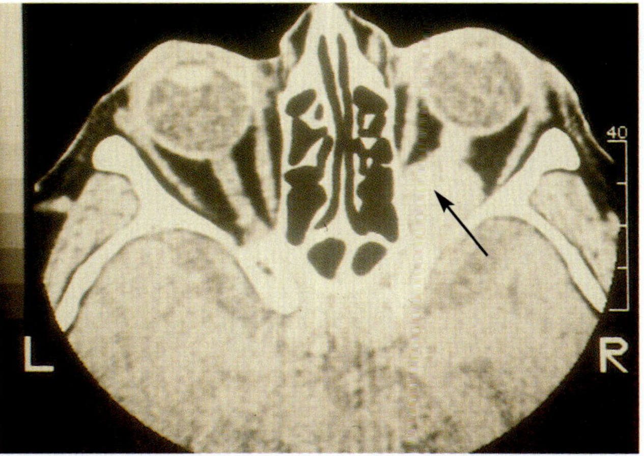

Figure 13.12   Axial CT scan of the patient shown in figure 13.11. An optic sheath meningioma takes up the complete apex of the right orbit.

Figure 13.13 Sagittal MRI scan of the head showing a pituitary tumor.

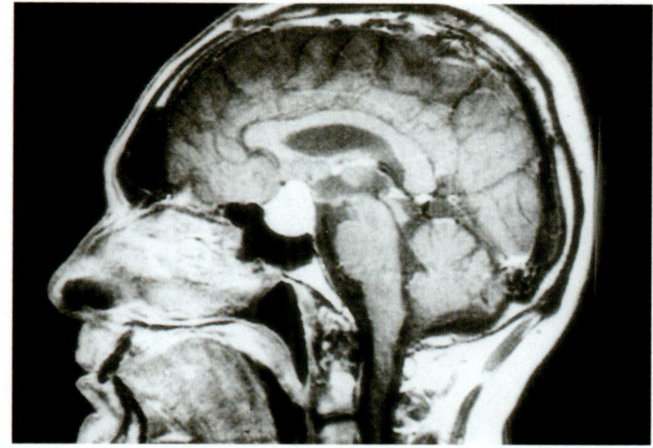

Figure 13.14 Pallor of the temporal and nasal portions of the optic disc resulting from descending optic atrophy. Same patient as shown in figure 13.13.

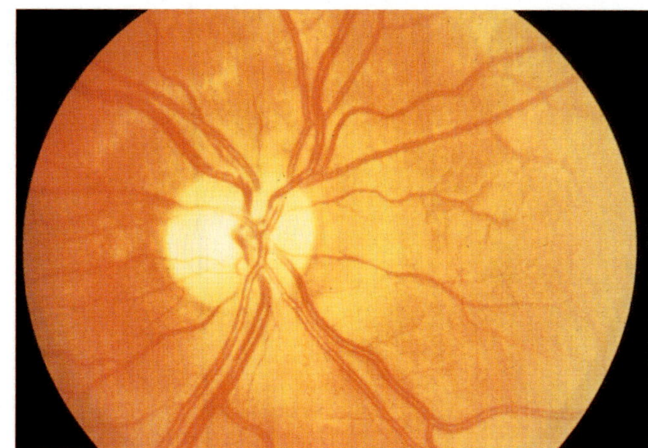

Figure 13.15 Perimetric presentation of a temporal hemianopic visual field defect evaluated with kinetic perimetry *(left)*, computer perimetry, neuro-ophthalmic testing pattern *(middle)* and computer assisted screening test of the central 15 degree field *(right)*. All three perimetric testing techniques reveal a loss of the temporal quadrants of the visual field.

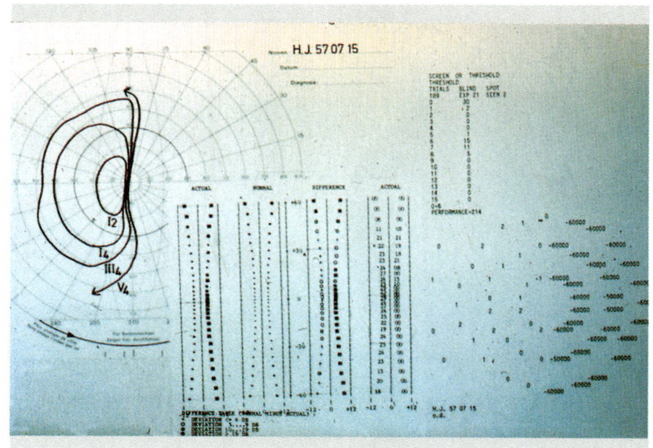

13.3 Lesions of the optic chiasm

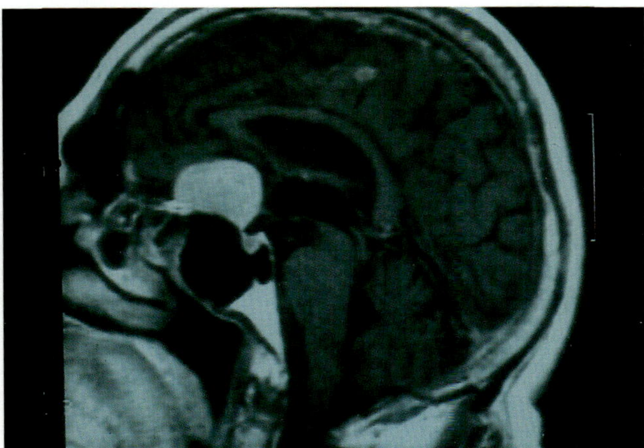

Figure 13.16 Sagittal MRI scan of an advanced pituitary tumor.

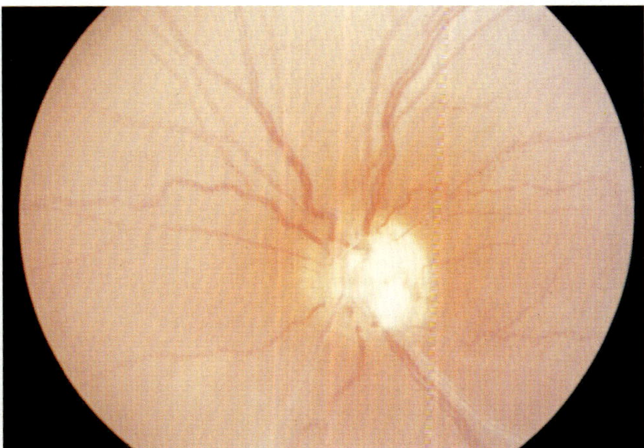

Figure 13.17 Subtotal optic atrophy in the patient shown in figure 13.16. Note the white, atrophic optic disc with advanced pseudoglaucomatous cupping.

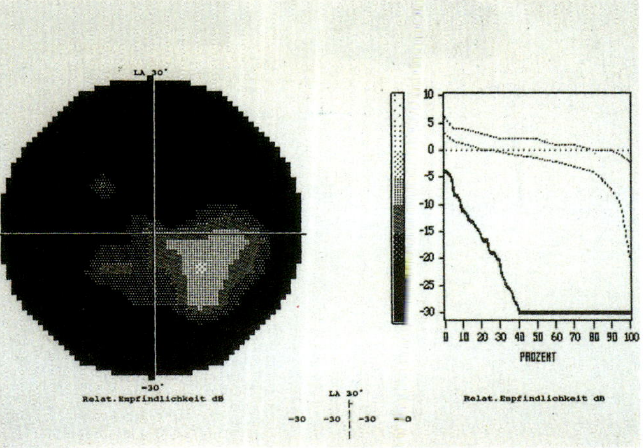

Figure 13.18 Central visual field of the eye shown in figure 13.17. The grey scale printout *(left)* shows preservation of a small eccentric island of vision. The cumulative defect curve on the *right* exhibits an absolute scotoma in the majority of test points.

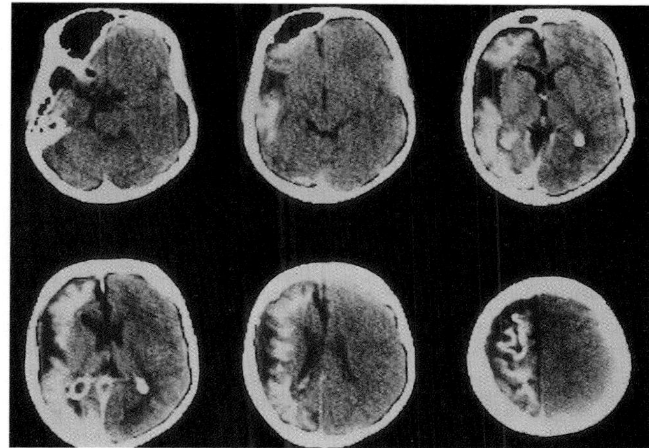

Figure 13.19 Axial CT scans of a patient with Sturge-Weber disease (encephalofacial cavernous hemangiomatosis). This neuroectodermal dysplasia, one of the phacomatoses, is characterized by facial hemangiomas in segmental distribution in association with calcified hemangiomas of the meninges with corresponding cortical lesions. The axial sequences show calification and atrophy of large portions of the left hemisphere, affecting the posterior visual pathways.

13.4 Postchiasmal lesions

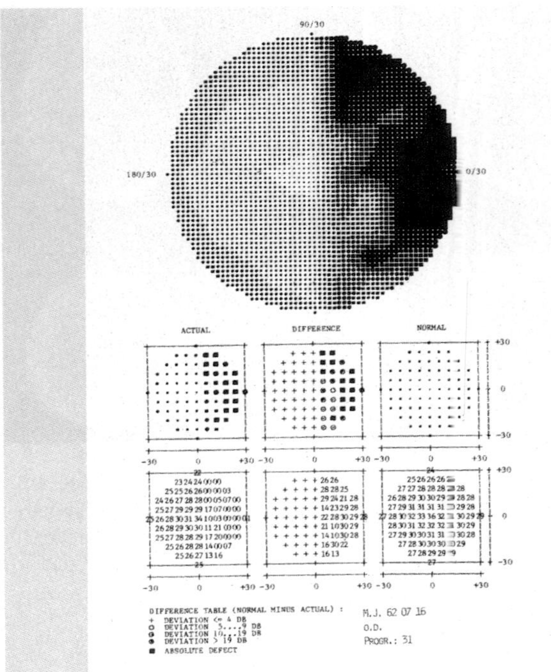

Figure 13.20 Hemianopic visual field defects in the same patient shown in figure 13.19. The *top* frame shows the grey-scale printout of the central 30 degree visual field of the right eye with almost complete loss of the temporal quadrants due to the lesion in the posterior visual pathways of the left hemisphere. The *bottom* frames depict the measured differential light thresholds of the retina in the central visual field, the age-corrected normal values and the differences between measured and age-corrected normal values.

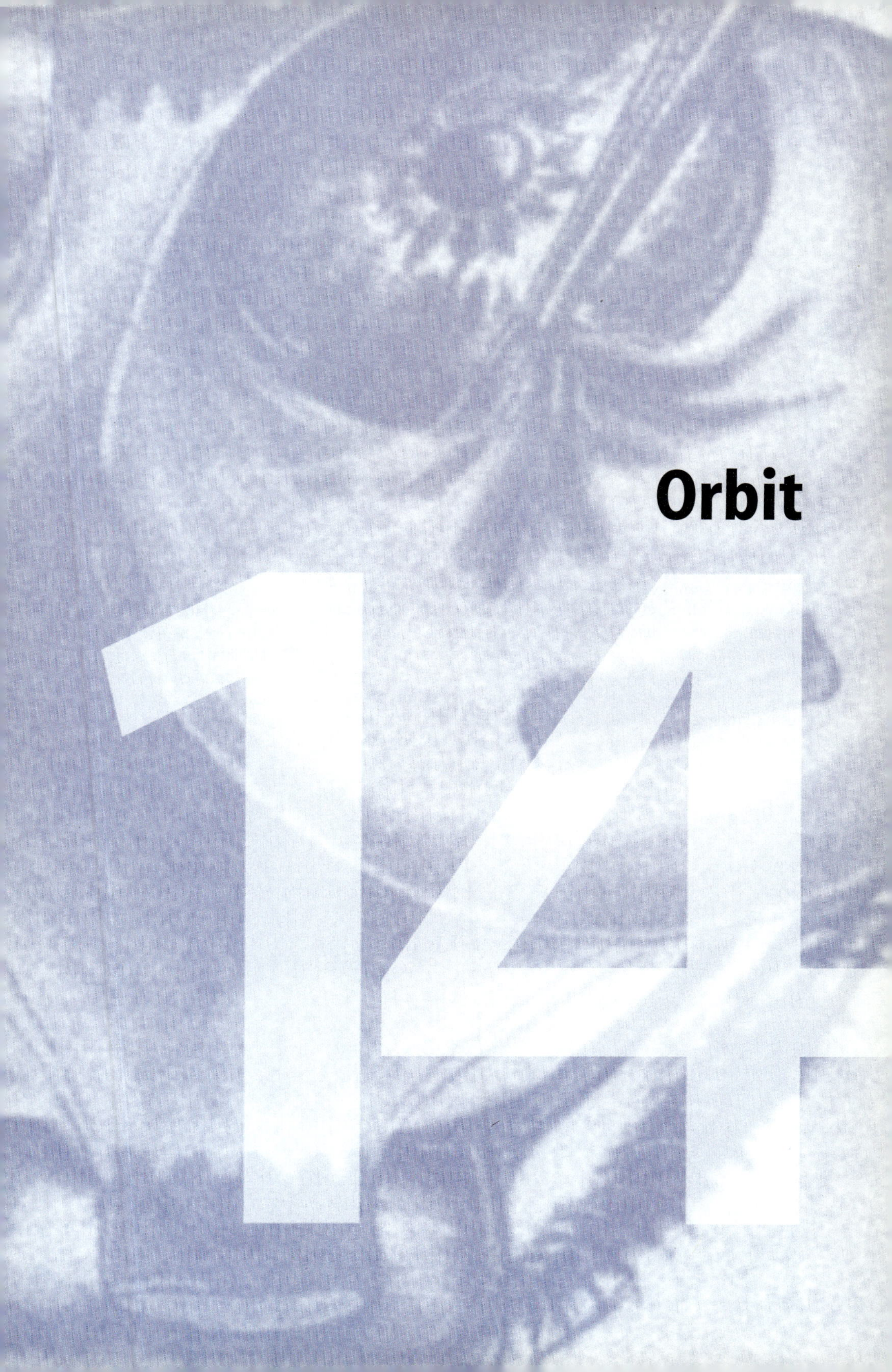

Orbit
14

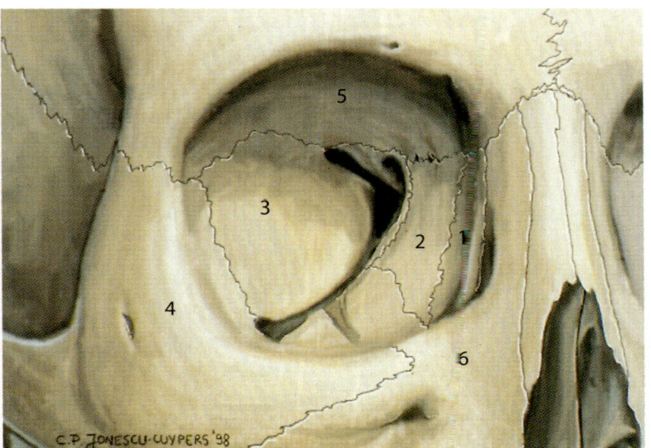

Figure 14.1 Bony orbit. The orbit has the shape of a pyramid with an open base, it is approximately 40-50 mm deep. At its apex lies the optic canal. Its posterior openings (optic foramen, superior and inferior orbital fissures, foramen rotundum and infraorbital canal) transmit various nerves and vessels. Processes in this area can involve different nerves at the same time (orbital apex syndrome, compare with figure 14.2). With the exception of the robust orbital rim, the bones which form the orbital walls are extremely thin. An invasion of pathological processes is possible (compare with figure 14.4). Adherent to the periost of the orbit is the so-called periorbit, which forms connective tissue septa, stabilizing the orbital content and enclosing the intraorbital muscles and vessels. Tenon´s capsule forms the inner limit of the orbit, the fibrous membrane covers the globe and the extraocular muscles. The anterior limit of the orbit is the orbital septum (compare with chapter 1). (1) lacimal bone; (2) ethmoid bone; (3) sphenoid bone; (4) zygomatic bone; (5) frontal bone; (6) maxillary bone.

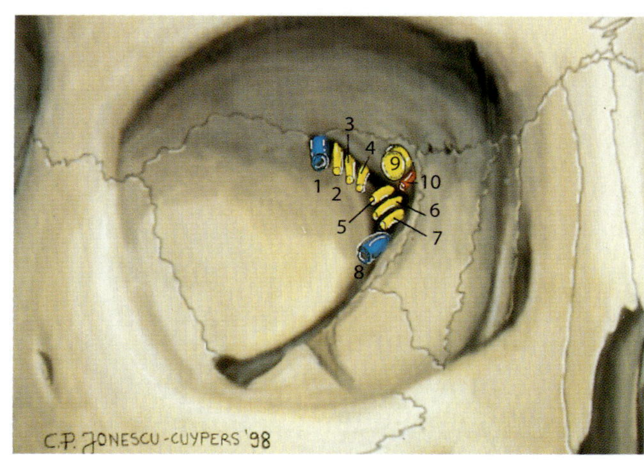

Figure 14.2 Posterior orbital openings with nerves and vessels, schematic drawing. Optic foramen: optic nerve, ophthalmic artery (branches of the internal carotid artery perfuse the entire orbit). Superior orbital fissure: superior ophthalmic vein, oculomotor nerve, trochlear nerve, branches of trigeminal nerve and abducens nerve. Inferior orbital fissure: inferior ophthalmic vein (communicates with cavernous sinus and pterygoid plexus). The orbital fissure is subdivided into a superior and inferior portion by a tendon. (1) superior ophthalmic vein; (2) lacrimal nerve; (3) frontal nerve; (4) trochlear nerve; (5) oculomotor nerve; (6) abducens nerve; (7) nasociliary nerve; (8) inferior ophthalmic vein; (9) optic nerve; (10) ophthalmic artery.

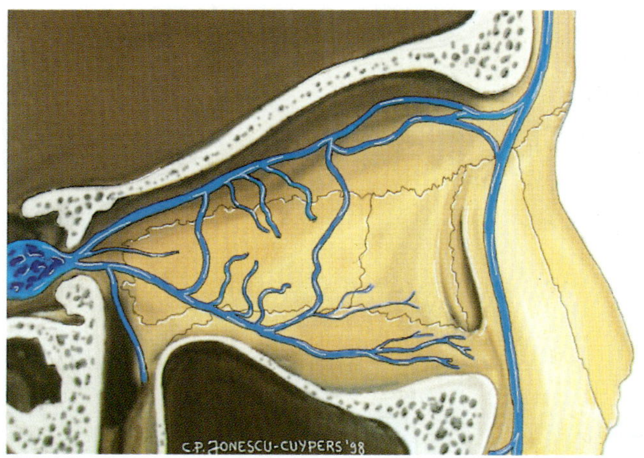

Figure 14.3 Venous drainage, schematic drawing. The orbit is provided with a dense vascular net. The valveless orbital veins anastomose with facial veins and empty into the cavernous sinus and pterygoid plexus (spread of infection!).

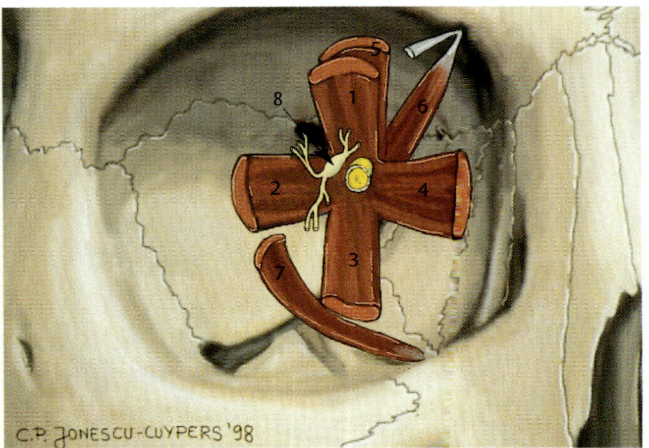

Figure 14.4 Muscle cone, schematic drawing. The four rectus muscles (1-4) and the levator muscle (5) originate in the orbital apex from a ring-shaped tendon, the annulus of Zinn, which is attached to the periorbit. The 4 rectus muscles are covered with a thin fascia and insert 5-8 mm posteriorly to the corneal limbus. The superior oblique muscle (6) originates from the superotemporal portion of the ring, passes the trochlea and arcs to its insertion at the anterior temporal portion of the globe behind the equator. The inferior oblique muscle (7) originates from below the lacrimal fossa, courses backward and temporally and inserts at the temporal aspect of the globe just anterior to the macular area. The origin and insertion of the muscles determine their function. Testing of ocular motility is indispensable for evaluation of orbital processes. The ciliary ganglion (8) contains parasympathetic fibers, sympathetic fibers and sensory fibers of the trigeminal nerve.

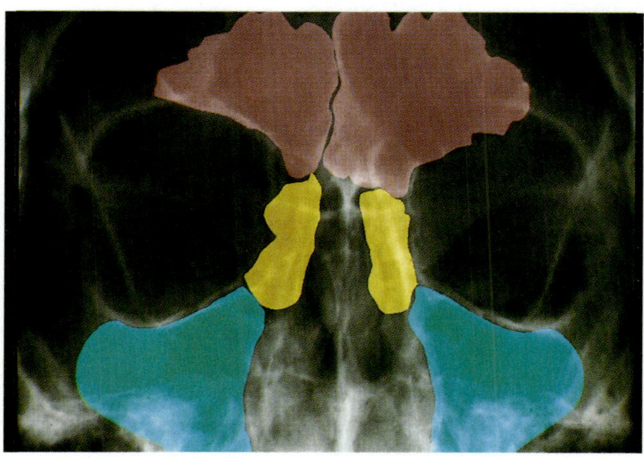

Figure 14.5 Radiograph demonstrating the orbits and the paranasal sinuses. Plain film radiography is mainly used for evaluation of the bony orbital structures. The paranasal sinuses are often primarily or secondarily affected in orbital processes. The thin orbital roof borders on the frontal sinus and the anterior cranial fossa, the medial orbital wall borders on the ethmoidal cells and the ethmoidal sinus (spread of infection, possibility of intraoperative injury!). Fractures mostly involve the paper-thin orbital floor and the medial orbital wall. Different radiographic projections are applied in order to visualize different bony details of the orbit and face. Soft tissue changes cannot be sufficiently evaluated with plain x-ray studies.

14.1 Anatomy and examination techniques

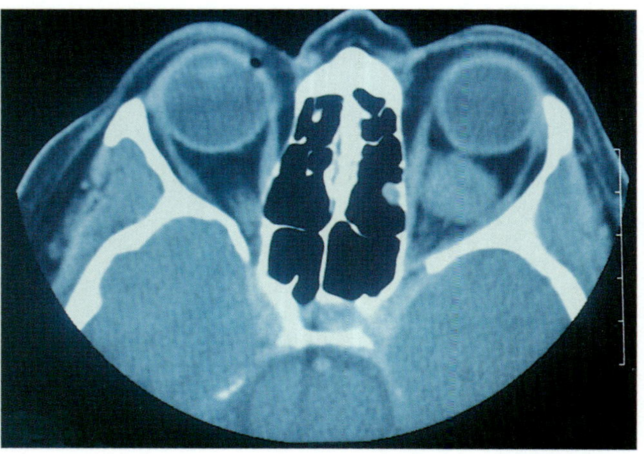

Figure 14.6 Computed tomography (CT) and magnetic resonance imaging (MRI) are essential examination techniques for the diagnosis of diffuse inflammatory, localized inflammatory processes and tumorous lesions of the orbit.

Any suspicion of an orbital process is an indication for CT or – particularly for the differentiation of soft tissue changes – MRI. The assessment of the studies should always be made in cooperation with a radiologist. On the *right* side of the figure note a round, sharply delineated mass in the depth of the orbit. The histologic evaluation after surgical removal gave the diagnosis of a dermoid cyst (benign tumor with slow growth).

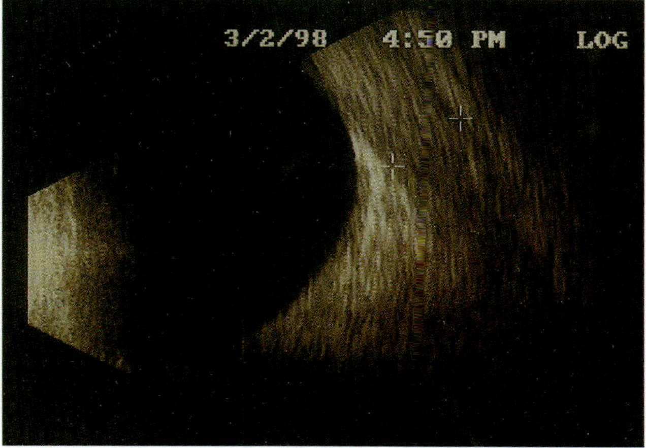

Figure 14.7 Ultrasonography (echography). This examination technique, along with CT and MRI, is an important tool for orbital evaluation, especially in soft tissue changes, e.g. endocrine ophthalmopathy. The one-dimensional A-scan and the two-dimensional B-scan are distinguished. The technique demands special training and extensive experience. The figure shows a thickened extraocular muscle (in between the white crosses) from endocrine ophthalmopathy.

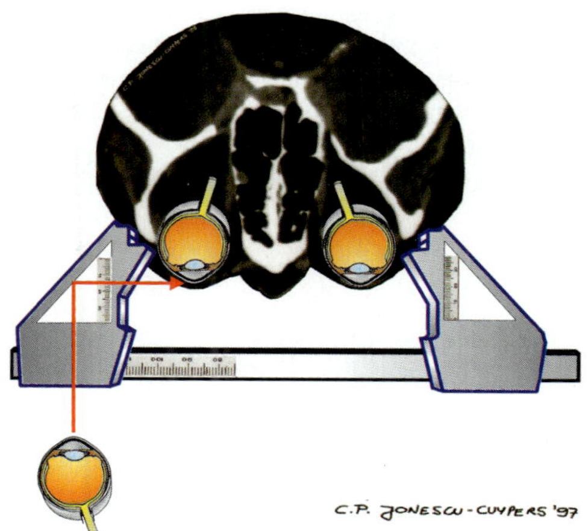

Figure 14.8 Exophthalmometry with Hertel instrument. This instrument is used for the measurement of proptosis. It is placed against the orbital rim. The position of the corneal apex of the patient is determined by means of mirrors. A difference betwen the two eyes of more than 2 mm is considered pathologic. Although variation of measurements often occurs with inexperienced observers, the technique provides important information on eye position in the course of orbital disease. On follow-up examinations, the instrument has to be adjusted to a constant baseline gauge.

14.2 Developmental anomalies

General: In congenital or early acquired changes of the globe (anophthalmos, microphthalmos, enucleation at early age), the growth of the orbit is hindered. An abnormally small orbit results. On the other hand, changes in shape and size of the orbit can also be due to abnormal development of the cranial bones.

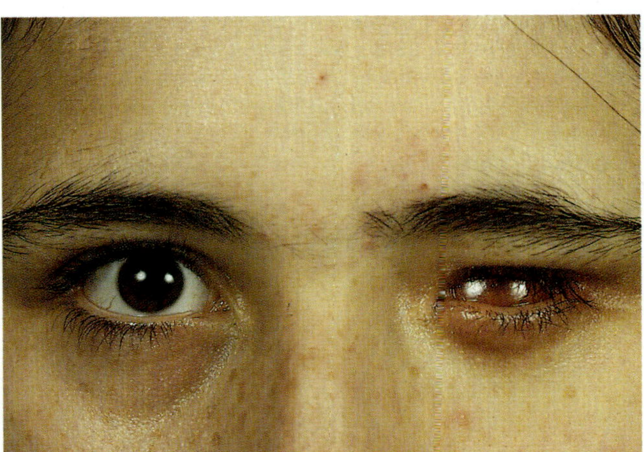

Figure 14.9   Small orbit due to congenital anomaly of the globe. Note the left orbit is significantly smaller than the right. The condition is caused by congenital anomaly of the left globe. The surgical creation of an orbit suitable for an ocular prosthesis is difficult.

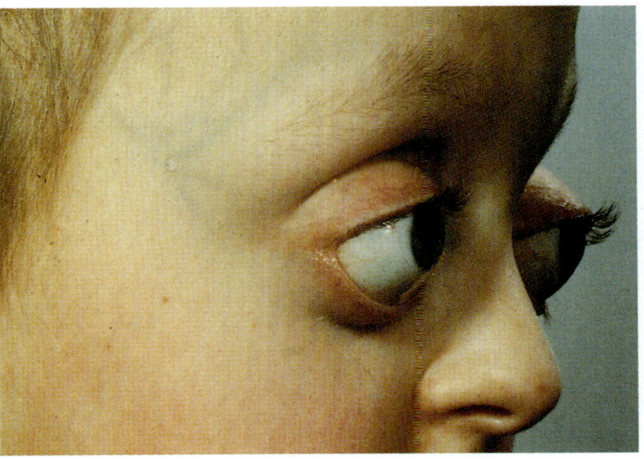

Figure 14.10   Exophthalmos from craniostenosis (dysostosis craniofacialis, Crouzon´s syndrome). The underlying pathology is a premature closure of the coronal and sagittal cranial sutures. A characteristic tower skull (turricephaly) with shallow orbits results. The figure shows bilateral exophthalmos with retraction of the lower eyelids. The turricephaly is not shown. Associated findings include raised intraocular pressure, optic atrophy as well as other facial anomalies.

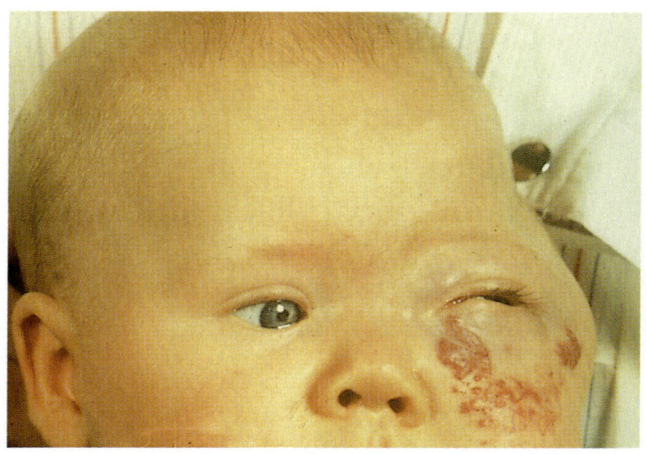

Figure 14.11 Capillary hemangioma (compare with chapter 1). Capillary hemangioma mostly affects eyelids and skin, rarely the orbit. In such cases, the diagnosis can be difficult. A bluish tinge of the eyelids and sponge-like consistency are suggestive of orbital hemangioma. The tumor typically grows during the first 6 weeks, then spontaneous regression can occur. If displacement of the globe results, surgical removal should be considered. The surgical intervention is difficult and carries a high risk of severe hemorrhage. The figure shows a capillary hemangioma in an infant located in the temporal portion of the orbit and eyelids with involvement of the skin. Note the bluish tinge in this area.

14.3 Vascular processes

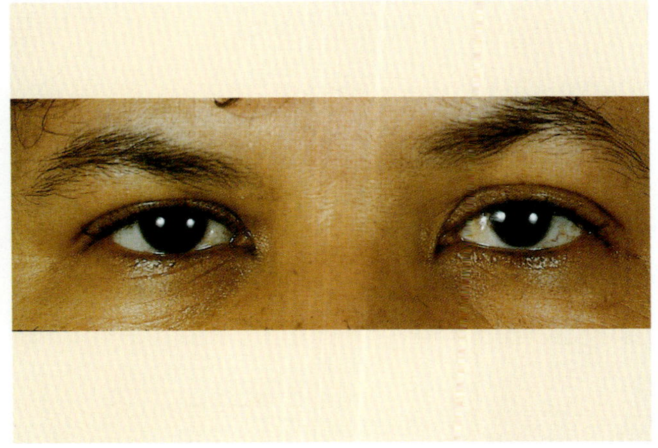

Figure 14.12 Intraorbital cavernous hemangioma. Cavernous hemangioma is a benign, vascular tumor typically seen in adults. Growth is usually slow, malignant transformation does not occur. The clinical picture includes slight proptosis and restriction of motility. The diagnosis is made by CT or MRI. The tumor is encapsulated and can therefore usually be surgically removed in toto. Recurrent hemorrhages into the orbit may occur. In such cases, surgical removal is indicated. The figure shows a patient with an intraorbital hemangioma in the left eye, located in the upper nasal portion of the orbit.

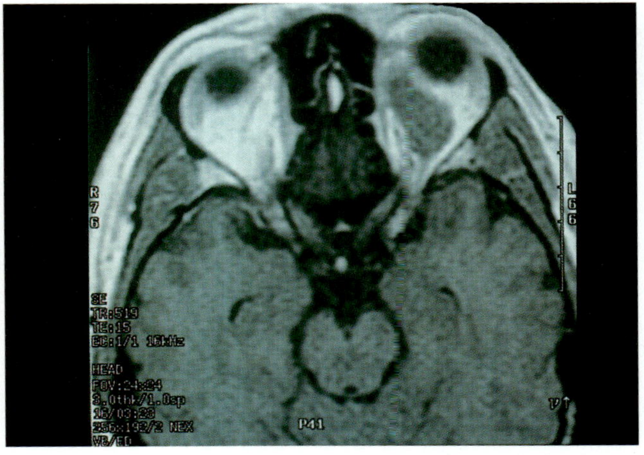

Figure 14.13 Axial MRI scan showing intraorbital cavernous hemangioma (same patient as in figure 14.12). The vascular tumor presents as a grey mass behind the left globe.

Figure 14.14 Carotid-cavernous sinus fistula. There is a pathologic communication between the carotid artery and the cavernous sinus. The clinical picture is characterized by mild exophthalmos, increased filling of conjuctival vessels with cork-screw-like appearance, increased filling of retinal vessels, sometimes with retinal hemorrhages and a pulse-synchronous bruit in the orbit. The fistulas mostly result from trauma and are rarely congenital vascular malformations. Surgical intervention with vascular ligature or cautery must be considered. Neurologic complications can occur.

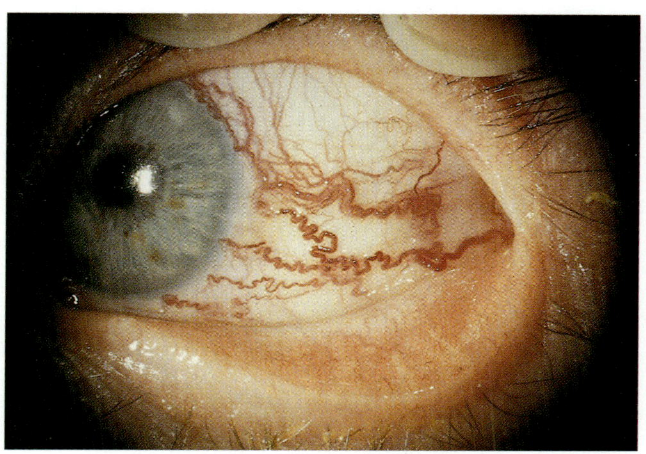

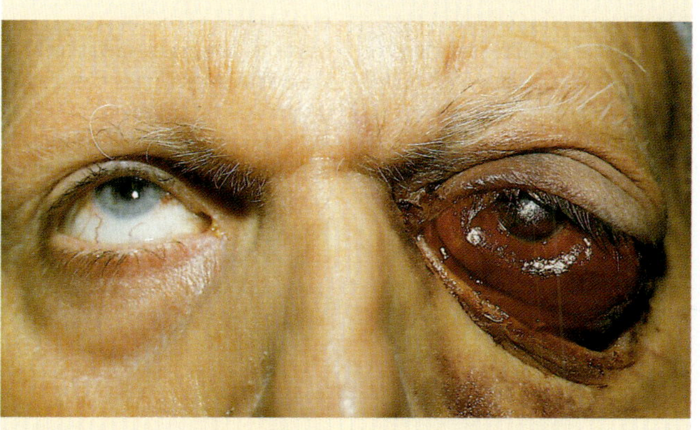

Figure 14.15 Retrobulbar hematoma. The orbit contains numerous vessels. Major retrobulbar hemorrhages can occur due to vascular malformation, hemorrhagic diathesis or following trauma – including surgery. The rise in intraorbital pressure can produce an ischemic optic neuropathy with irreversible visual loss. The figure shows a status post retrobulbar hematoma. Note the proptosis and the marked subconjunctival hematoma. Immediate ophthalmoscopy as well as testing of pupillary light reflex are mandatory. In case of subnormal or loss of direct pupillary light response, attenuated or absent perfusion of the optic nerve head, decompression incisions have to be performed at once (incision of the orbital septum, lateral canthotomy, lysis of the lateral canthal tendon). Any time consuming diagnostic procedures should be omitted in this emergency situation.

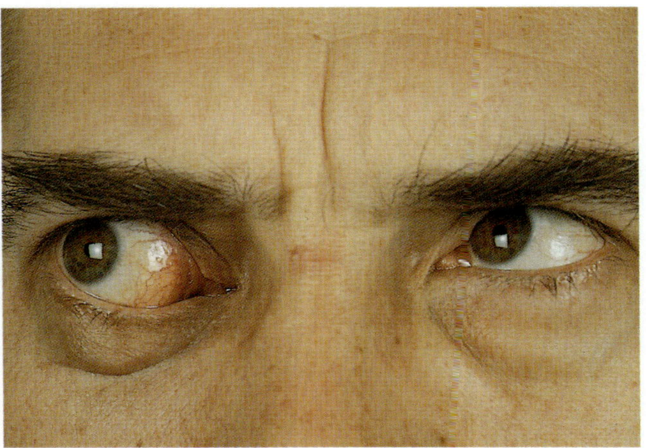

Figure 14.16   Orbital pseudo-tumor/ idiopathic orbital inflammation. The characteristic clinical signs of this disorder, which primarily affects adults, are: pain, restricted ocular motility, swelling, proptosis and sometimes loss of vision. The inflammatory process can involve different portions of the orbit. In the anterior orbit, there is an association with scleral thickening and thickening of the extraocular muscles. An isolated involvement of the muscles (myositis) is possible. Invasion of the orbital apex carries the worst prognosis. The disorder is of autoimmune origin. An association with other autoimmune disorders like lupus erythematosus, dermatomyositis and polyarteritis nodosa has been described. The clinical presentation can be confused with orbital lymphoma. Muscular and scleral thickening indicates the presence of pseudotumor. Lymphoma appears more circumscribed. The figure shows mild left-sided exopthalmos with inflammatory changes of the internal rectus muscle indicating myositis. Corticosteroids are the treatment of choice and lead to a rapid clinical remission. Recurrences are possible.

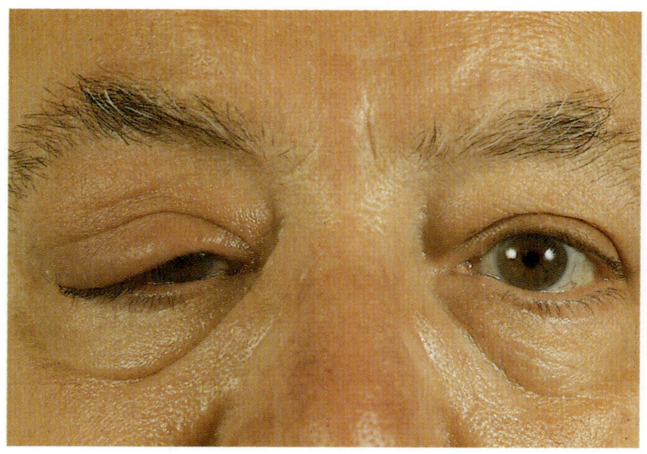

Figure 14.17   Wegener´s granulomatosis / orbital involvement. Wegener´s granulomatosis can involve different ocular areas. Orbital involvement is the most common eye finding with restriction of ocular motility, eyelid swelling, ptosis and granulomatous infiltration of the orbit. The disorder is of autoimmune origin and can involve all organs. Ocular manifestation may be the presenting manifestation. The figure shows a patient with right-sided swelling of the upper and lower eyelids. The CT revealed a mass in the superior lateral aspect of the right orbit without signs of bony erosion. Histologic evaluation (biopsy) confirmed the diagnosis. A test for antineutrophil cytoplasmatic antibodies (ANCA) is of great help for the diagnosis. C-ANCA are specifically found with orbital involvement. Immunosupressive treatment with a combination of corticosteroids and cyclophosphamide can control the disease. Without treatment, the mortality is very high.

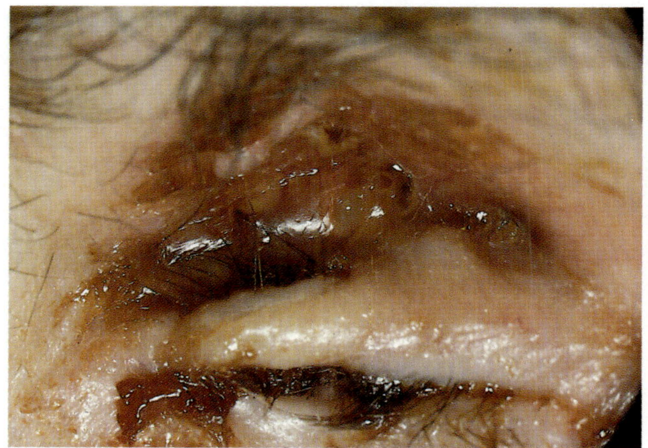

Figure 14.18   Wegener´s granulomatosis, necrotic changes of upper eyelid and orbit. In every inflammatory orbital process, particularly with necrotic changes, Wegener´s granulomatosis must be considered. Orbital inflammation may be the first manifestation of the disease. Early diagnosis and immediate treatment are crucial for the prognosis.

14.4 Orbital involvement in immunologic disease

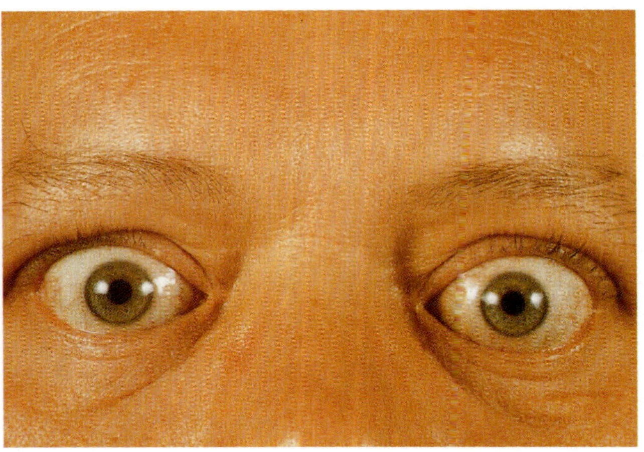

Figure 14.19 Exophthalmos due to endocrine ophthalmopathy. The classic signs of endocrine ophthalmopathy are bilateral exophthalmos (10% unilateral), eyelid retraction and restriction of ocular motitlity as a result of infiltration of the orbital fat pad and the extraocular muscles, including the levator muscle. Involvement of the optic nerve with consequential visual loss is possible. Eyelid retraction (Dalrymple´s sign), delay of upper eyelid following globe movement in downward gaze (Graefe´s sign) and reduced blinking (Stelwag´s sign) are pathognomonic. The figure shows bilateral exophthalmos with visible rims of sclera superiorly and inferiorly due to eyelid retraction. This is the characteristic picture of endocrine ophthalmopathy. The diagnosis can be made without further examination. CT and ultrasonography are important diagnostic tools. Both can detect thickened extraocular muscles in endocrine ophthalmopathy (compare with figure 14.7). The disorder can be associated with hypo- or hyperfunction of the thyroid gland or even euthyroidism. During the active stage of the disease (lymphocytic infiltration and deposition of glycosaminoglycans), the treatment consists of retrobulbar irradiation and systemic corticosteroids. In the end stage (fibrosis), surgical treatment is indicated with orbital decompression by reduction of orbital fat. Severe exophthalmos can cause strangulation of the conjunctiva, corneal ulceration due to exposure and compressive optic neuropathy.

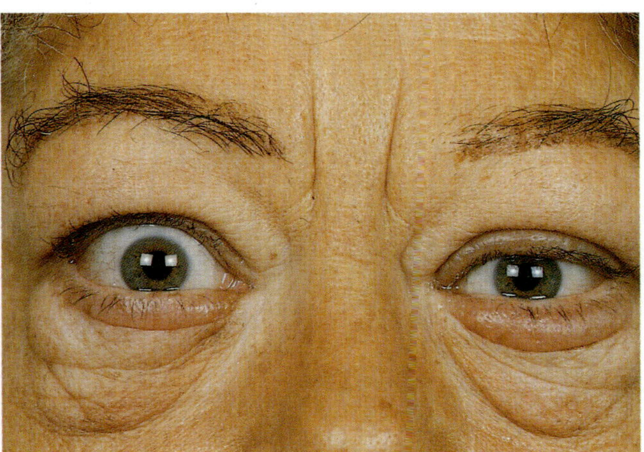

Figure 14.20 Endocrine ophthalmopathy, "unilateral" case. Note bilateral swelling of the upper and lower eyelids, upper lid retraction with visible superior rim of sclera and pronounced proptosis in the right eye. Marked eyelid swelling can be a symptom of endocrine ophthalmopathy. If exophthalmos is pronouced in one eye, the differential diagnosis includes orbital tumor and myopia.

Figure 14.21 Endocrine ophthal-mopathy, restriction of ocular motility. In this case, the medial and inferior rectus muscles are affected. Weakness of convergence results (sign of Möbius). Additional fibrosis of the lateral rectus muscles leads to esotropia. A characteristic viewing posture is sometimes assumed to compen-sate for the functional impairment of the inferior rectus muscles. At early stages, the misalignment can be treated with prisms, later on muscle surgery or orbital decom-pression is needed.

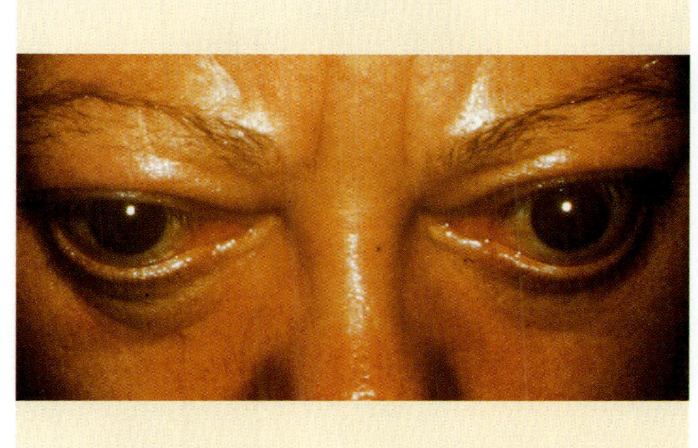

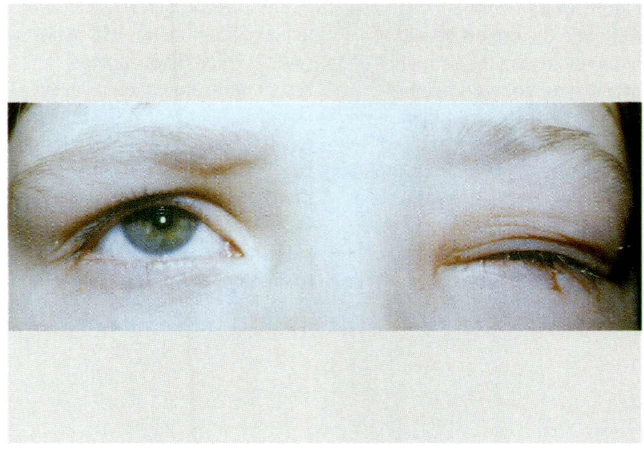

Figure 14.22 Orbital cellulitis. Bacterial orbital cellulitis usually arises from spread of infections from the paranasal sinuses (com-pare with figure 14.5) and via the valveless orbital veins (compare with figure 14.3). Early clinical signs are redness and swelling of the eyelids. Proptosis and restric-tion of ocular motility are distinct signs of orbital involvement. The infection can diffusely invade the entire orbit or form a localized abscess. CT or MRI are essential for the diagnosis. The most feared complication is spread of con-tiguous infection to the cavernous sinus (compare with figure14.3). Orbital cellulitis can thereby lead to life threatening thrombosis of the cavernous sinus. The work-up of inflammatory orbital disease includes monitoring of blood counts and body temperature. Antimicrobial therapy has to be initiated immediately, if cellulitis is suspected. A failure to institute further examinations and to start antimicrobial therapy is conside-red malpractice negligence.

14.5 Tumors

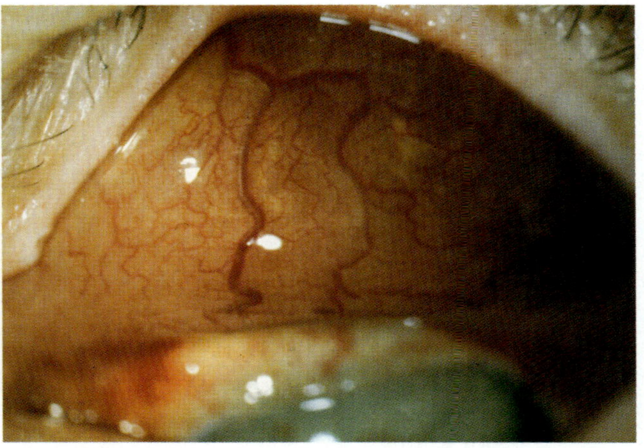

Figure 14.23 Orbital lymphoma. Although the orbit is devoid of lymphoid tissue, the ocurrence of orbital lymphomas is relatively frequent. The spectrum of diseases ranges from benign lymphoid hyperplasia to malignant lymphoma. Histologic differentiation is difficult. The process can be restricted to the orbit or affect other organs. Growth is usually slow. The figure shows hyperemic and swollen tarsal conjunctiva with a fleshy, salmon-colored appearance. Histologic examination revealed changes consistent with lymphoma. The marked vascularization suggests malignancy. Every salmon-colored conjunctival swelling should be biopsied. If orbital involvement is suspected, additional tissue samples must be taken from the orbit. Even a combination of benign conjunctival lymphoma and malignant lymphoma of the orbit has been described. A systemic evaluation for generalized lymphoproliferative disease should be performed. Treatment depends on the histologic diagnosis.

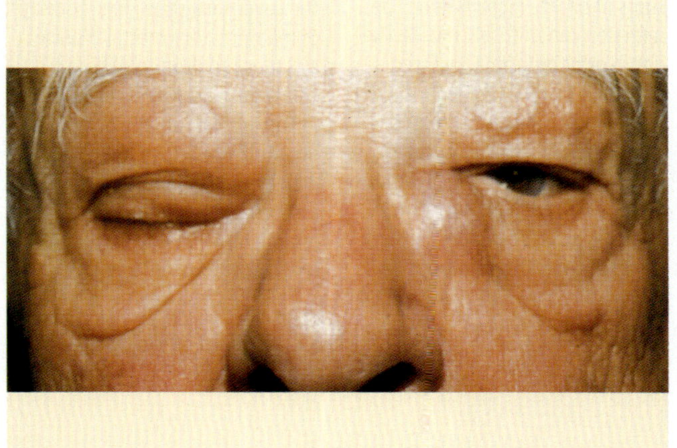

Figure 14.24 Bilateral lymphoma of the orbit. The figure shows bilateral eyelid swelling. Histologic evaluation gave the diagnosis of lymphoma. Clinically, slow growth and globe displacement without signs of inflammation are suggestive of lymphoma and practically rule out the diagnosis of pseudotumor (compare with figure 14.16). Lymphomas are mostly located in the antero-superior portion of the orbit. Globe displacement varies with the location of the tumor. Lymphomas appear better delineated on CT scans than pseudotumor. Malignancy or benignancy cannot be determined from a CT scan.

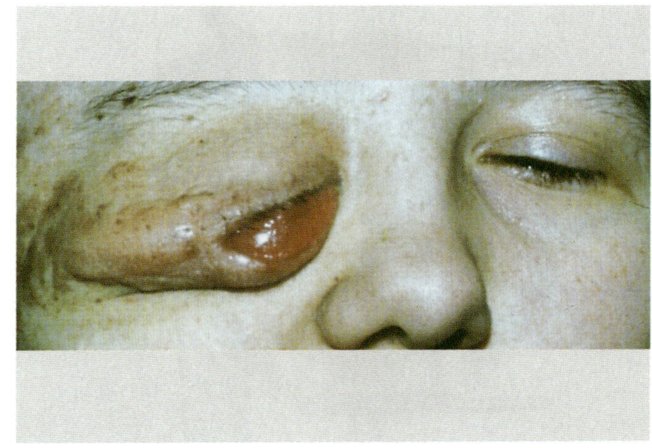

Figure 14.25 Orbital involvement in neurofibromatosis (von Recklinghausen´s disease). Another ocular manifestation of neurofibromatosis von Recklinghausen besides iris changes (compare with chapter 7) is a diffuse infiltration of the eyelids and orbit. The figure shows a large infiltrating tumor of the right upper and lower lids, orbit and temple. The neoplasm is benign, but has an infiltrative growth pattern. Surgical removal is therefore difficult. Recurrences after removal are common. The cosmetic result following multiple surgical procedures is often poor.

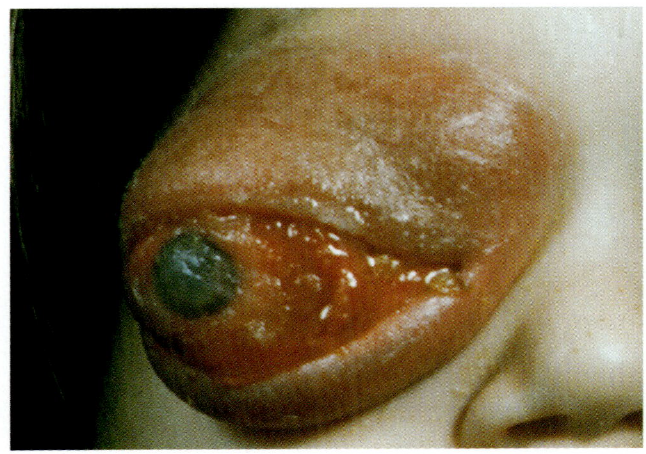

Figure 14.26 Rhabdomyosarcoma. This extremely malignant neoplasm often has a very early age of presentation (under 8 years). The rapidly growing tumor leads to an acute onset of proptosis. The figure shows marked proptosis. Chemotherapy and radiotherapy had been performed, but recurrence has occurred. Histologic evaluation of tissue obtained from orbital exenteration confirmed the diagnosis of rhabdomyosarcoma.

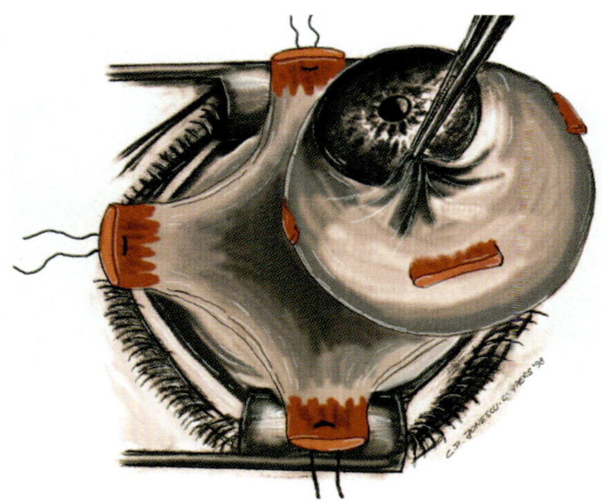

Figure 14.27   Enucleation of the eye. Certain malignant tumors, irreparable trauma or painful disorders that cannot be controlled otherwise require removal of the eye. If a pathologic process is restricted to the eye, an enucleation is sufficient. It is recommended to sever the optic nerve in its posterior portion. The figure shows an enucleated eye, the muscle stumps can later be sutured over an implant (compare with figure 14.28).

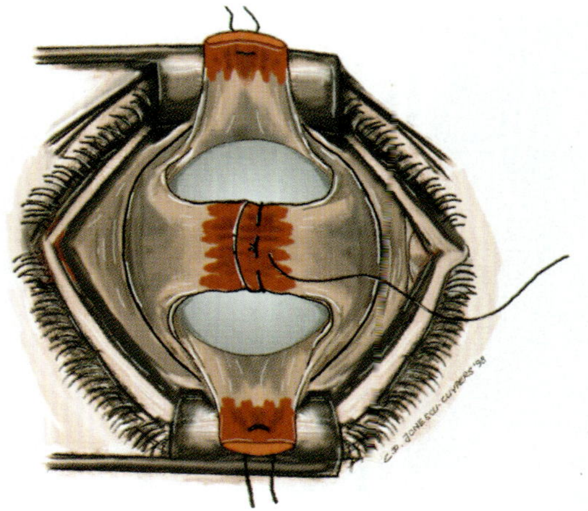

Figure 14.28   Orbital implant. After enucleation is performed, an implant is inserted and the preserved extraocular muscles are sutured over it. An ocular prosthesis, which can be fitted later on, shows good motility, due to the muscular fixation.

Figure 14.29 Orbital exenteration. Enucleation of the eye is not sufficient with malignant processes extending behind the globe (e.g. rhabdomyosarcoma). All orbital contents have to be removed (orbital exenteration). The resulting socket is lined with skin.

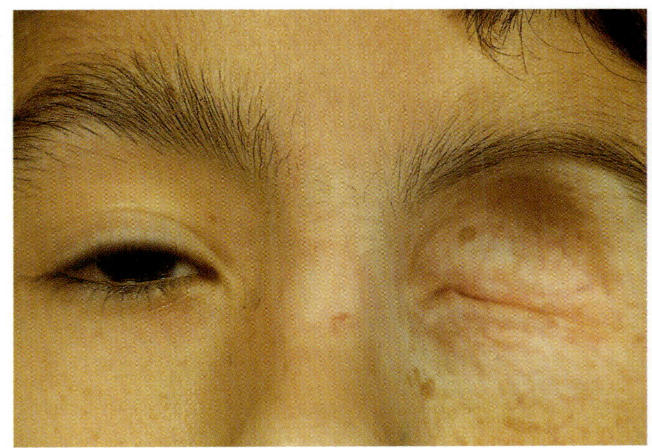

Figure 14.30 Orbital exenteration – epiprosthesis. An epiprosthesis, which is attached to an eyeglass frame, gives a satisfactory cosmetic appearance.

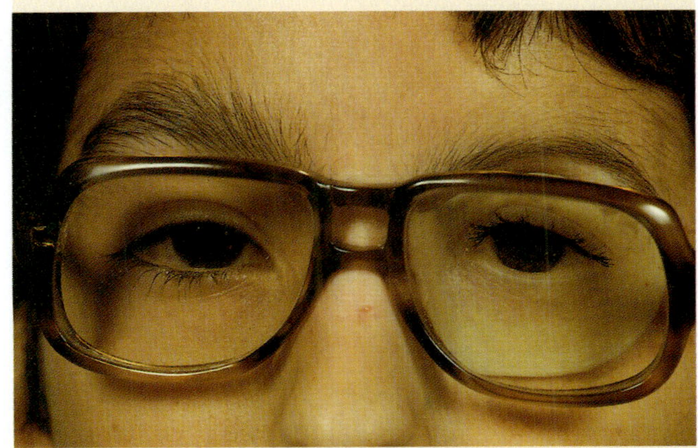

Optics and Refraction

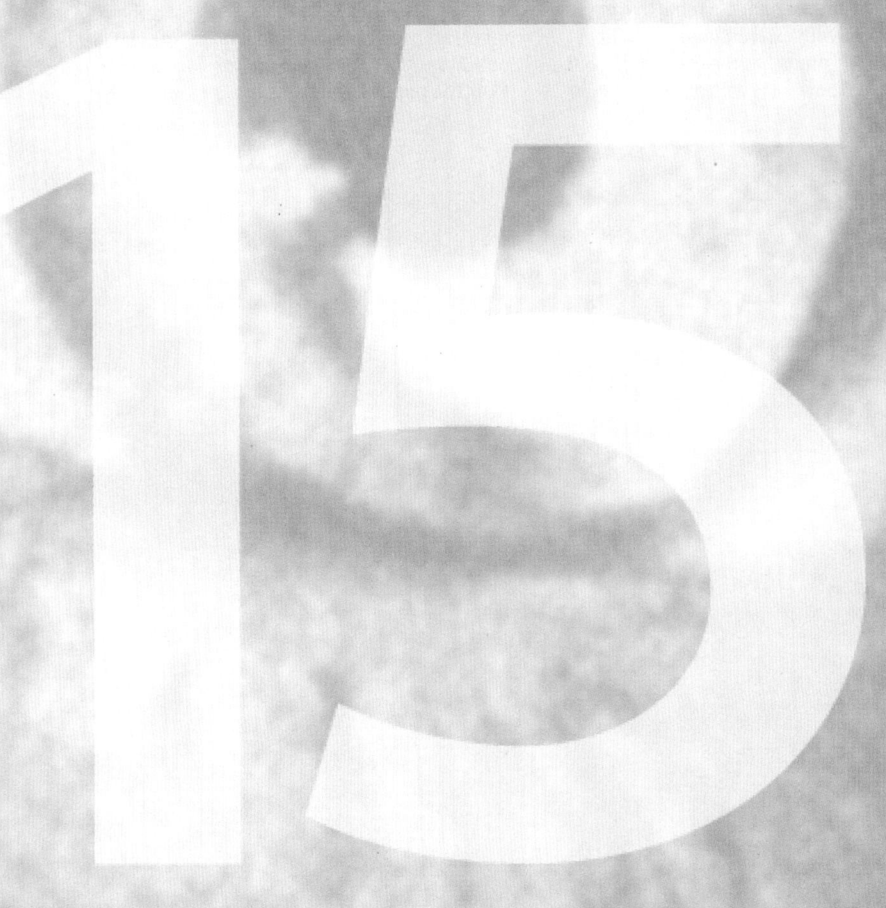

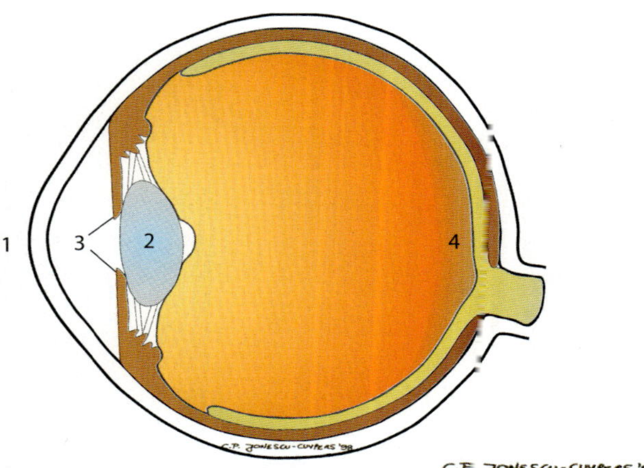

Figure 15.1 The human eye is a compound optical system consisting of multiple refractive media with axial arrangement. The cornea has the greatest refractive power (1) with approx. 43 diopters. The refractive power of the crystalline lens varies with accommodation (19-30 D), the total refractive power of the compound optical system amounts to approx. 61 D. The pupil (3) regulates the amount of entering light and is comparable to the diaphragm of a camera. In the emmetropic eye, parallel incident light rays are refracted in such a way, that they focus on the retina (4).

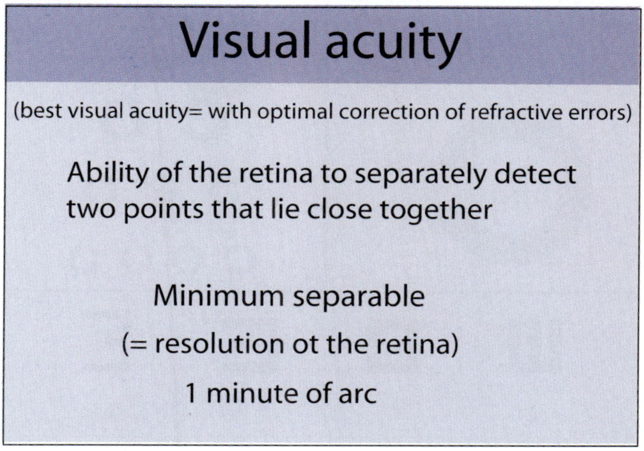

Visual acuity

(best visual acuity= with optimal correction of refractive errors)

Ability of the retina to separately detect
two points that lie close together

Minimum separable

(= resolution ot the retina)

1 minute of arc

Figure 15.2 Visual acuity describes one category of visual discrimination – the ability to separately detect two object points that lie close together. Best corrected visual acuity means with optimal correction of refractive errors. The lower limit of this spatial discrimination is the minimum separable, which is 1 minute of arc (in adolescents 0,5 minute of arc) for a visual acuity of 100%. Visual acuity is expressed in English speaking countries in the Snellen notation format based on a test distance of 20 feet (such as 20/20), while in other countries a decimal system of notation is used (such as 1.0). Any change in the refractive ocular media, the retina or other structures of the visual system can influence the visual acuity.

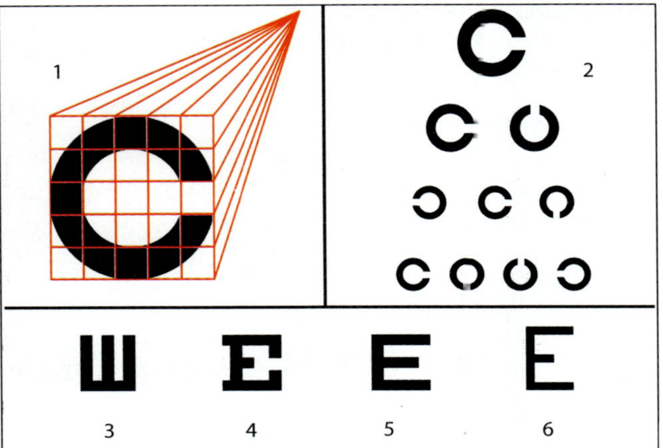

Figure 15.3 Visual acuity is tested with optotypes (test targets). The commonly used Snellen letters are configured in accordance to the one minute visual angle, they are subdivided into 25 squares, of which each subtends 1 arc minute in width (1), (3), (4). The fact that letter recognition is involved in testing with Snellen charts produces imprecision. Therefore, abstract optotypes were designed like the Landolt C (2) or the "tumbling E" (5).

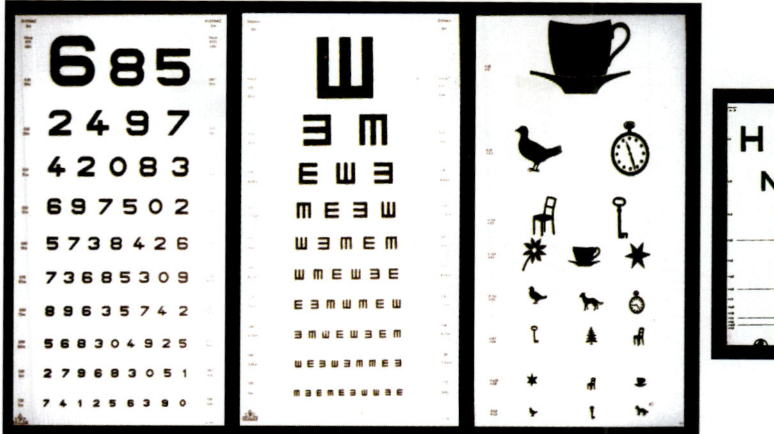

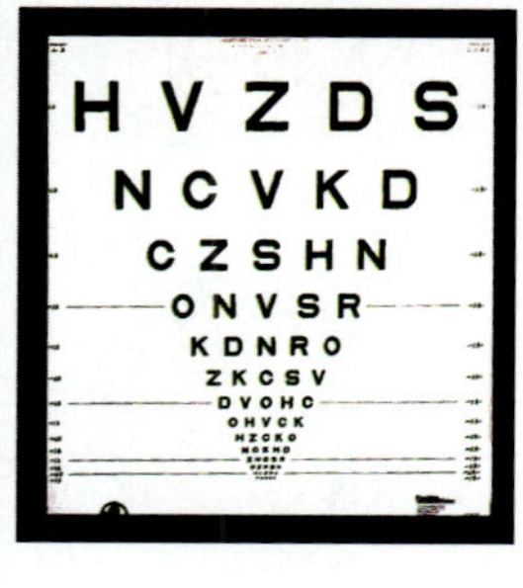

Figure 15.4 Examples of different standardized visual acuity charts: number and letter recognition, "tumbling E", picture recognition. The latter two tests are suitable for children or illiterates. In cases, where the shown charts cannot be employed, the recording of visually evoked cortical potentials (VECP) can sometimes provide information on visual acuity (compare with chapter 12).

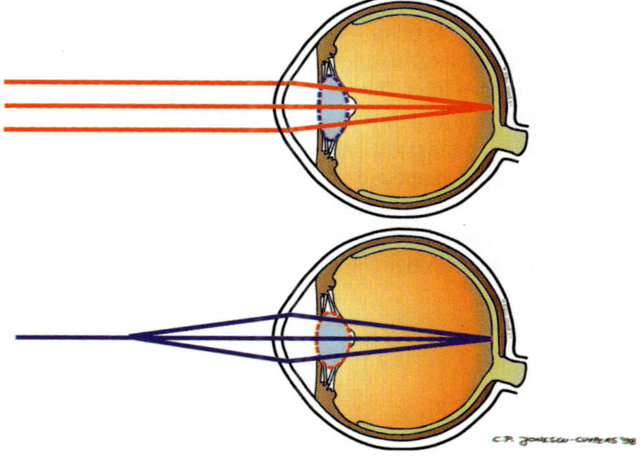

Figure 15.5 In the emmetropic eye parallel light rays (emerging from an object point at infinity) are sharply focussed on the retina *(top)*. The axial length of the eye and its refractive power are balanced. Light rays emerging from a close object are also sharply focussed on the retina *(bottom)* due to changes in the refactive power of the lens (accommodation).

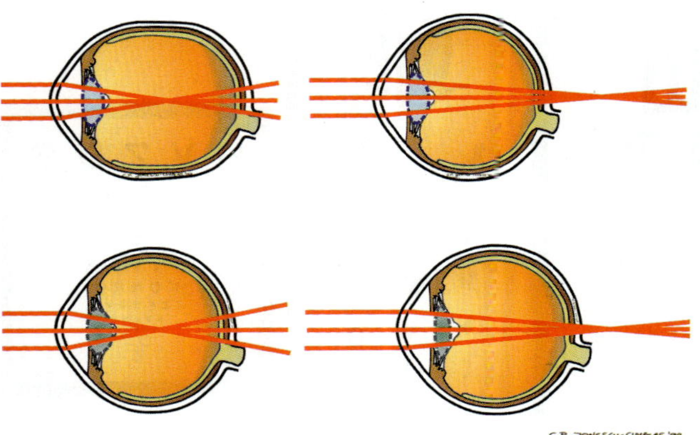

Figure 15.6 In the ametropic eye the axial length and the refractive power are not properly matched. Causes of ametropia can be changes in the refractive media [refractive myopia *(bottom left)*, refractive hypermetropia *(bottom right)*] or alterations of the axial lengh of the eye [axial myopia *(top left)*, axial hypermetropia *(top right)*].

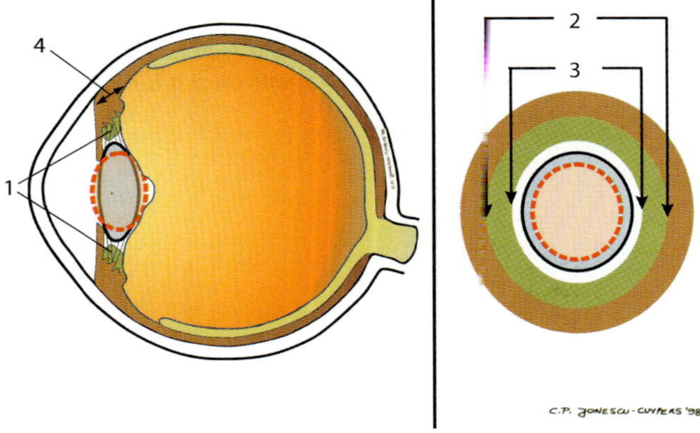

Figure 15.7 Accommodation is the ability of the eye to bring retinal images of objects in various distances into sharp focus. This is accomplished by varying the refractive power that the crystalline lens supplies to the compound optical system. The lens is fixated within the globe *(left* sagittal view; *right* frontal view) with elatic ligaments, the zonules (1), which in the periphery insert at the ciliary muscle. When the ciliary muscle is relaxed (2 *brown*), the zonules are under tension and the lens takes on a flattened form *(blue with black margin)*. With contraction of the ciliary muscle (3,4 *green*), the diameter of the ring-shaped muscle becomes smaller, the zonules become flaccid and the lens reforms to its relaxed spherical shape *(pink area with red interrupted margin)*. Condensation of the lens fibers, occurring with age, leads to a loss of elasticity and thereby to a loss of accommodation.

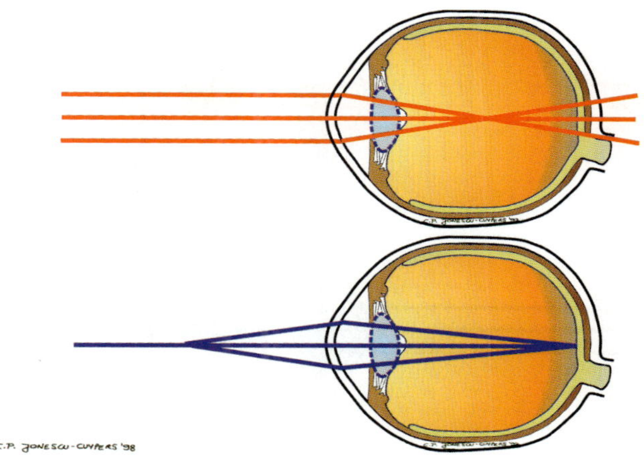

Figure 15.8   In the myopic eye parallel light rays (emerging from an object point at infinity) are focussed in front of the retina, so that the retinal image is blurred (*top*). The far point of the myopic eye is at a finite distance in front of the eye. Objects that lie at the far point of the myopic eye are sharply focussed on the retina *(bottom)* (compare with figure 15.6). Myopia is often a hereditary condition, it can be associated with diverse fundus changes, e.g myopic maculopathy, equatorial degeneration.

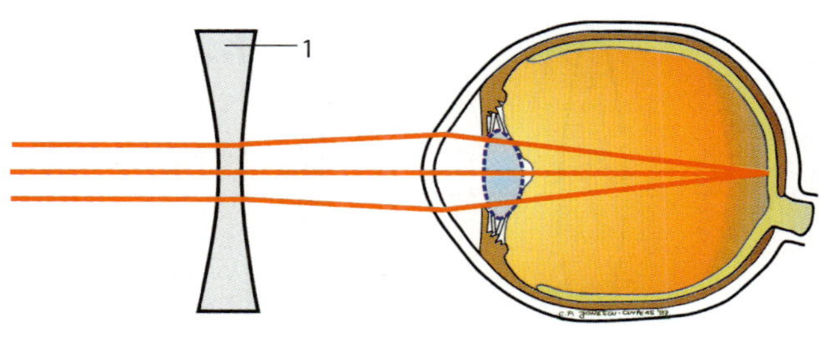

Figure 15.9   Myopia is corrected with concave lenses (1), which produce a sharply focussed retinal image by diffracting the light beams entering the eye. Myopic spectacle lenses produce image minification. Contact lenses, which are also used for the correction of myopia, have the advantage of a lesser degeree of image minification and visual field restriction, particularly in high myopia.

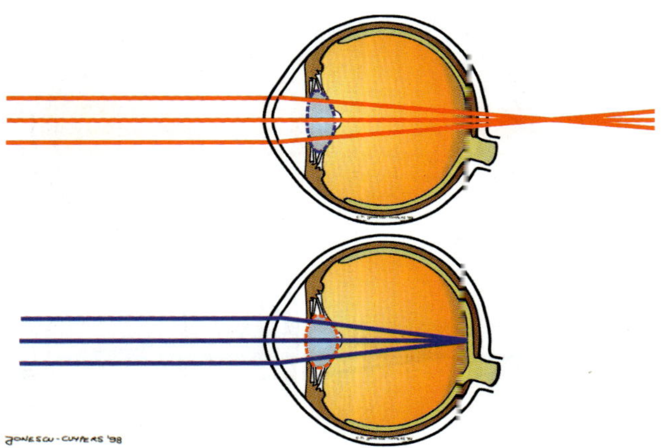

Figure 15.10   In the hypermetropic (hyperopic) eye parallel light beams (emerging from an object at infinity) entering the non-accommodated eye are focussed behind the retina *(top)*. Axial hypermetropia, i.e. the axial length is too short in relation to the refractive power of the media, is distinguished from refractive hypermetropia with a refractive power, which is too little in relation to the axial length (compare with figue 15.6). If the ability to accommodate is good *(bottom)*, i.e. particularly at young age, accommodation (changed shape of the lens is marked with *red interrupted line*) can compensate the hypermetropia, leading to latent hypermetropia. With high hypermetropia or decreased ability to accommodate, asthenopic symptoms occur, first during near vision, then also during far vision. Accommodation is normally coupled to convergence (compare with chapter 16). An abnormally increased convergence in hyperopia can produce disturbances in binocular vision.

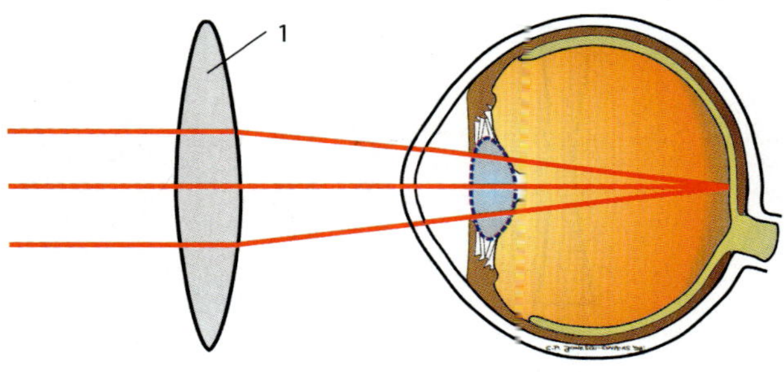

Figure 15.11   Hypermetropia is corrected with convex lenses (1), which produce a sharply focussed retinal image by converging the light beams entering the eye.

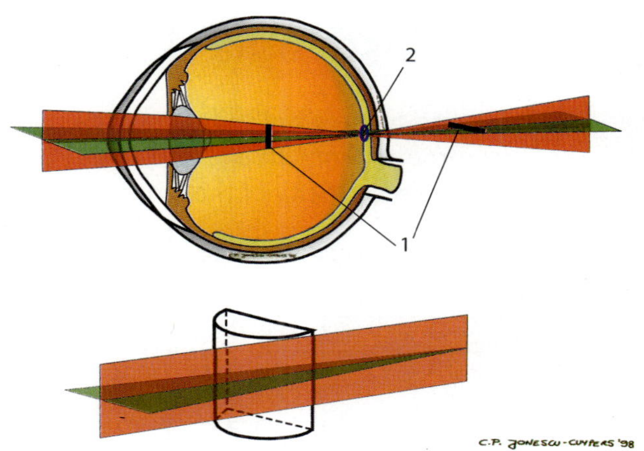

Figure 15.12 Astigmatism arises from different curvatures in different meridians of a refracting surface, i.e the cornea (the lens to a lesser degree). An object point is formed into two line images (1) at right angles to each other and at different distances along the axis. In between the line images lies the circle of least confusion (2).

Regular astigmatism, in which the meridians of dissimilar curvature are at right angles to each other, is distinguished from irregular astigmatism. An irregular astigmatism results mostly from uneven optical surfaces (e.g. corneal ulcer, scar). Regular astigmatism is subclassified into with-the-rule astigmatism (corneal curvature of greatest refractive power is vertical) and against-the-rule astigmatism (corneal curvature of greatest refractive power is horizontal). Astigmatism is corrected with cylindric lenses, of which the refractive power is greatest in a determined axis (*bottom*).

Figure 15.13 Anisometropia is the common condition in which both eyes have different refractive errors. The higher the amount of ametropia, the more often anisometropia occurs. Aniseikonia results from different retinal image sizes in both eyes with correction of ametropia, e.g. following unilateral lens extraction or with myopia in one eye and hypermetropia in the other eye. Problems with spectacle correction occur if the difference between the two eyes is more than 3 diopters. An aniseikonia of larger than 5% produces disturbances in binocular vision.

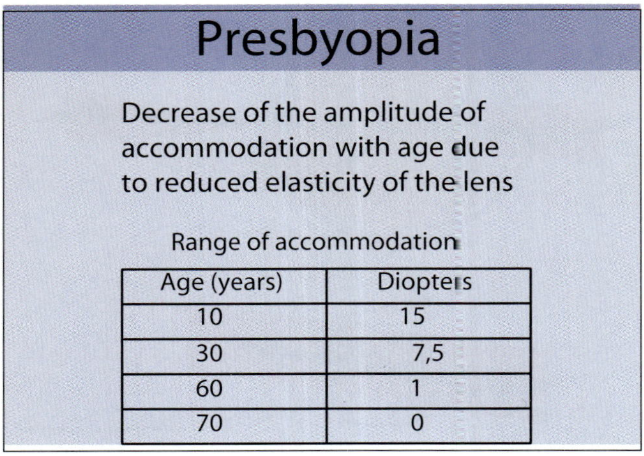

Presbyopia

Decrease of the amplitude of accommodation with age due to reduced elasticity of the lens

Range of accommodation

Age (years)	Diopters
10	15
30	7,5
60	1
70	0

Figure 15.14 Due to the condensation of lens fibers and the associated loss of elasticity of the lens that occurs with age, the range of accommodation continuously decreases. Presbyopia affects virtually all individuals above the age of 45, according to the progressive loss of the ability to accommodate. The range of accommodation comprises approx. 15 diopters at age 10, approx. 1 diopter at age 60 and vanishes around the age of 70. Presbyopia is corrected with convex lenses (plus lenses), of which the refractive power varies with age.

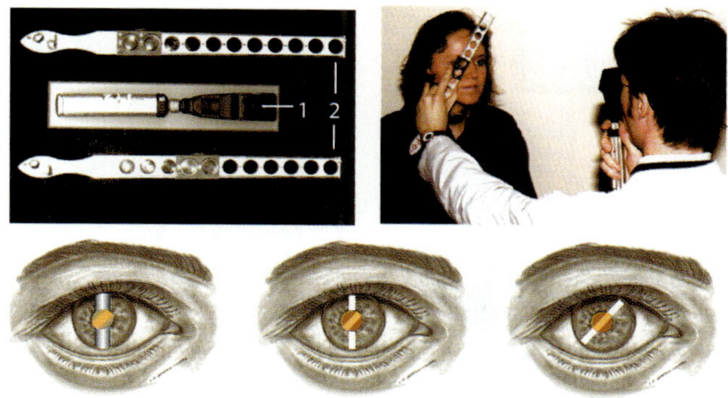

Figure 15.15 Various techniques have been developed in order to objectively assess the refractive error of an eye. One of them is streak retinoscopy (skiascopy). The streak retinoscope (1) is held in front of one of the examiner´s eyes, it projects a slit beam onto the eye of the patient that is examined *(top right)*. Various phenomena are observed, when the slit beam is moved across the pupil. The slit beam reflected from the retina may move in the same direction as the beam reflected fom the iris (with movement) or in the opposite direction (against movement). Plus and minus lenses of progressive power are held in front of the patient´s eye. The lens power is adjusted until the entire pupil lights up when moving the slit beam across it (neutral point). The slit beam can be rotated in order to take into account astigmatism *(bottom)*. There are various types of automated devices, so called auto-refractometers, used for objective refraction. Subjective refraction is performed with optotypes (compare with figures 15.3, 15.4). First, the best spherical correction is measured, then the cylindrical, e.g. with the cross-cylinder.

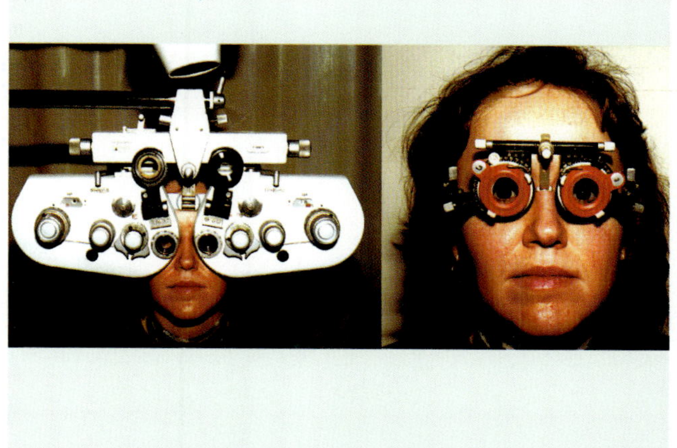

Figure 15.16 Phoropters *(left)* are widely used today for clinical refraction. These instruments incorporate spherical and astigmatic trial lenses as well as filters and diaphragms, which can be interposed by changing various dials, and have virtually replaced the trial frame *(right)*.

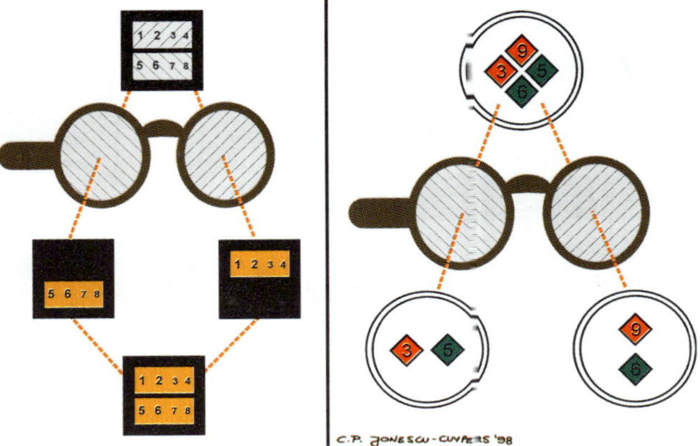

Figure 15.17 In order to balance the refraction obtained with monocular testing, binocular refraction is performed. Different techniques are applied to dissociate the eyes, i.e. different test targets are presented to each eye. The most widely used are polarizing filters. Osterberg´s red-green test uses polarizing filters in creating an individual red-green test for each eye (test types 9 and 6 for the right eye; test types 3 and 5 for the left eye). The refraction is balanced, if all four test types are seen equally.

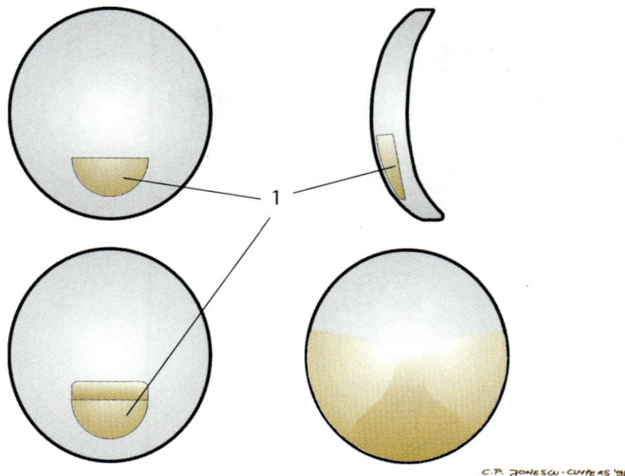

Figure 15.18 Refractive errors can be corrected with spectacle lenses. Multifocal lenses are used for the correction of ametropia in combination with presbyopia. Bifocal lenses *(top left)* are distinguished from trifocal lenses *(bottom left)*. The image jump at the dividing line of the reading segment (1) is eliminated in progressive multifocal lenses *(bottom right)*, they also have a cosmetic advantage. Patients are sometimes unable to adjust to progressive multifocal lenses, due to the amount of image distortion inherent in this type of lens.

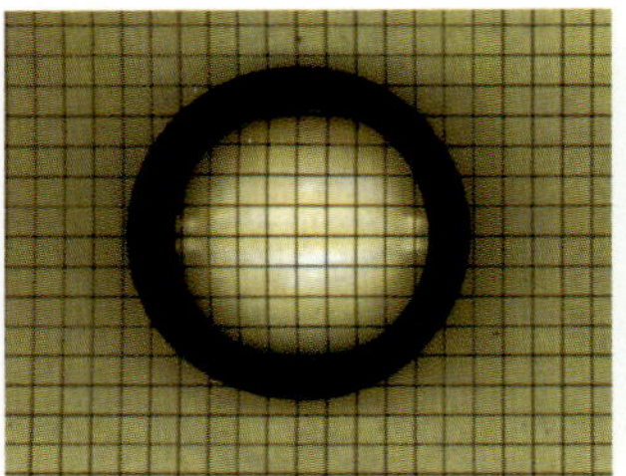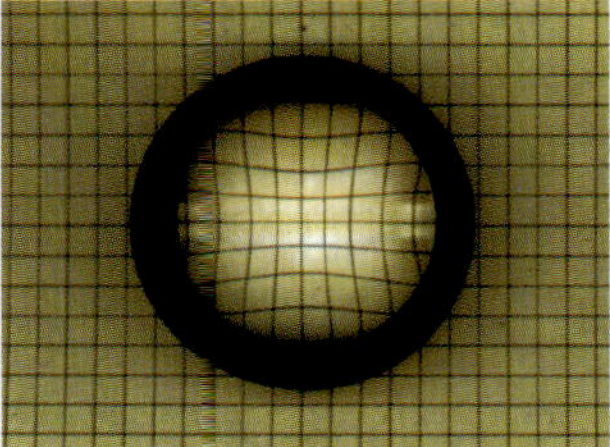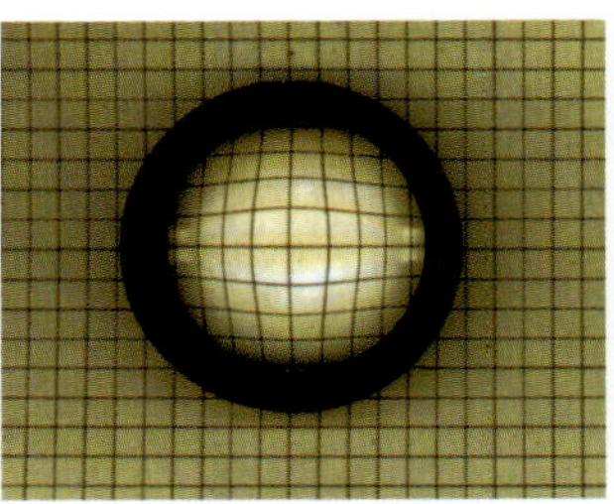

Figure 15.19 Spectacle lenses produce so-called distortion, i.e. an alteration of images caused by different magnification in the center and the edge of a lens. A square pattern is used to demonstrate this form of lens aberration. If magnification is uniform throughout a lens, no distortion is created *(left)*. A minus power lens exhibits a "barrel" distortion *(right)*, while a plus power lens produces a "pincushion" distortion of an image *(center)*. Other types of optical corrections are prisms, which are prescribed in heterophoria and heterotropia and high power convex lenses, which are used to enhance visual performance by magnification, if central visual acuity is severly impaired (compare with chapter 19).

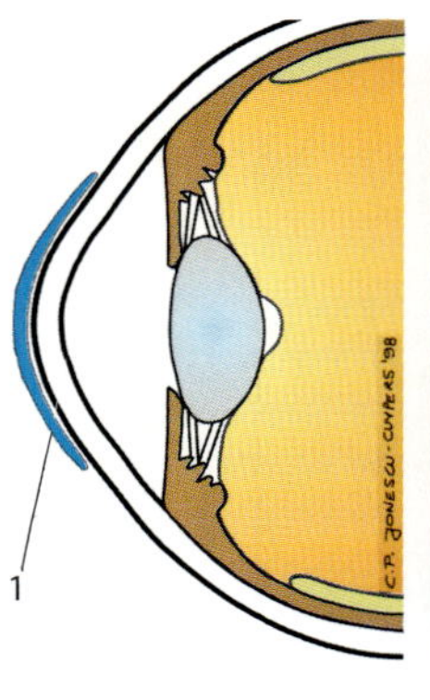
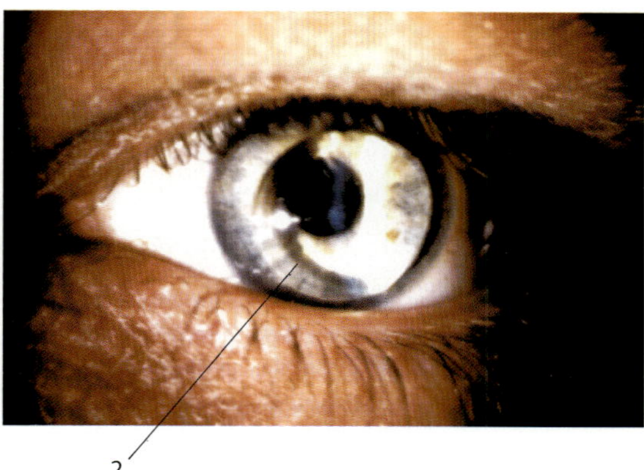

Figure 15.20   A correction of refractive errors can also be achieved with contact lenses. Hard and soft contact lenses are distinguished. Soft contact lenses (*left*) (1) have a diameter larger than the corneal diameter and mold to the corneal surface. Wearing comfort is the major advantage of soft contact lenses. They carry an increased risk of corneal infection, if care regimens are not strictly followed. Furthermore, they can induce allergic conjunctival changes and corneal neovascularization. For that reason, frequent eye exams are indispensable. Hard contact lenses (*right*) (2) have a diameter smaller than the corneal diameter, do not mold to the shape of the cornea and can therefore be used for the correction of astigmatism or other corneal anomalies such as keratoconus. Lens care is easier with hard contact lenses, but adaptation takes longer than with soft contact lenses. Unlike spectacle lenses, contact lenses do not produce image magnification or minification and visual field restriction (compare with figure 15.9).

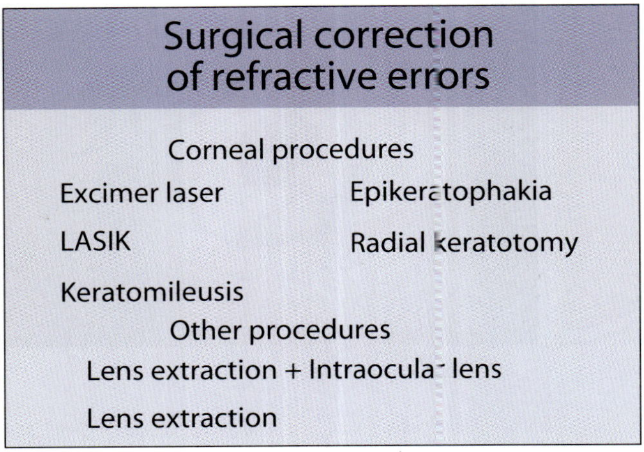

Surgical correction of refractive errors

Corneal procedures

Excimer laser   Epikeratophakia

LASIK   Radial keratotomy

Keratomileusis

Other procedures

Lens extraction + Intraocular lens

Lens extraction

Figure 15.21   There are numerous surgical procedures for the correction of refractive errors. Today, excimer laser photorefractive keratotomy (PRK) and laser in-situ keratomileusis (LASIK) are widely used for the correction of myopia. A postoperative complication, particularly following correction of high myopia, is stromal opacification. Other techniques include keratomileusis, which is accomplished by performing a lamellar keratectomy, resecting stromal tissue and replacing the "carved" corneal button on the bed, as well as keratophakia and epikeratophakia, where a prelathed tissue lens of donor corneal stroma is employed. In radial keratotomy (RK), flattening of the cornea and thereby reduction of myopia is achieved by making radial incisions (compare with chapter 4).

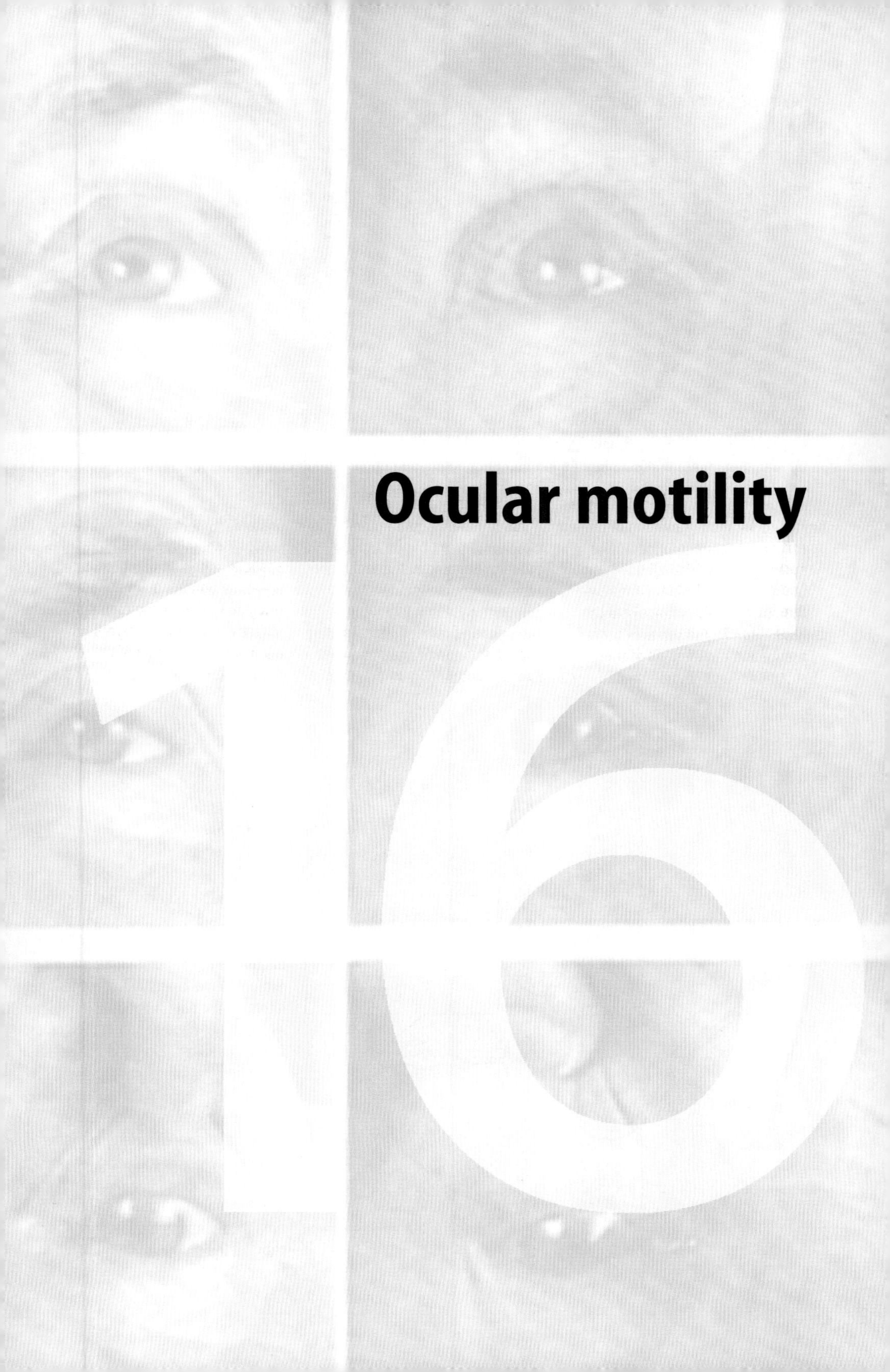

Ocular motility

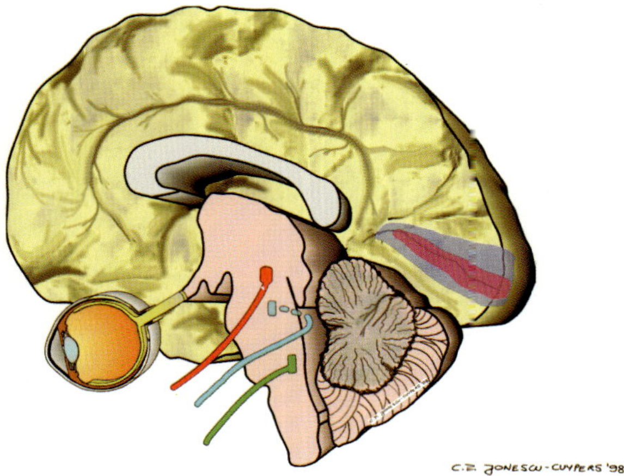

Figure 16.1 Innervation of the extraocular muscles. *Red* oculomotor nerve with nucleus in the brain stem, exit into the interpeduncular fossa, entrance into the orbit through the superior orbital fissure and innervation of the superior rectus muscle, medial rectus muscle, inferior rectus muscle, inferior oblique muscle and levator muscle. *Blue* trochlear nerve with nucleus in the brain stem, entrance into the orbit through the superior orbital fissure and innervation of the superior oblique muscle. *Green* abducens nerve with nucleus in the brain stem, exit laterally at the transition of pons and medulla oblongata, entrance into the orbit through the superior orbital fissure and innervation of the lateral rectus muscle.

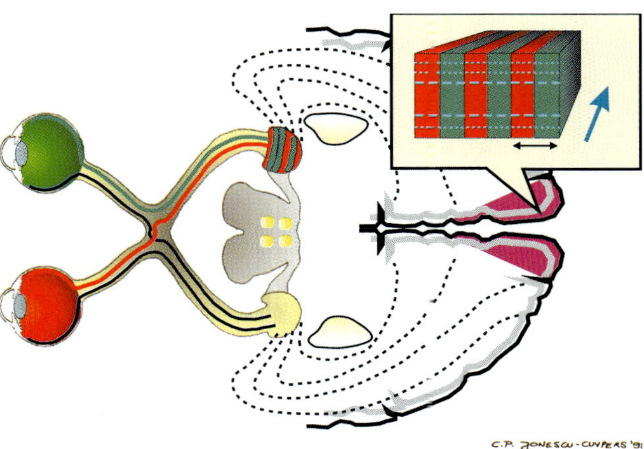

Figure 16.2 Cortical organization of binocularity. The axons from the temporal halves of the retinas do not decussate in the optic chiasm and project to the layers 2, 3, 5 in the lateral geniculate nucleus (*green*). The axons of the nasal retinal halves cross to the contralateral side in the optic chiasm and approach the layers 1, 4, 6 in the lateral geniculate nucleus (*red*). The visual radiation connects the lateral geniculate nucleus with the cortical area 17 in the occipital lobe. The nerve fibers of the visual radiation terminate in the layer IV of the area 17. The overyling layers contain most of the synaptic organization of binocularity.

Figure 16.3 *Top:* Normal retinal correspondence. The fixated object (A) projects to the fovea in both eyes. *Bottom:* Anomalous retinal correspondence. The left eye is esodeviated, the fixated object is projected nasally.

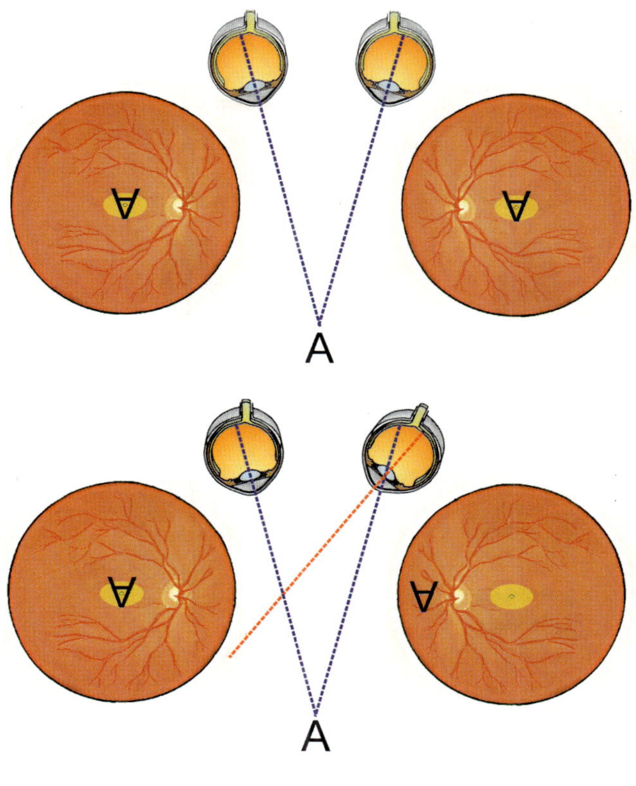

Figure 16.4 Visual acuity as a function of field angle. Visual acuity *(ordinate)* is greatest at the fovea and decreases exponentially with increasing distance from the fovea *(abscissa:* degrees of eccentricity).

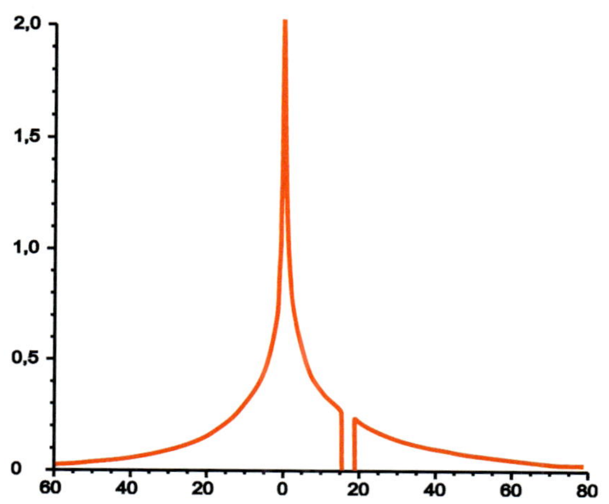

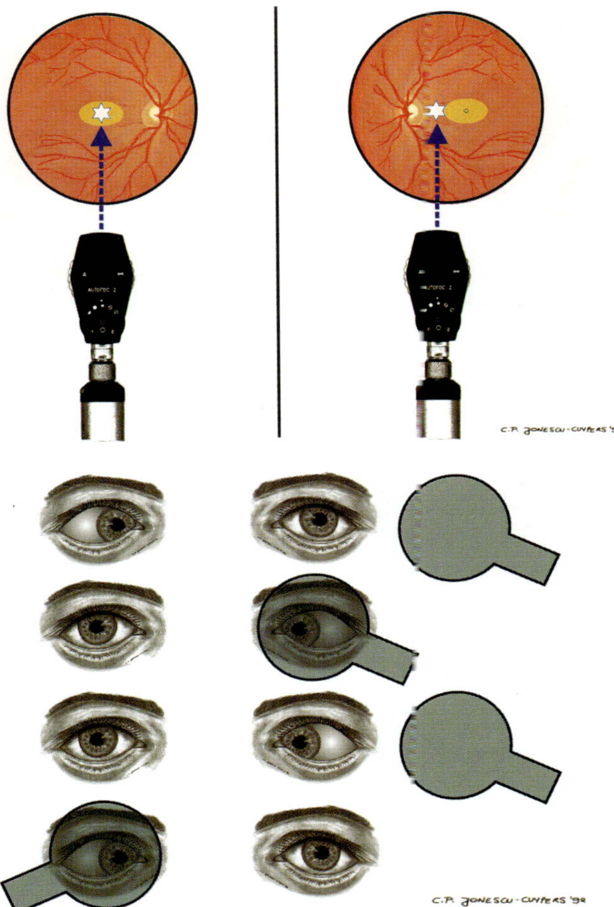

Figure 16.5 Evaluation of fixation with the direct ophthalmoscope. *Left:* Central fixation. The fixation star is projected on the fovea. *Right:* Nasal paramacular fixation.

Figure 16.6 Cover-uncover test. A patient with alternating esotropia (inward deviation) is examined *(top to bottom)*. The patient fixates a distant target. Before covering, the right eye is in a convergent position *(top)*. When the left (nonconvergent eye) is covered, the right eye moves outward and assumes fixation. When the left eye is uncovered, the initially deviated eye does not move and continues fixating. An outward movement of the left eye to assume fixation can be observed, when the right eye is covered *(bottom)*.

Figure 16.7 Cover-uncover test in a patient with alternating esotropia (compare with figure 16.6).

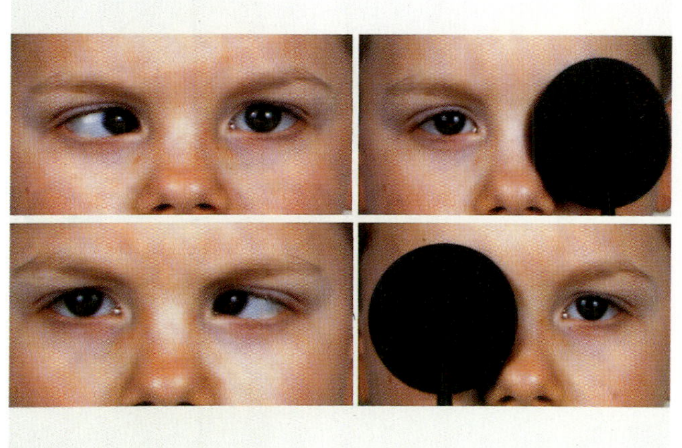

Figure 16.8 Cover-uncover test in esophoria (latent convergent strabismus). In the primary position *(top),* no manifest deviation can be observed. When one eye is covered, the uncovered eye does not move. Binocularity is denied. Removal of the cover reveals an outward movement of the convergent eye to assume fixation *(bottom).*

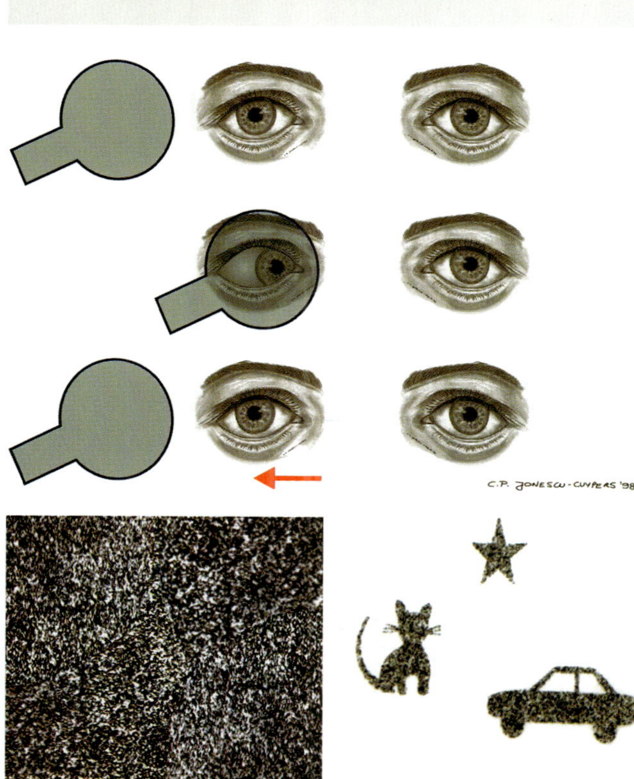

Figure 16.9 Stereoscopic test (Lang´s test). The test is based on the angular disparity phenomenon. Various objects (star, cat, car) are concealed by a grey pattern. Identification of the objects indicates stereopsis.

16.2 Examination techniques

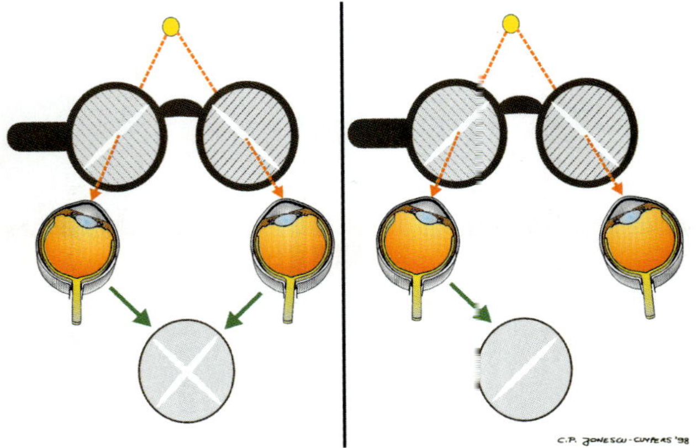

Figure 16.10 Bagolini striated glasses test. The *left frame* shows normal retinal correspondence and parallel alignment. A point light source is viewed through striated glasses as two perpendicular streaks of light. The *right frame* shows esotropia (inward deviation) in the right eye with exclusion of visual input. Only the streak of the left eye is viewed.

Figure 16.11   Testing for heterophoria. Binocular vision is dissociated by the use of a polarizing filter. The horizontal line is made visible to one eye, while the vertical line is made visible to the other. The *left frame* shows the binocular visual perception with parallel alignment, orthophoria. The *right frame* shows the binocular visual perception in heterophoria.

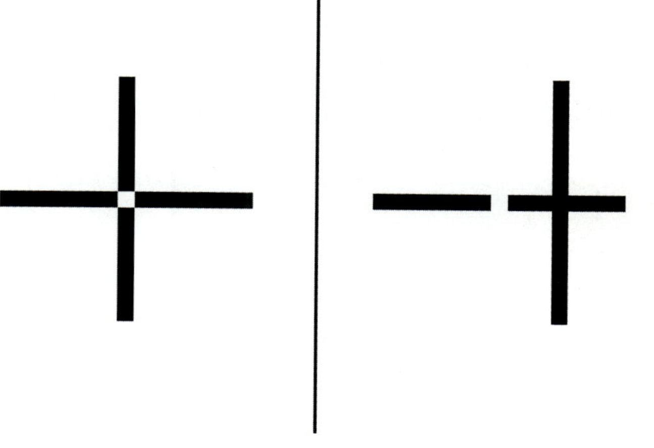

16.4 Heterotropia (manifest strabismus)

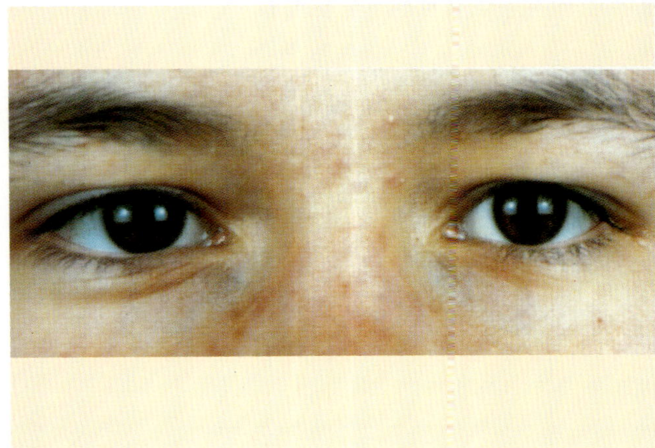

Figure 16.12 Microstrabismus. The figure shows a patient with microesotropia (inward deviation) of the right eye with small strabismus angle.

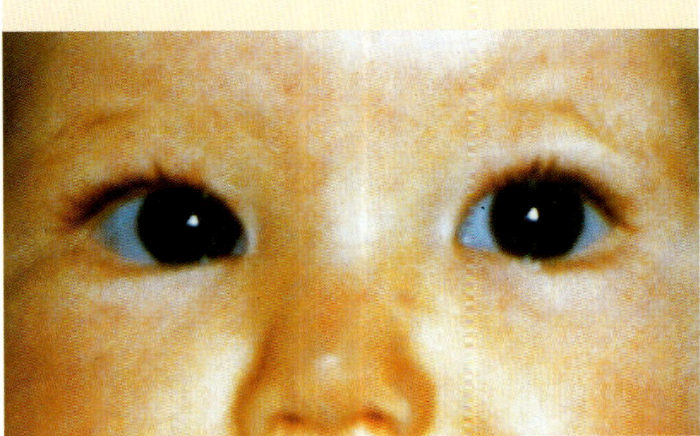

Figure 16.13 Pseudostrabismus due to epicanthus. A broad nasal bridge in combination with marked epicanthal folds, which cover the caruncle, are frequently apparent in infancy and give the impression of inward deviation, despite parallel alignment, so-called "pseudostrabismus". Note the central corneal reflex in both eyes.

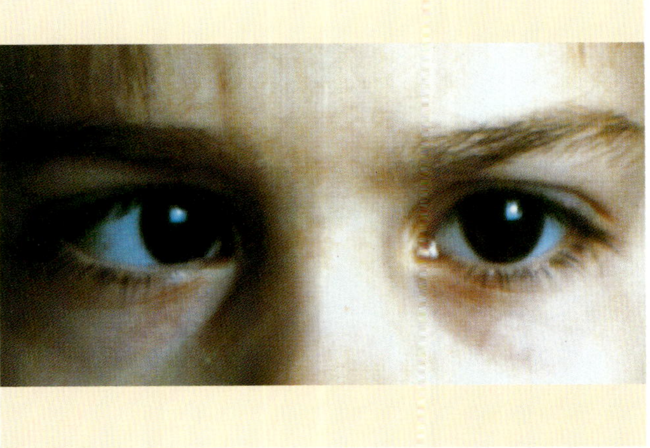

Figure 16.14 Convergent strabismus. There is a manifest inward deviation of the right eye. The corneal reflex in the right eye is displaced temporally from the pupillary center.

Figure 16.15   Divergent strabismus. There is an outward deviation of the right eye. The corneal reflex is displaced medially from the pupillary center.

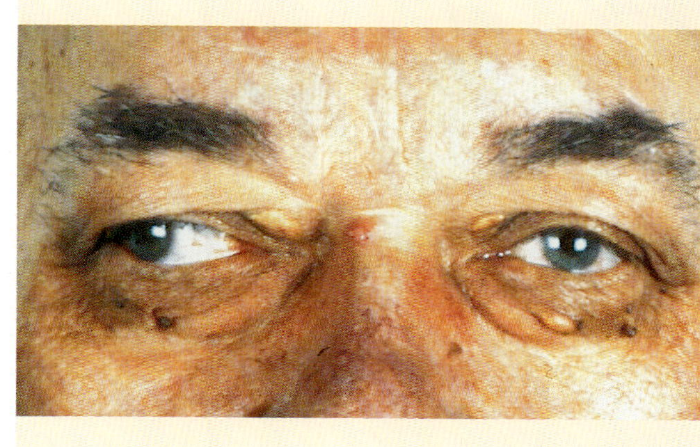

Figure 16.16   Congenital esotropia, V-pattern. In upgaze position *(top left),* there is almost parallel alignment. The inward deviation in the primary position *(top right)* increases on downgaze *(bottom).*

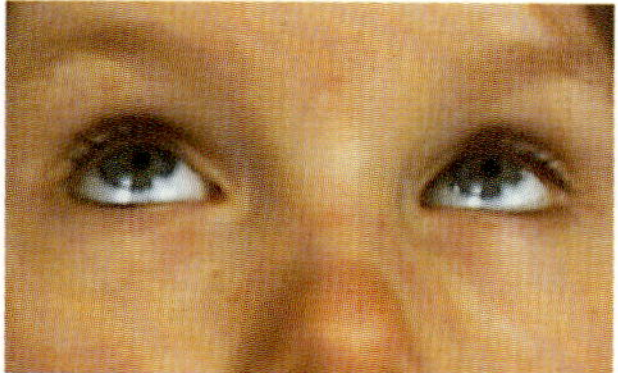
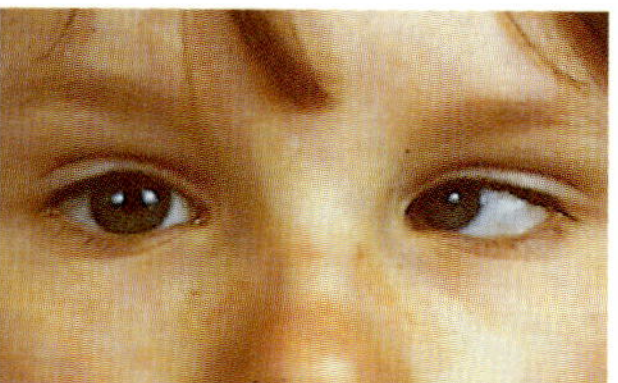
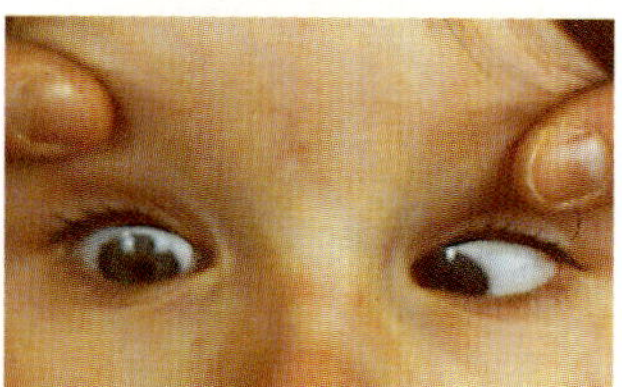

16.5 Cranial nerve palsies (paralytic strabismus)

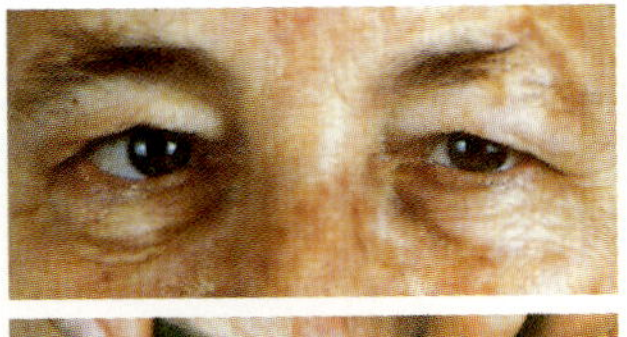
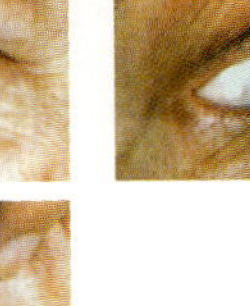
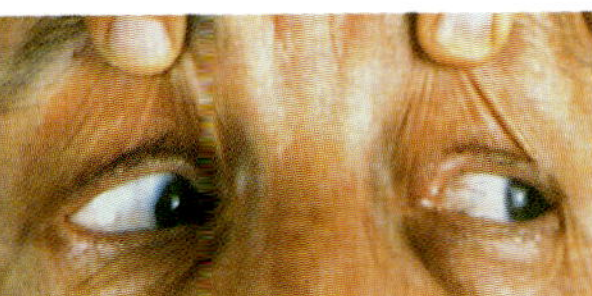
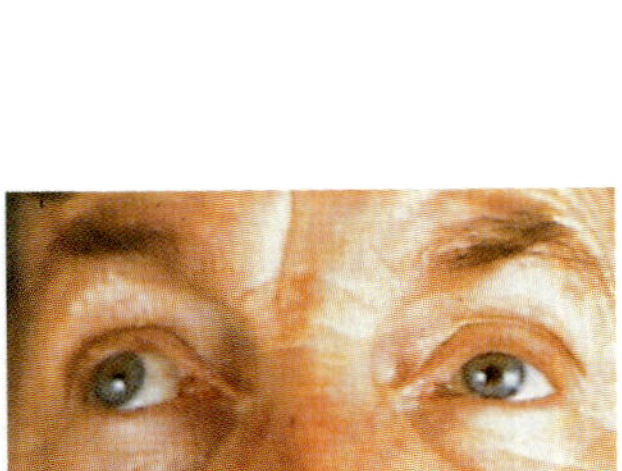

Figure 16.17 Paralytic strabismus of the right eye due to abducens nerve palsy. In the primary position *(top left)*, there is an inward deviation of the paretic right eye. In right gaze *(bottom right,)* abduction is absent in the paretic eye, while the sound eye shows normal adduction. In left gaze *(right),* horizontal ductions (adduction and abduction) are normal in both eyes.

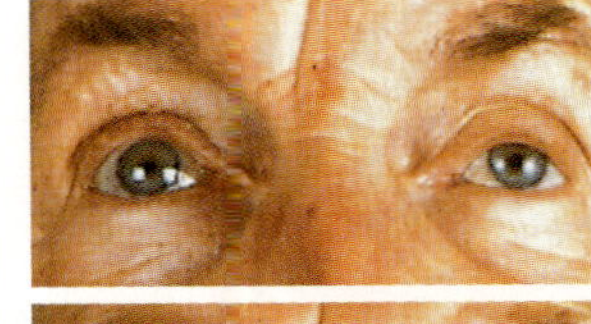
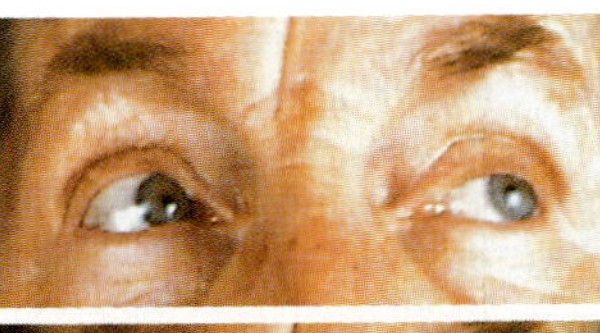
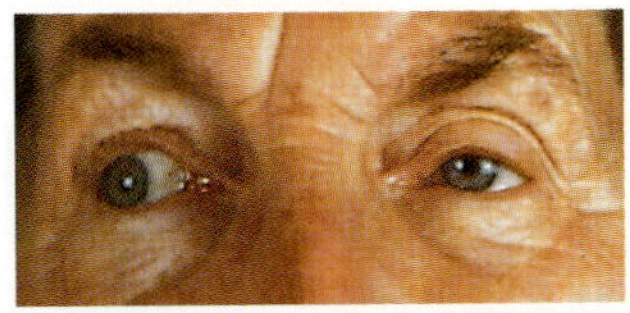
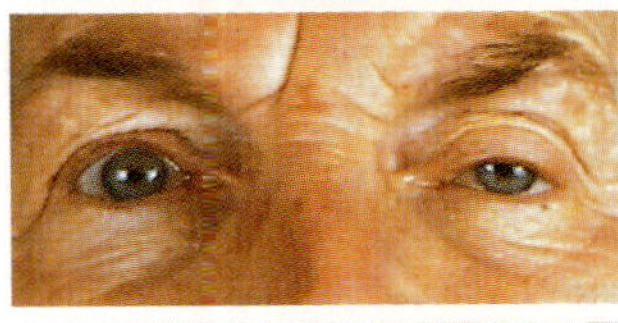
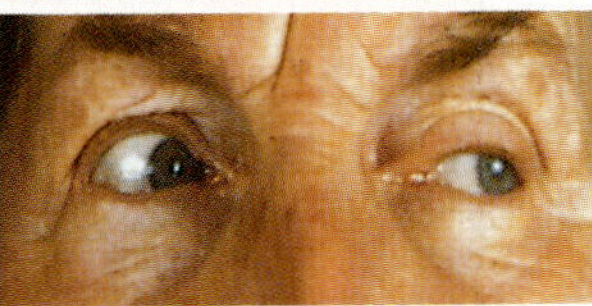
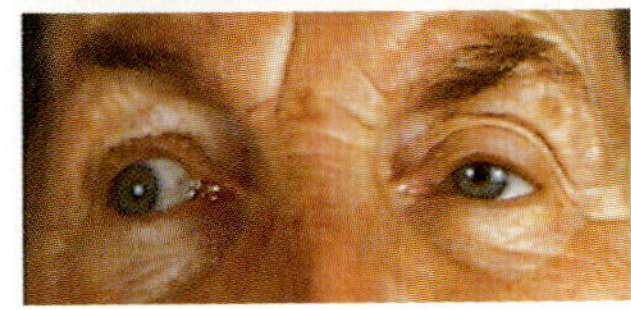
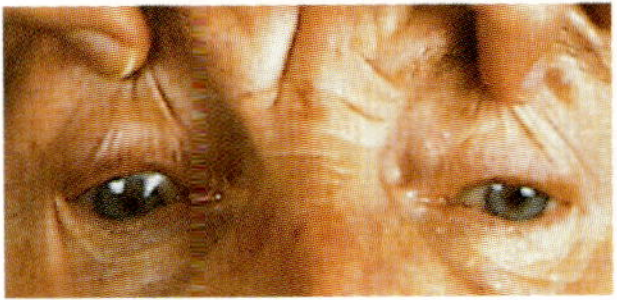
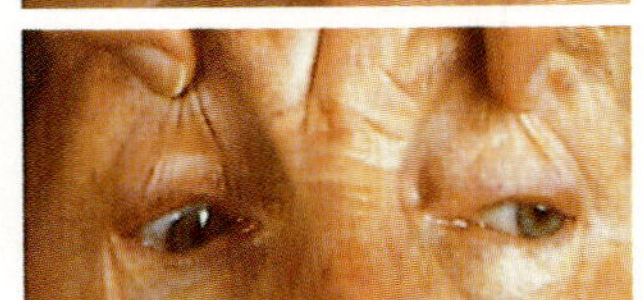

Figure 16.18 Paralytic strabismus of the left eye due to oculomotor nerve palsy. Involvement of the levator muscle results in mild ptosis in the left eye. The pupil in the paretic eye is moderately dilated due to involvement of the pupillary constrictor muscle. The nine cardinal positions are shown. The four extraocular muscles innervated by the oculomotor nerve are affected to various extents. Adduction is almost absent, elevation and depression are limited in the left eye. Abduction is intact, since the abducens nerve is not involved.

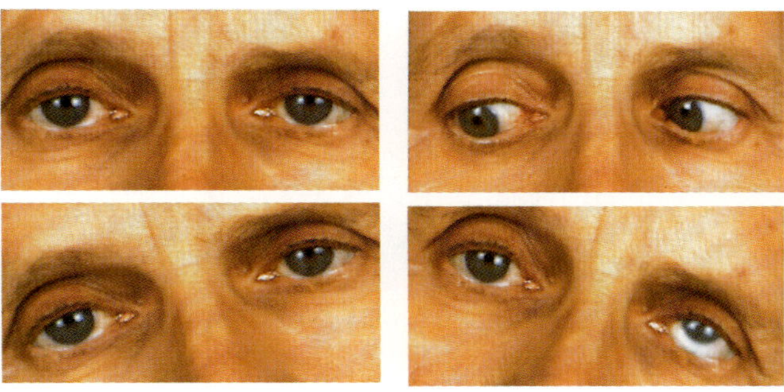

Figure 16.19 Paralytic strabismus of the left eye due to trochlear nerve palsy. There is no deviation in the primary position *(top left)*. In right gaze *(top right)*, adduction is limited in the left eye due to palsy of the superior oblique muscle. A compensatory viewing posture of head tilt to the right is assumed *(bottom left)*. As the head is tilted to the left (paretic) side, the left eye shows an upward deviation (positive Bielschowsky head tilt test). Defective incyclotorsion and depression due to palsy of the superior oblique muscle account for a positive head tilt test result.

16.6 Ocular myopathy

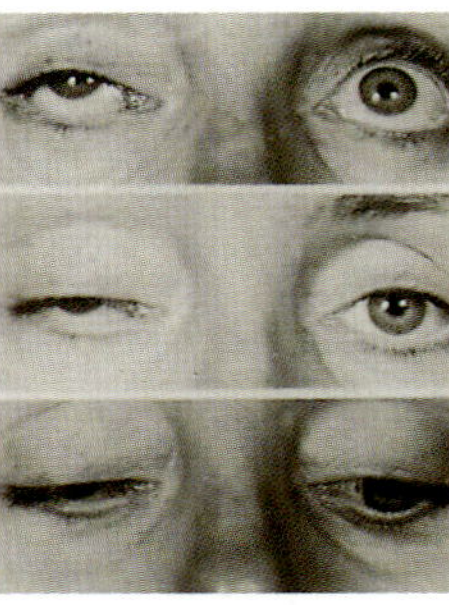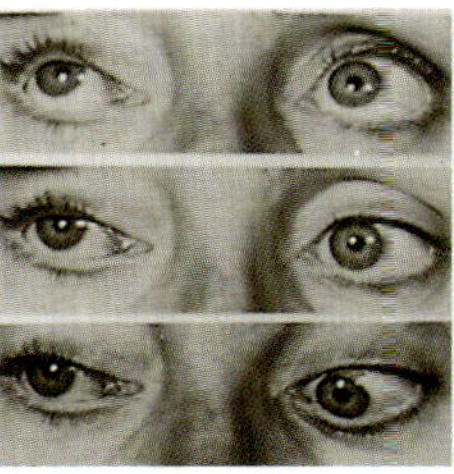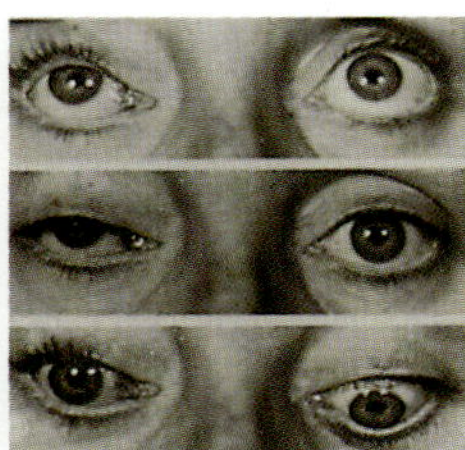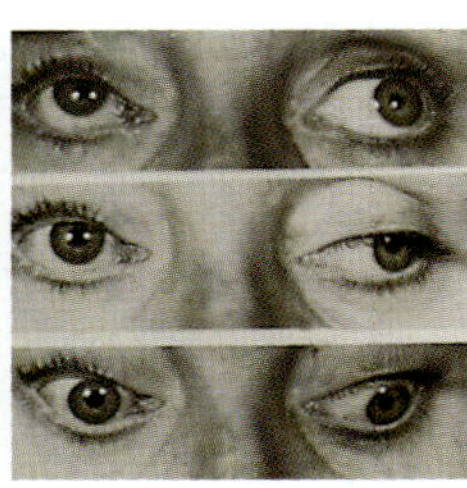

Figure 16.20 Palsy of extraocular muscles due to myasthenia gravis. The right eye shows ptosis (levator muscle) as well as limited depression (inferior rectus muscle), limited abduction (lateral rectus muscle) and limited adduction (medial rectus muscle). The left eye shows moderately limited elevation as well as moderately limited abduction and adduction. The palsies cannot be assigned to a particular ocular motor nerve, they result from defective neuromuscular transmission.

Figure 16.21 Overview of disorders affecting the ocular muscles.

Disorders of ocular muscles

Ocular myositis

Ocular myopathies
due to metabolic defects
(carnitine deficiency, amyloidosis, Refsum disease)

hereditary generalized muscular dystrophies

mitochondrial myopathies
(CPEO, Kearns-Sayre syndrome)

Ocular myotonia

Myasthenia

Endocrine ophthalmopathy

Traumatic restrictive myopathy

Figure 16.22 Various types of ocular nystagmus. The slow phase of the nystagmus is marked with a *blue arrow*, the fast (saccadic) phase is marked with a *red arrow*. The direction of the fast phase defines the nystagmus direction. *Top left* jerk-right nystagmus; *bottom left* jerk left nystagmus; *top middle* pendular nystagmus; *bottom middle* circular nystagmus; *top right* upbeat nystagmus; *bottom right* downbeat nystagmus.

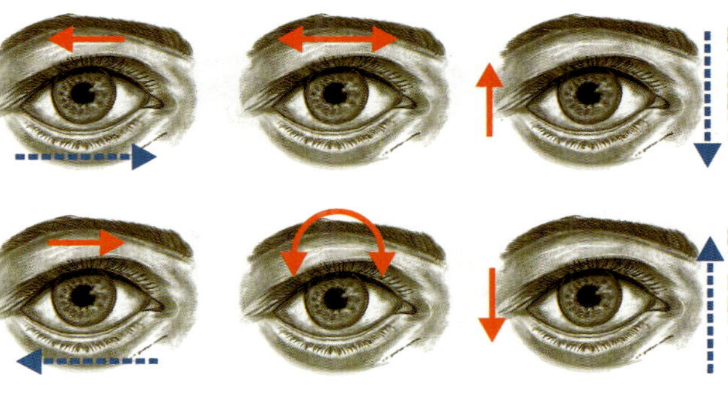

Figure 16.23 Overview of different causes of nystagmus and associated disorders.

Nystagmus		
Causes / associated disorders		
Congenital		
Ocular	Albinism; aniridia congenital cataract ROP	Optic nerve hypoplasia retinal dystrophies central retinal scars (e.g. toxoplasmosis) colobomas

Acquired	Peripheral-vestibular
	  Infectious-inflammatory
	  Toxic
	  Vascular
	  Tumor
	  Acoustic neurinoma
		Central
		  Toxic
		  Vascular
		  Inflammatory (demyelination)
		  Tumor
		  Spasmus nutans
		  Arnold-Chiari syndrome

16.8 Gaze palsies

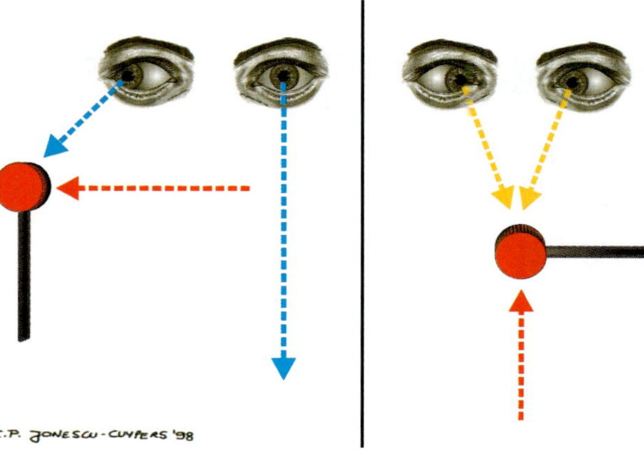

Figure 16.24　Gaze palsy. In right gaze, there is no adduction of the left eye *(left)*. Adduction however occurs with convergence associated with near fixation *(right)*. This impairment of binocular gaze coordination is caused by a lesion in the brainstem.

Gaze palsies		
Causes / types		
Vertical	Pineal gland tumor Vascular Inflammatory demyelination (MS) Infection (syphilis) Parinaud syndrome	
Horizontal	**Unilateral** *Pontine lesion* Vascular Inflammatory Tumor *Hemispheric lesion* Vascular	**Bilateral** *Pontine lesion* Vascular Inflammatory Tumor

Figure 16.25　Overview of different causes of various types of gaze palsies.

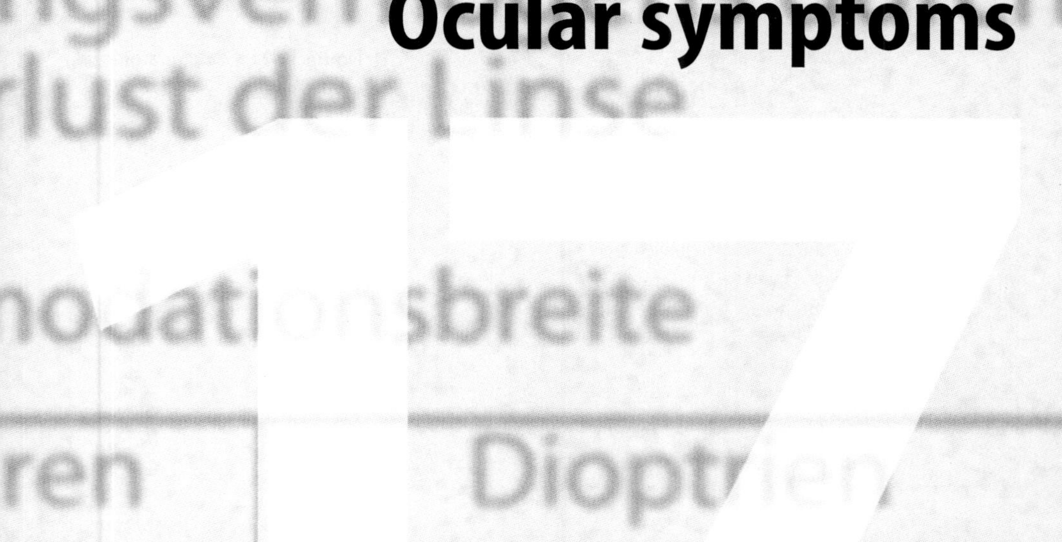

Ocular symptoms

17

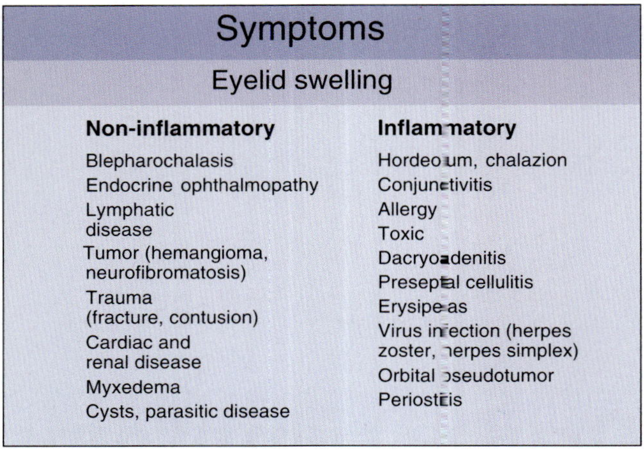

Symptoms

Eyelid swelling

Non-inflammatory

Blepharochalasis
Endocrine ophthalmopathy
Lymphatic
disease
Tumor (hemangioma,
neurofibromatosis)
Trauma
(fracture, contusion)
Cardiac and
renal disease
Myxedema
Cysts, parasitic disease

Inflammatory

Hordeolum, chalazion
Conjunctivitis
Allergy
Toxic
Dacryoadenitis
Preseptal cellulitis
Erysipelas
Virus infection (herpes
zoster, herpes simplex)
Orbital pseudotumor
Periostitis

Figure 17.1 Overview of common causes of eyelid swelling.

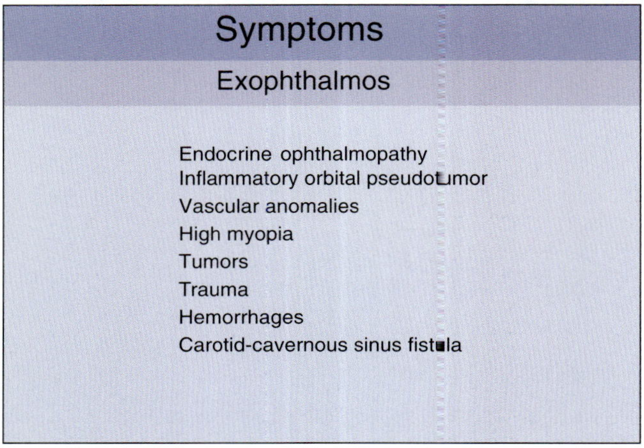

Symptoms

Exophthalmos

Endocrine ophthalmopathy
Inflammatory orbital pseudotumor
Vascular anomalies
High myopia
Tumors
Trauma
Hemorrhages
Carotid-cavernous sinus fistula

Figure 17.2 Common causes of exophthalmos.

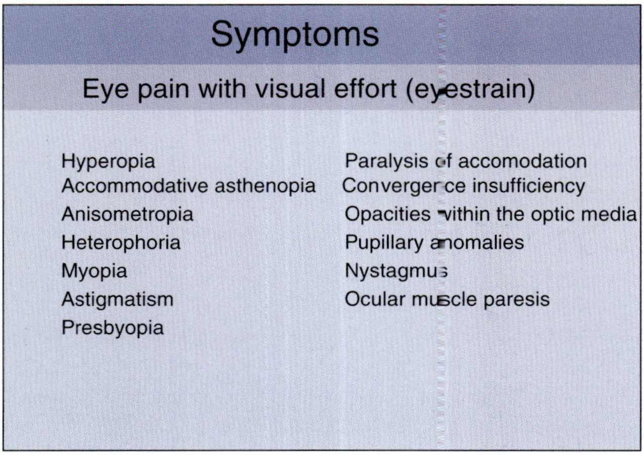

Symptoms

Eye pain with visual effort (eyestrain)

Hyperopia
Accommodative asthenopia
Anisometropia
Heterophoria
Myopia
Astigmatism
Presbyopia

Paralysis of accomodation
Convergence insufficiency
Opacities within the optic media
Pupillary anomalies
Nystagmus
Ocular muscle paresis

Figure 17.3 Overview of common causes of eye pain with visual effort (eyestrain).

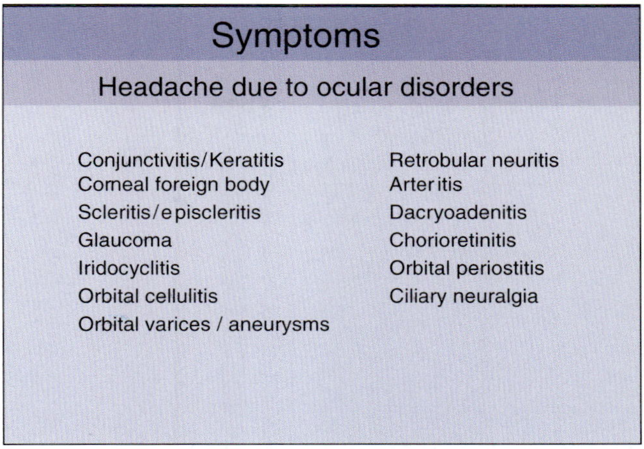

Figure 17.4 Common causes of headache in association with various ocular disorders.

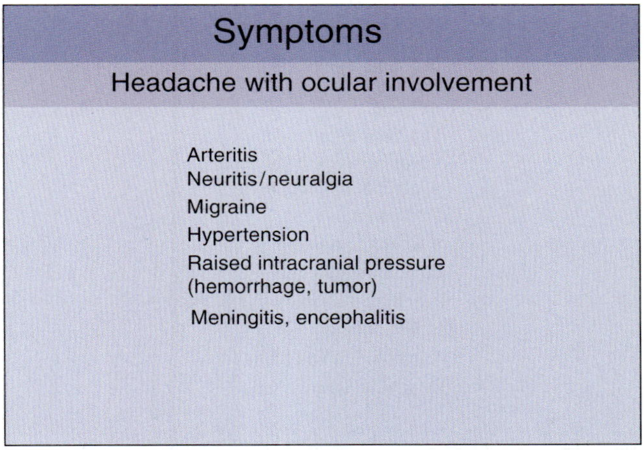

Symptoms

Headache due to ocular disorders

Conjunctivitis/Keratitis	Retrobular neuritis
Corneal foreign body	Arteritis
Scleritis/episcleritis	Dacryoadenitis
Glaucoma	Chorioretinitis
Iridocyclitis	Orbital periostitis
Orbital cellulitis	Ciliary neuralgia
Orbital varices / aneurysms	

Figure 17.5 Common causes of headache with ocular involvement.

Symptoms

Headache with ocular involvement

Arteritis

Neuritis/neuralgia

Migraine

Hypertension

Raised intracranial pressure
(hemorrhage, tumor)

Meningitis, encephalitis

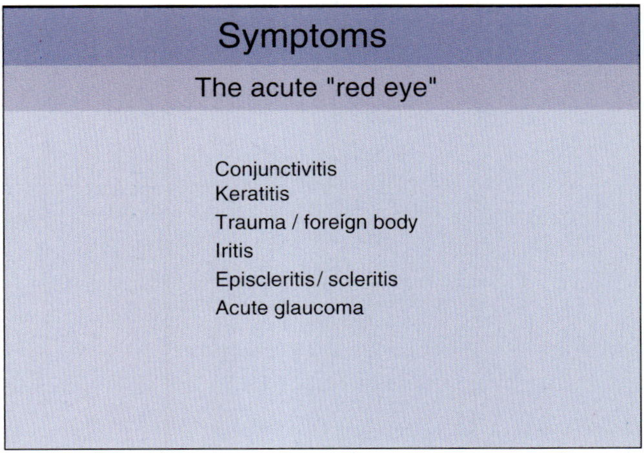

Figure 17.6 Common causes of the acute „red eye".

Symptoms

The acute "red eye"

Conjunctivitis

Keratitis

Trauma / foreign body

Iritis

Episcleritis / scleritis

Acute glaucoma

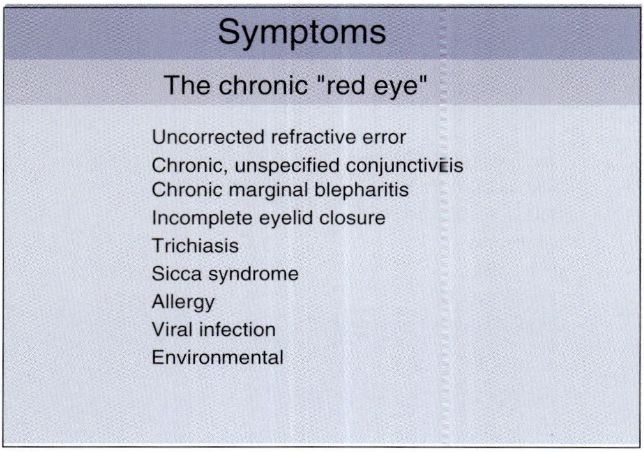

Symptoms

The chronic "red eye"

Uncorrected refractive error
Chronic, unspecified conjunctivitis
Chronic marginal blepharitis
Incomplete eyelid closure
Trichiasis
Sicca syndrome
Allergy
Viral infection
Environmental

Figure 17.7 Common causes of the chronic „red eye".

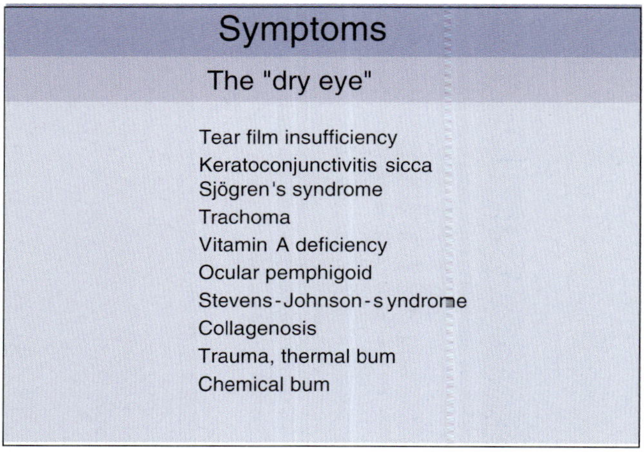

Symptoms

The "dry eye"

Tear film insufficiency
Keratoconjunctivitis sicca
Sjögren's syndrome
Trachoma
Vitamin A deficiency
Ocular pemphigoid
Stevens-Johnson-syndrome
Collagenosis
Trauma, thermal bum
Chemical bum

Figure 17.8 Common causes of the „dry eye".

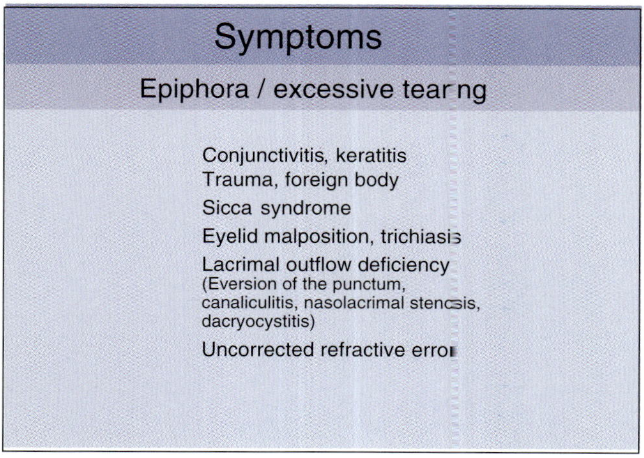

Symptoms

Epiphora / excessive tearing

Conjunctivitis, keratitis
Trauma, foreign body
Sicca syndrome
Eyelid malposition, trichiasis
Lacrimal outflow deficiency
(Eversion of the punctum,
canaliculitis, nasolacrimal stenosis,
dacryocystitis)
Uncorrected refractive error

Figure 17.9 Differential diagnosis of epiphora / excessive tearing.

Figure 17.10   Common causes of an acute loss of vision.

Symptoms

"Sudden" loss of vision

Central retinal vein occlusion
Central retinal artery occlusion
Acute glaucoma
Vitreous hemorrhage
Retinal detachment
Retrobulbar neuritis
Ischemic optic neuropathy
Central chorioretinitis
Homonymous hemianopia

Figure 17.11   Common causes of an insidious loss of vision.

Symptoms

"Insidious" loss of vision

Refractive error
Cataract
Macular degeneration
Chronic glaucoma
Diabetic retinopathy
Retinitis pigmentosa
Choroidal tumor
Optic neuropathy
Chiasmal tumors

Figure 17.12   Common causes of a temporary loss of vision.

Symptoms

"Temporary" loss of vision

Amaurosis fugax
Migraine
Subacute glaucoma
Retinal embolization
Optic disc edema
Circulatory disorders

Symptoms

Diplopia

Binocular

Paralytic strabismus
Myasthenia
Ocular myopathy
Endocrine ophthalmopathy
Orbital tumor
Orbital hematoma
Blow-out-fracture
Internuclear
ophthalmoplegia

Monocular

Cataract
Corneal scars
Iridodialysis
Polycoria

Figure 17.13 Common causes of binocular and monocular diplopia.

Symptoms

Glare / photophobia

Mydriasis
Aniridia
Iris colomba
Albinism
Opacities
within the optic media
Conjunctivitis, keratitis, iritis
Retrobulbar neuritis

Achromatopsia
Infectious disease
(measles, rabies)
Cranial trauma
Trigeminal neuralgia
Migraine
Bright artificial light

Figure 17.14 Common causes of glare / photophobia.

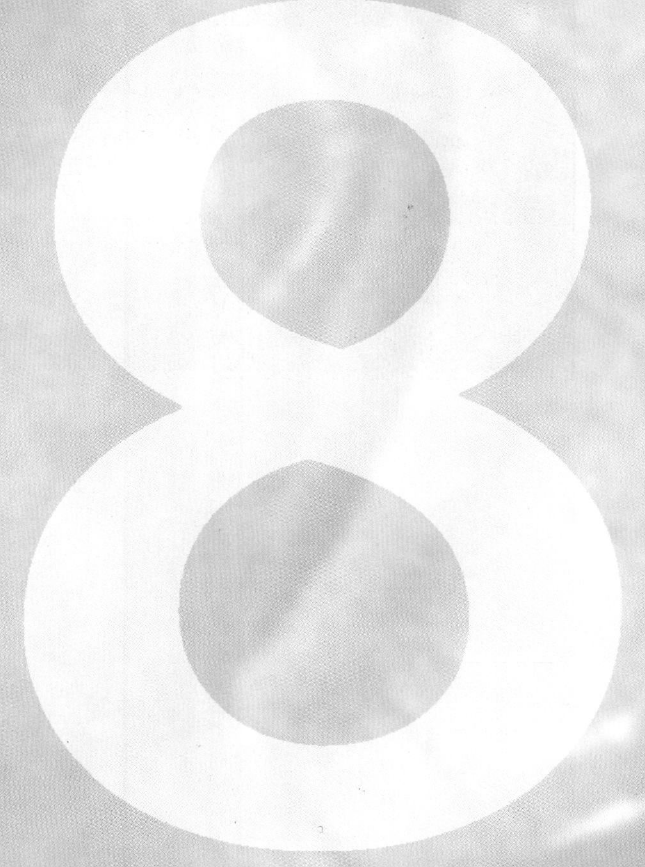

Trauma

18

18.1 Trauma to the eyelids and orbit

General: Injuries involving the eyelids can result from blunt trauma (lacerations) or penetrating trauma (cut). Periorbital and eyelid trauma requires careful examination in order to rule out injury to the globe, the orbit and the anterior cranial fossa. Antibiotic prophylaxis is necessary, since the orbital veins empty into the cavernous sinus and pteryoid plexus (compare with chapter 14). A detailed anatomic knowledge (compare with chapter 1) is needed for surgical repair of injured eyelids in order to obtain good functional results. In orbital trauma, radiographic examination has to be conducted to rule out fractures of the orbit and neighboring cranial structures. Antibiotic prophylaxis is mandatory, if the orbital septum is opened (compare with chapter 14). Essential procedures are the assessment of visual acuity, ocular motility testing (to rule ot e.g. blow-out fracture, compare with figures 18.10, 18.11), pupillary testing (to rule out optic nerve injury) and the exclusion of intracranial injuries (neurologic consultation).

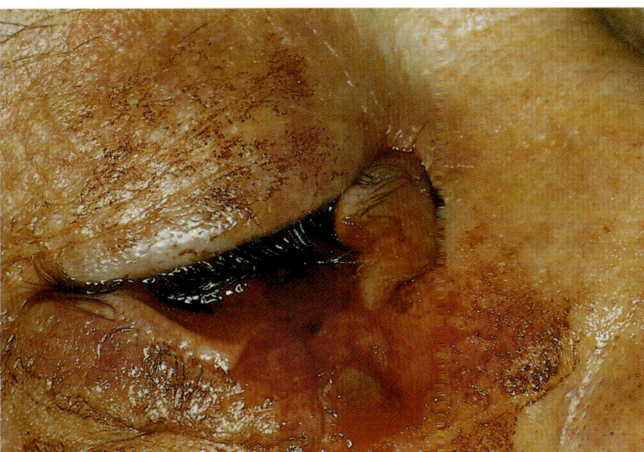

Figure 18.1 Cut to the lower eyelid. The figure shows an injury, which affects the full thickness of the lower eyelid and extends to the inferior periocular area.

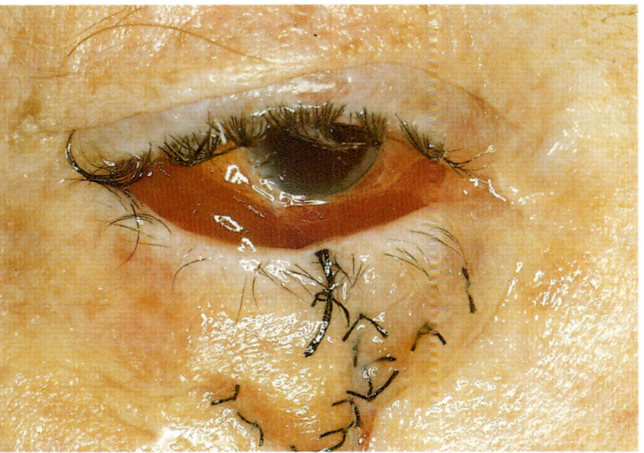

Figure 18.2 Status post surgical repair (compare with figure 18.1) with exact reapproximation of the eyelid margin and the deeper layers. Intact eyelid position postoperatively.

Figure 18.3 Status post windshield injury and surgical repair. The figure shows a typical wound presenting in windshield injury. The cut to the upper eyelids and the nose bridge is so characteristic that the mechanism of injury can be concluded from the wound. The frequency of injuries of this kind has decreased significantly since seat-belts have become mandatory. Note that eyelid position is good following surgical repair, there is incomplete eyelid closure in downgaze in the left eye.

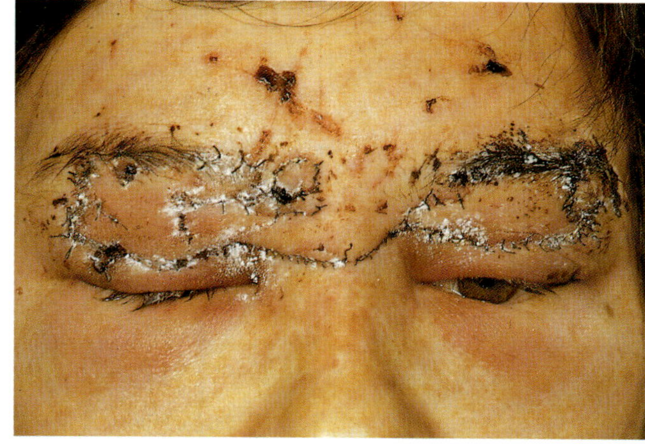

Figure 18.4 Status post windshield injury, incomplete eyelid closure. Avulsions with loss of tissue frequently occur in severe windshield injuries. In such cases, surgical repair is extremely diffcult. Tissue defects asociated with extensive scarring can lead to significant incomplete eyelid closure following primary surgical repair.

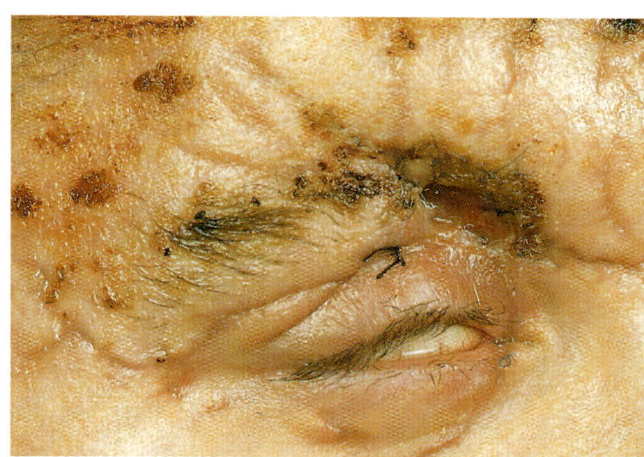

Figure 18.5 Status post severe facial injury (cut). Note the lagophthalmos due to scar formation in the upper lid in the left eye. The upper eyelid is retracted in downgaze. Eyelid closure is incomplete, the cornea is exposed. Scar revision has to be performed.

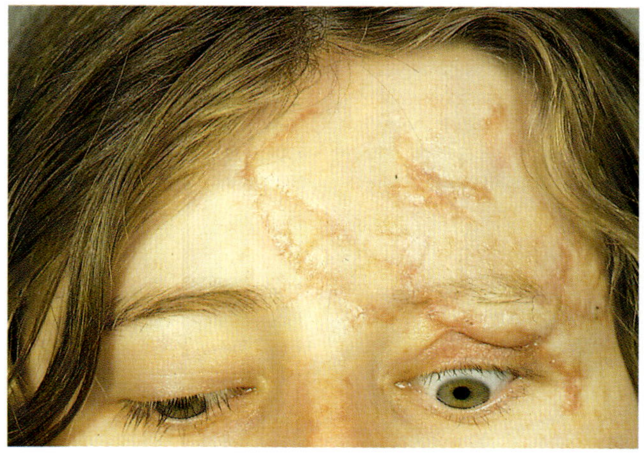

18.1 Trauma to the eyelids and orbit

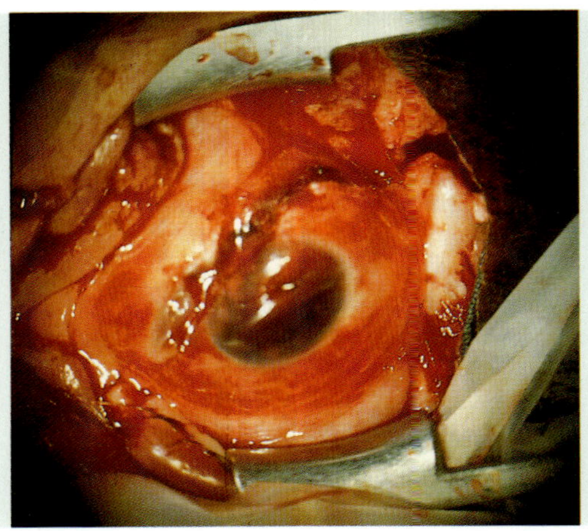

Figure 18.6   Injury to the eyelids and the globe (windshield). The figure shows multiple full-thickness lacerations of the eyelids and a penetrating globe injury at the limbus extending from the 9 to 12 o´clock position and to the periphery. The surgical reconstruction of the eyelids and the globe is one of the most challenging tasks. The patient has to be admitted immediately. If possible, radiographic studies should be conducted before surgery.

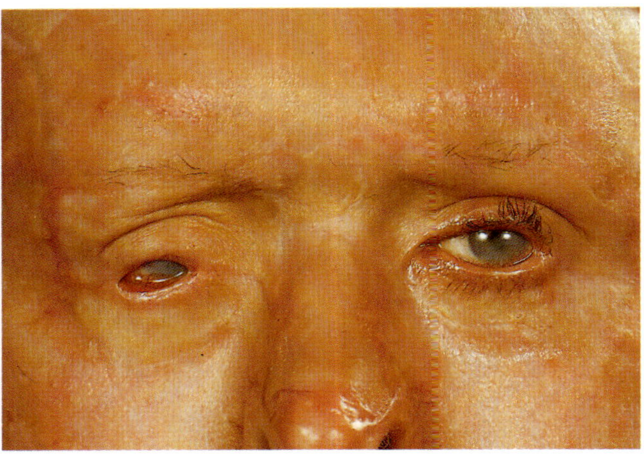

Figure 18.7   Status post thermal facial burn. Burns lead to coagulation necroses with susbsequent scar formation and progressive shrinkage of the skin. If the eyelids are affected, significant incomplete eyelid closure can ensue. Scar revisions, including skin grafting, are necessary. Severe corneal complications occur, if sufficient eyelid closure cannot be achieved. The figure shows a status post facial burn. Note the bilateral corneal opacification due to incomplete eyelid closure, lack of blink reflex and reduced tear secretion. The right palpebral fissure was surgically reduced in size (tarsorraphy) in order to protect the cornea.

Figure 18.8 Status post explosion injury with severe thermal burn, status post implantation of skin grafts in the upper eyelids. As a result, the upper lids are relatively rigid, however, they provide sufficient protection of the globe. The lower eyelids are retracted, exposing the inferior third of the cornea and the inferior sclera. Multiple surgical revisions were necessary in the later course.

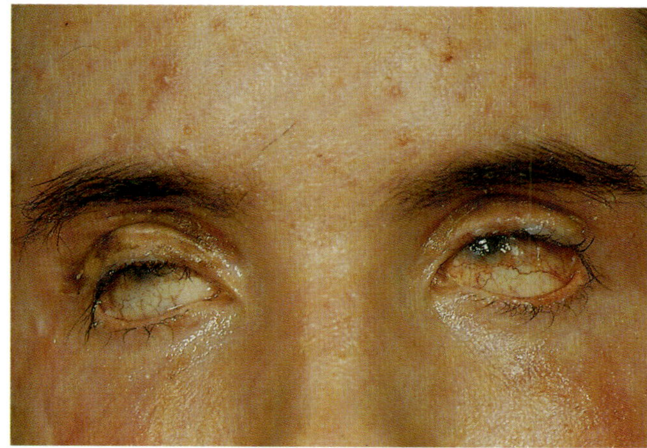

Figure 18.9 Hematoma of the upper and lower eyelids following closed head trauma. Skull fracture has to be ruled out in the presence of bilateral periocular hematoma.

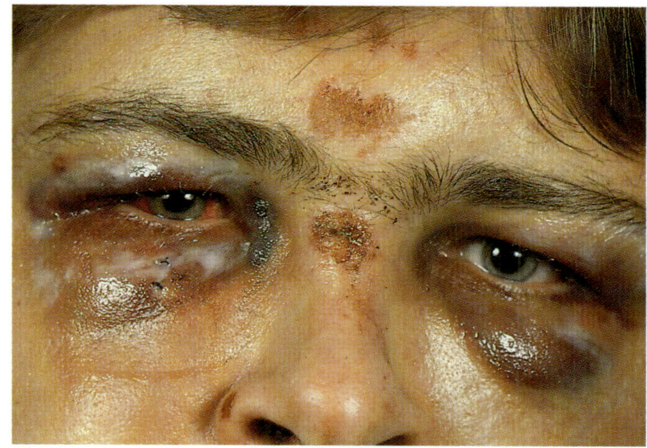

Figure 18.10 Left-sided blow-out fracture, restricted elevation of the globe. The bony walls of the orbit are extremely thin in places (compare with chapter 14). Blunt trauma to the globe and the orbital rim frequently results in fractures of the orbital floor and the medial orbital wall. The inferior rectus muscle can become entrapped within a fracture of the orbital floor. In such a case, the motility findings include restricted elevation and depression of the globe. The figure shows the characteristic picture of restricted elevation in the left eye due to blow-out fracture of the orbital floor. Involvement of the infraorbital nerve results in sensory abnormality in the supplied area.

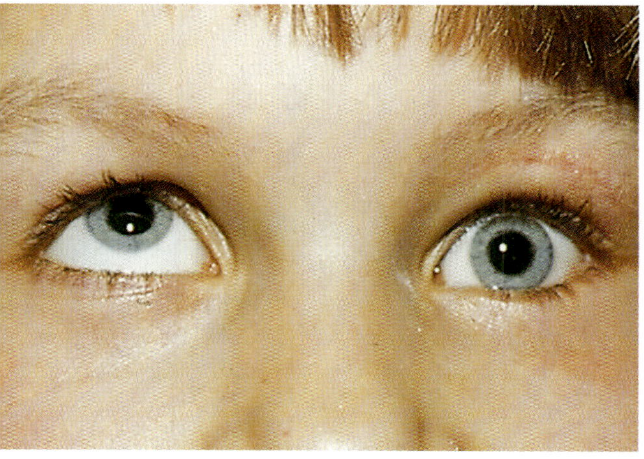

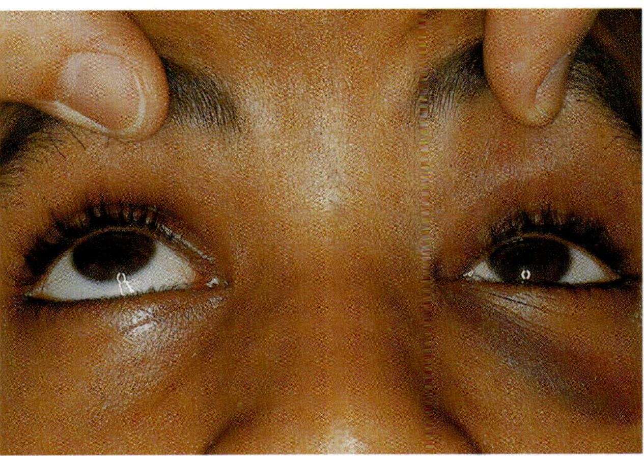

Figure 18.11 Blow-out fracture, enophthalmos. In fractures of the orbital walls, orbital tissue can be incarcerated within the fracture site. Extraocular muscles and orbital fat can be displaced to the neighboring sinuses (mostly maxillary sinus), resulting in enophthalmos. The figure shows left-sided enophthalmos and restricted elevation of the globe due to blow-out fracture of the orbital floor. The diagnosis of a blow out fracture is determined by:

1. plain x-ray studies or CT (visible fracture or opacification of the maxillary sinus),
2. motility status (almost always restricted elevation and depression),
3. test of facial sensation (hypesthesia or anesthesia in the supplied areas by the infraorbital nerve).

Surgical repair is indicated in severe blow-out fractures like this.

General: Every chemical burn can induce severe complications. The amount of complications depends on the pH of the damaging agent, the time of exposure and the rapidity with which therapy is initiated. The severity of an alkali burn (colliquative necrosis) cannot be determined until several hours after the accident. The classification and assessment of prognosis is based on the degree of damage to the perilimbal vessels, the corneal changes (erosion, opacification) and involvement of deeper ocular structures. Alkalies rapidly destroy cells. Penetration into deeper ocular structures causes a rise in pH of the aqueous. Ammonium hydroxide can be found in the anterior chamber within a few seconds of contact. The damage caused by acid burns is limited by the coagulation of proteins in the epithelium and superficial corneal stroma. In general, acid burns have a better prognosis than alkali burns. In any case of chemical eye burn, immediate flushing - preferably with Ringer lactate solution, otherwise with water, is mandatory. The eyelids should then be everted. Large lime particles should be removed with a moistened swab. Subsequent treatment demands immediate hospitalization. Conservative measures as well as surgical interventions (conjunctiva, cornea) may be required.

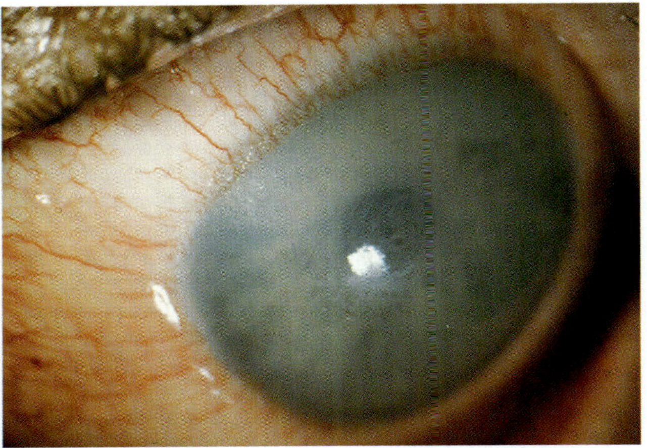

Figure 18.12   Calcium hydroxide (lime) burn, stage II. Note the discrete corneal opacification, the iris and the round pupil are fairly well visible. There is no apparent damage to the deeper ocular structures. The assessment of the perilimbal vessels is crucial. An impaired circulation in this area (blanching) is important in determination of the prognosis. The degree of blanching can only be measured upon slit lamp examination with suitable magnification. The evaluation may be hindered by concomitant conjunctival chemosis. The figure shows moderate conjunctival chemosis and localized conjunctival blanching. Superficial melting may in the later course occur in the adjacent portions of the cornea.

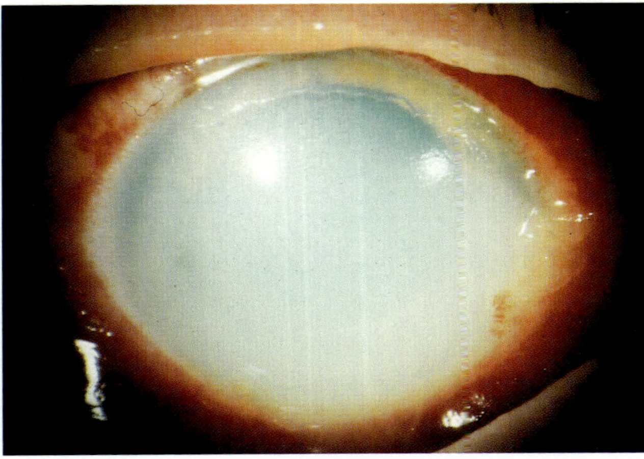

Figure 18.13   Status post alkali burn, stage III. Severe alkali burns are characterized by opacification of the entire corneal thickness, so that pupillary outline is blurred. The conjunctiva appears anaemic at the limbus (in this case obscured by subconjunctival hemorrhage). The extent of injury to the perilimbal area (half of the circumference in stage III) ist the most important prognostic factor. Damage to the corneal stem cells impedes normal epithelization of the corneal surface (compare with chapter 4).

Figure 18.14 Status post severe calcium hydroxide (lime) burn with corneal melting (stage IV). The figure depicts the cornea in high magnification. Centrally, the stroma is melted, the remaining thin membrane is perforated in places. The iris *(inferior half)* is attached to the posterior corneal surface.

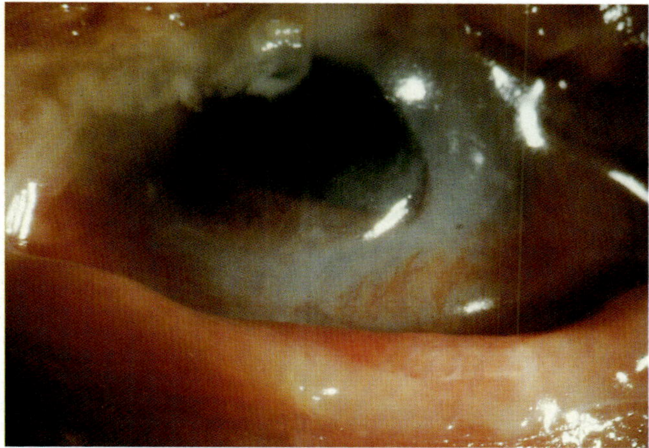

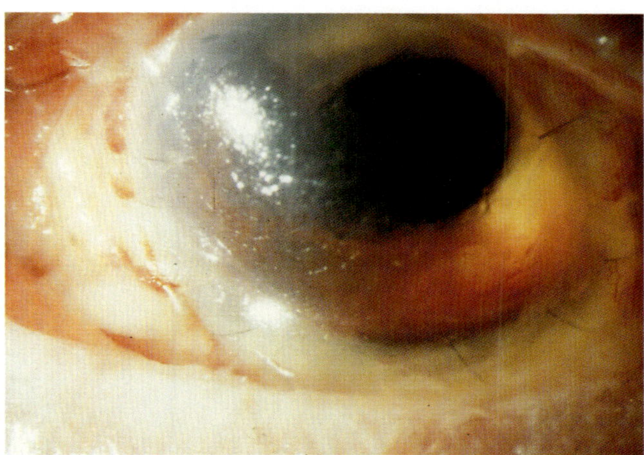

Figure 18.15 The same patient as shown in figure 18.14, status post penetrating keratoplasty with scleral ring. A corneal graft with a ring of adjacent sclera was sutured in place to treat the extensive corneal melting. The figure shows the postoperative status, the anterior chamber is deep. In the lower portion, clots of blood lie on the iris. The pocedure was performed for globe preservation . Immuno- logic problems and secondary glaucoma must be expected and further surgical interventions may be needed. The final prognosis is very poor.

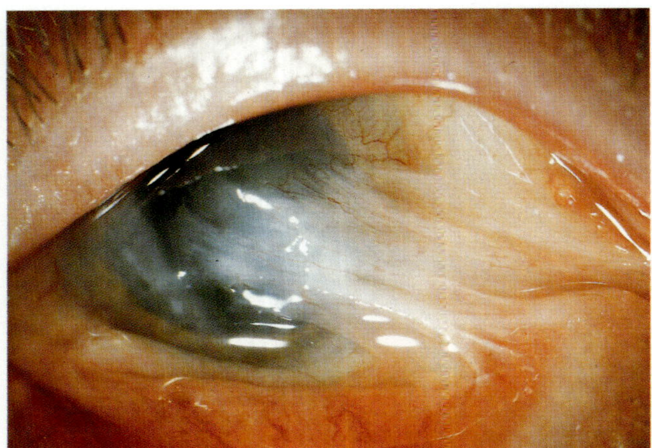

Figure 18.16 Sequels of a calcium hydroxide (lime) burn, symblepharon. Following severe chemical burns, formation of symblepharon may occur, i.e. fusion of the bulbar and tarsal conjunctiva with restriction of ocular motility and sometimes corneal involvement. Treatment is surgical: lysis of the synechiae, lining of the resulting defect with either conjunctiva harvested from the contralateral eye or buccal mucosa (difficult procedure).

General: Contusion is defined as a closed globe injury, which is caused by blunt force. All ocular segments can be involved. Since intraocular hemorrhages are frequently produced, the retina and optic nerve head can often not be visualized. The following examination techniques may be referred to:

1. visual field testing (to rule out retinal detachment and optic nerve damage),
2. ultrasonographic examination (to rule out retinal detachment and lens luxation),
3. testing for pupillary light reaction (to rule out severe optic nerve damage).

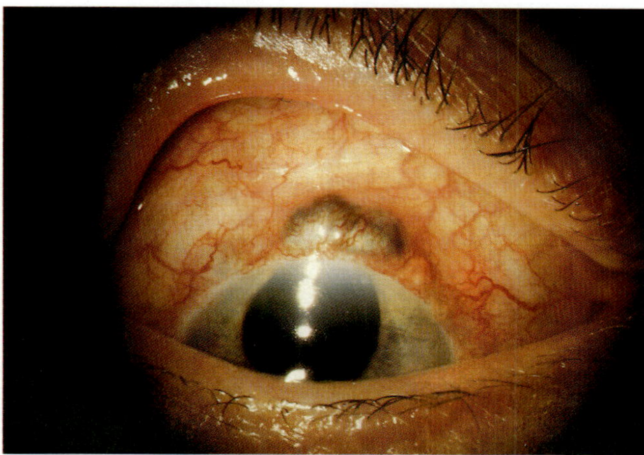

Figure 18.17   Subconjunctival iris prolapse following contusion. Severe contusions can lead to rupture of the globe with extensive prolapse of ocular contents. The corneal limbus marks the point of least resistance, it is the most common location of scleral ruptures. They may be covered by intact conjunctiva, which decreases the risk of infection. Subconjunctival hemorrhages make the diagnosis more difficult. Surgical repair, including conjunctival incision and reposition of the iris, has to be conducted in order to prevent late complications (high IOP).

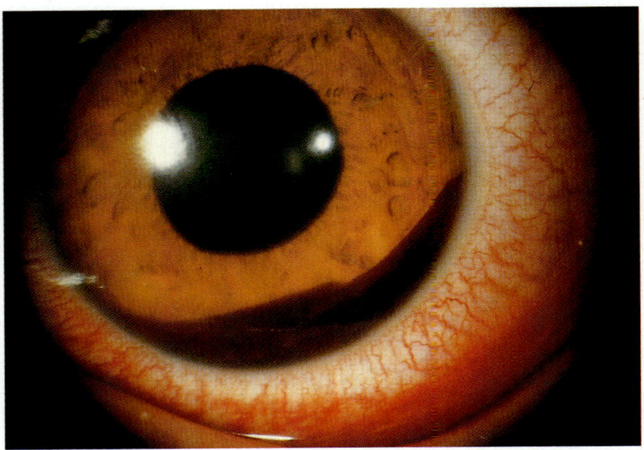

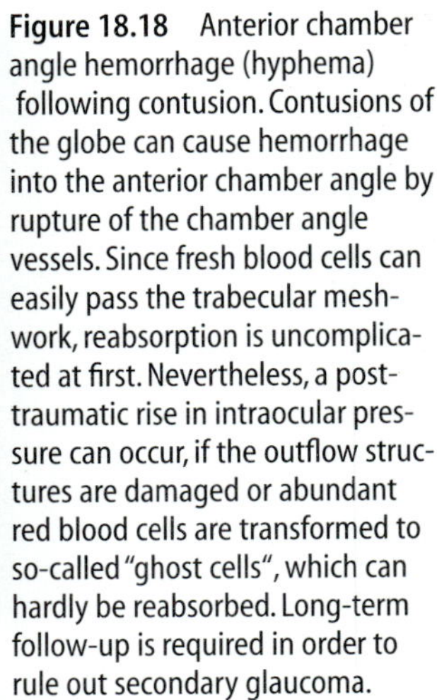

Figure 18.18 Anterior chamber angle hemorrhage (hyphema) following contusion. Contusions of the globe can cause hemorrhage into the anterior chamber angle by rupture of the chamber angle vessels. Since fresh blood cells can easily pass the trabecular meshwork, reabsorption is uncomplicated at first. Nevertheless, a post-traumatic rise in intraocular pressure can occur, if the outflow structures are damaged or abundant red blood cells are transformed to so-called "ghost cells", which can hardly be reabsorbed. Long-term follow-up is required in order to rule out secondary glaucoma.

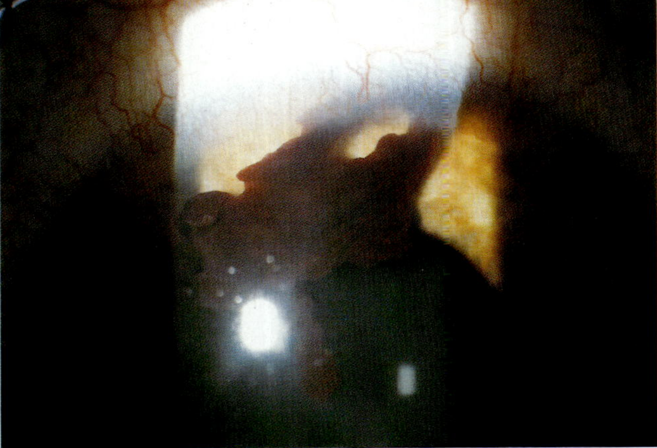

Figure 18.19 Anterior chamber hemorrhage (hyphema) following contusion. The figure shows a circumscribed hemorrhage from the superior portion of the anterior chamber angle. The reabsorption of such hemorrhages is usually fast, recurrence can occur. If the entire anterior chamber is filled with blood (total hyphema), surgical removal is recommended to prevent corneal blood staining as a result of suffusion of hemoglobin into the corneal stroma with elevated intraocular pressure (and metabolization into hemosiderin). Recurrence can occur in such cases as well. The intraocular pressure has to monitored during long-term follow-up.

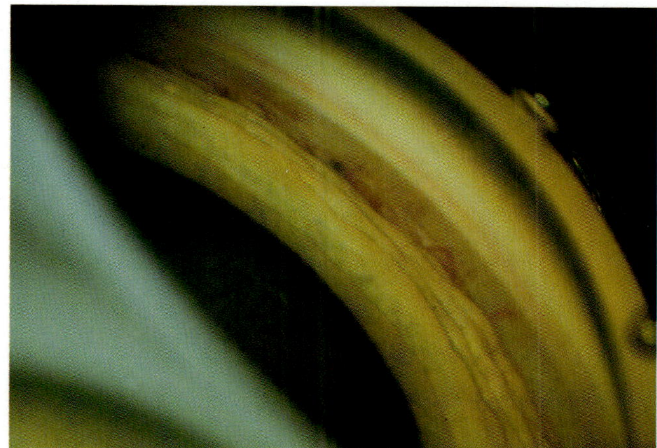

Figure 18.20 Recession of the anterior chamber angle following contusion. Tearing of the ciliary body can create a recession of the anterior chamber angle (so-called pseudo chamber angle) with decreased outflow facility. The figure shows a gonioscopic appearance of a traumatic anterior chamber angle recession with visible vessels at the iris root. Since a particularly wide, normal anterior chamber angle may resemble this condition, gonioscopy has to be performed bilaterally before the diagnosis is made. A rise in intraocular presure can still occur years after the contusion.

Figure 18.21 Iridodialysis following contusion. Every contusion can cause a rupture of the iris at its root. Note that with retroillumination the area of iridialysis, the ciliary processes and the lens equator are well visible. Since the iridodialysis is located within the palpebral fissure, the condition may be associated with monocular diplopia. Surgical repair with refixation of the iris is indicated. A postoperative rise in intraocular pressure may occur. Long-term follow-up is required.

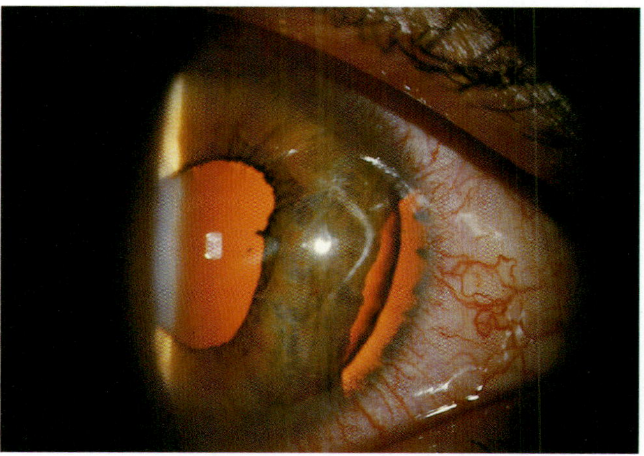

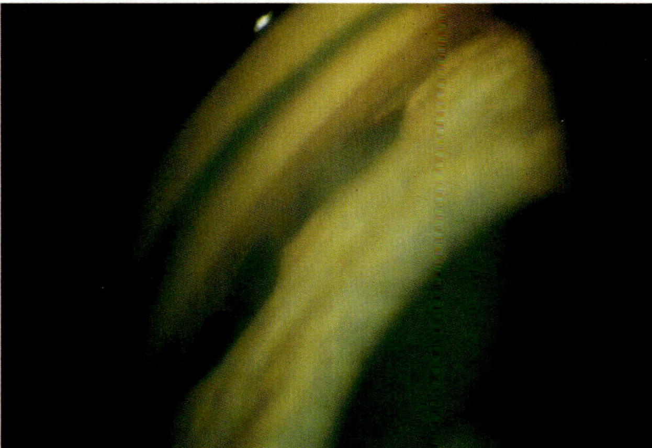

Figure 18.22 Incomplete iridodialysis. With incomplete rupture of the iris at its root, the anterior segment may look inconspicuous. An impairment of pupillary motility suggests traumatic changes in the corresponding sector. The changes can only be detected by gonioscopy. No treatment is needed, if the intraocular pressure is normal.

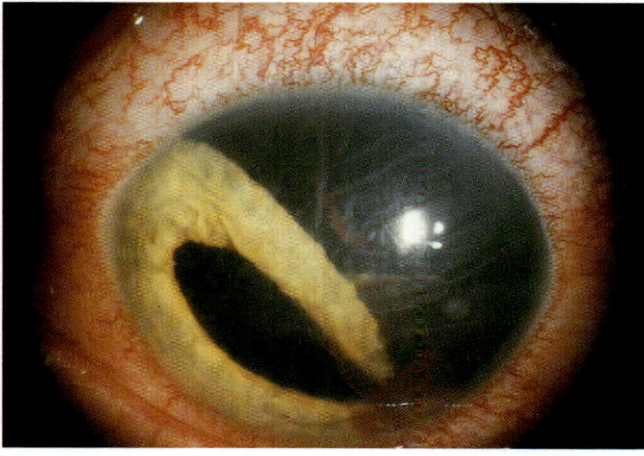

Figure 18.23 Iris rupture following severe contusion. A contusion can cause a rupture of large portions of the iris. Delayed consequences include disturbances of intraocular pressure regulation resulting in ocular hypo- or hypertension, glare and visual impairment. The examiner must keep in mind that the contusion can also cause damage in the posterior ocular segment. Surgical repair with refixation of the iris at the its root has to be consisdered. The procedure is technically difficult. The risk of a postoperative rise in intraocular pressure remains, despite successful refixation.

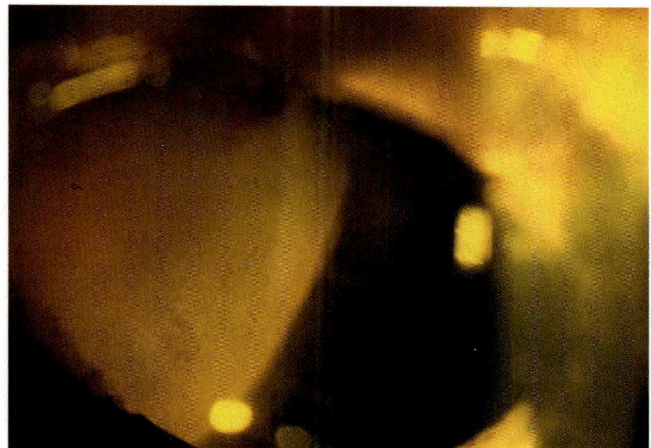

Figure 18.24 Partial luxation of the lens following blunt trauma. A contusion can cause a rupture of the zonular fibers with displacement of the lens. Note the stretched remaining zonular fibers, the opaque lens is luxated temporally upwards, there is blood on the iris and the lens. The complications, apart from visual impairment, can be elevated intraocular pressure, phacolysis and complete luxation of the lens into the vitreous cavity. The lens has to be removed. Aphakia can later be corrected with a contact lens or by implantation of an intraocular lens (compare with chapter 6).

Figure 18.25 Luxated lens following blunt trauma. The figure shows the opaqe lens, which is luxated backwards. In this particular case, the zonular apparatus was completely ruptured and the lens has sunk into the vitreous cavity. The lens has to be removed in order to prevent secondary complications (phacolysis, glaucoma, retinal changes). The procedure includes vitrectomy.

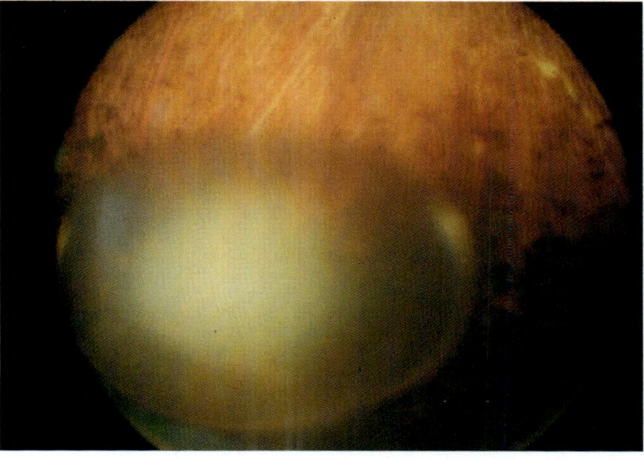

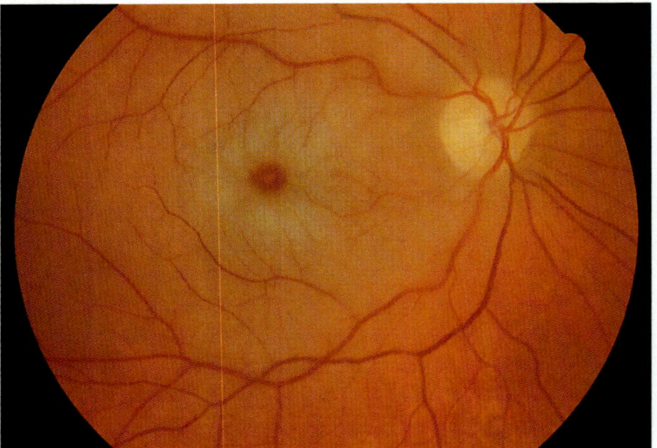

Figure 18.26   Retinal edema ("Berlin´s edema") following contusion. Every contusion can cause retinal edema, either in the periphery or the posterior pole. Peripheral edema remains unnoticed at first, but may later on result in a retinal hole and cause retinal detachment. More than 60% of all retinal dialyses in children are due to trauma (compare with chapter 11). Long-term follow-up is necessary. The figure shows a contusional retinal edema in the posterior pole (Berlin´s edema). Visual acuity is significantly diminished. As opposed to central retinal artery occlusion, which gives a similar ophthalmoscopic picture, retinal circulation is normal. The edema spontaneously resolves within few days. Systemic corticosteroids may accelerate the resorption. The prognosis for complete visual rehabilitation is very good.

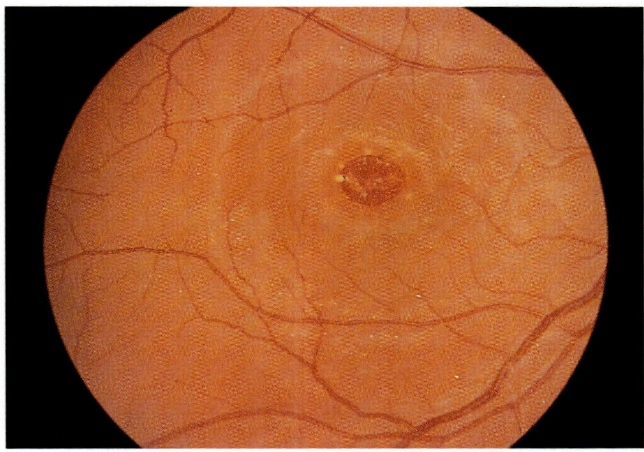

Figure 18.27 Macular hole following contusion. After resolution of a contusional retinal edema, the destruction of the photoreceptors can lead to formation of a retinal hole in the periphery as well as in the posterior pole. Peripheral retinal holes frequently cause retinal detachment (follow up). The formation of a retinal hole in the posterior pole leads to severe visual impairment. The figure shows a central, sharply delineated area of intense red color (choroid) and surrounding retinal opacification (shallow retinal detachment, compare with chapter 11). A macular hole usually does not cause extensive retinal detachment.

18.3 Contusion

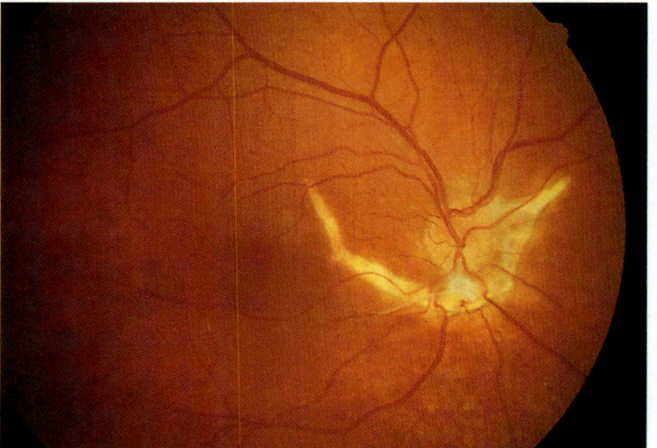

Figure 18.28 Choroidal rupture. Ocular contusion can cause posterior choroidal ruptures. The ruptured area is characteristically concentric to the optic disc. The figure shows the opthalmoscopic appearance of a postcontusion choroidal rupture. The overlying retina is intact (see retinal vessels). The choroid is ruptured and the white sclera is bared. Late complications are hyperplasia of retinal pigment epithelium and proliferation of choroidal vessels. The extent of functional impairment correlates with the extent of injury to the sensory retina. There is no known treatment.

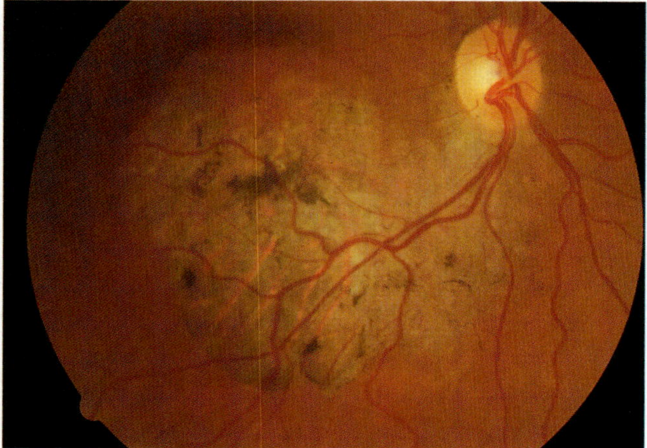

Figure 18.29 Choroidal infarction following contusion. Apart from the damage caused by the direct concussive effect, blunt trauma can lead to a rupture of the posterior ciliary arteries. The figure shows an area inferior to the optic disc, in which the pigment epithelium is absent and the choriocapillaris is partially atrophied.

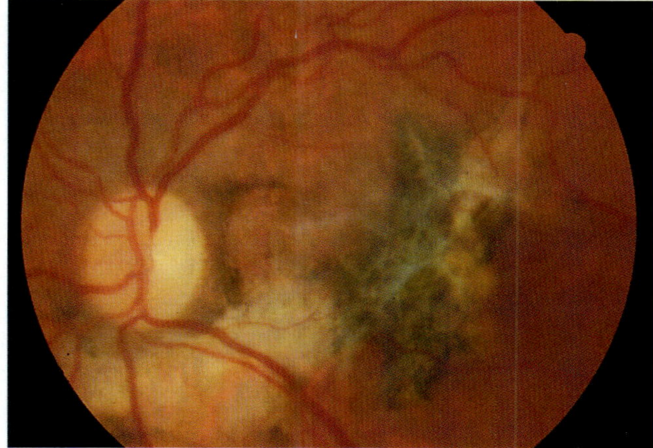

Figure 18.30   Retinopathia sclopetaria. Hyperplasia of the retinal pigment epithelium and formation of fibrous scars occur as a late complication of traumatic choroidal rupture. Note the grey-whitish area inferior to the optic disc and the hyperplasia of retinal pigment epithelium temporally with overlying fibrous proliferation. In the superotemporal portion of the darkly pigmented area, the white streak representing the choroidal rupture is visible. The proliferations can progress.

18.4 Corneal injuries

General: There is risk of infection in all corneal injuries. Severe infections (e.g. Pyocyaneus) can originate from minor injuries when there is a specific predisposition (compare with chapter 4). For that reason, local antibiotic treatment is mandatory in corneal injuries. Symptomatic treatment with local anaesthetics or corticosteroids is considered malpractice. (For healing of corneal defects / corneal scarring see chapter 4.)

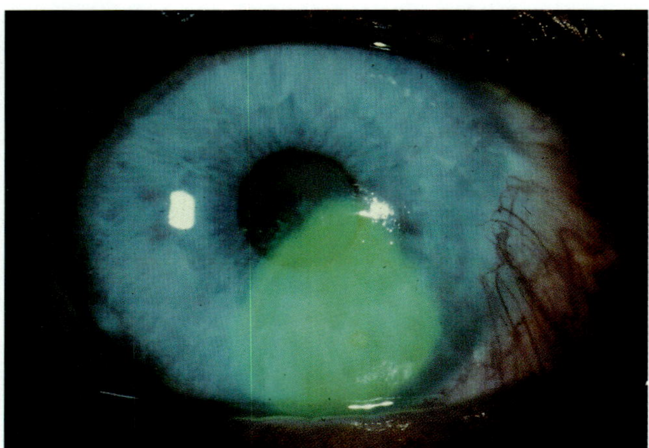

Figure 18.31   Corneal erosion. The figure shows an epithelial defect in the inferior half of the cornea that stains with fluorescein dye. An erosion can be caused by various kinds of mechanical trauma. Usually fast resolution without scar formation (compare with chapter 4). Topical antibiotics are necessary in order to prevent corneal infection.

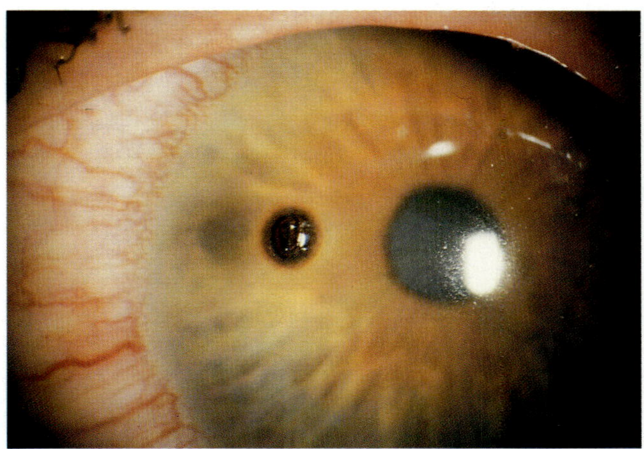

Figure 18.32 Corneal foreign body. Corneal foreign bodies may lie on the corneal surface or be "burned" into the superficial corneal layers (frequently as a consequence of grinding or welding without protective goggles). Some corneal foreign bodies can be removed with a swab. Burned-in iron containing foreign bodies usually rust. They have to be dislodged with a fine metal spatula or removed with a foreign body drill (compare with figure 18.33). Deep stromal foreign bodies are difficult to remove and may require repeated manipulation. In the interim, antibiotic ointment and a patch are applied.

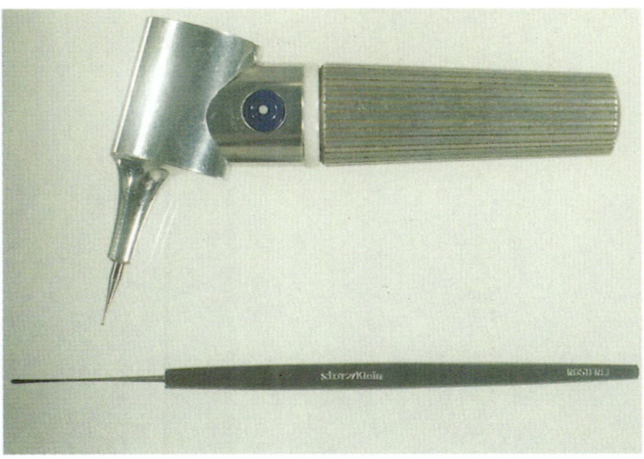

Figure 18.33 Foreign body drill and foreign body spatula.

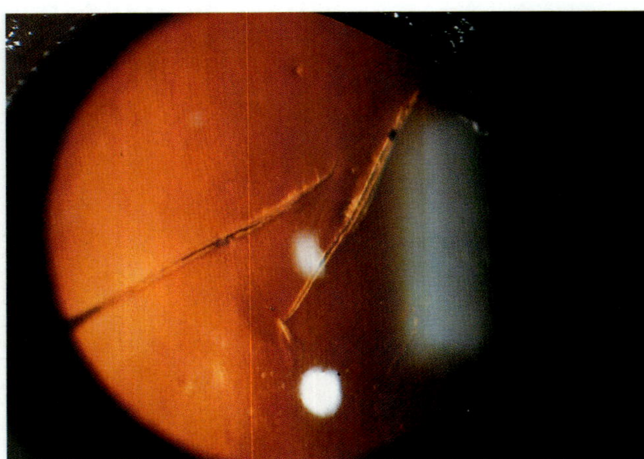

Figure 18.34 Lamellar incision wounds in the cornea. The figure shows two cuts, which do not penetrate the cornea. The anterior chamber is deep. The wound edges show good apposition and alignment. In such cases, no corneal sutures are needed. A soft contact lens is used to maintain apposition and to shield the healing epithelium.

General: Open-globe injuries involving solely the cornea are managed with topical antibiotics and sometimes antimycotics (injuries caused by vegetable matter). In such cases, topical treatment is more effective than systemic administration of drugs. With involvement of deeper ocular structures (uvea, vitreous, retina), systemic antibiotic (antimycotic) treatment is needed for the prevention of endophthalmitis. A fulminant course indicates bacterial infection (most frequently isolated germs are Pneumococcus, hemolytic Streptococcus, Staphylococcus and Pseudomonas), a more "silent", protracted course suggests fungal infection. The most feared complication of open-globe injury is sympathetic ophthalmia. It is defined as bilateral granulomatous uveitis mainly affecting the choroid. The inflammation starts in the injured eye, the noninjured eye then follows, showing all clinical signs of uveitis. The disease is very uncommon. Nevertheless, every patient suffering from a penetrating injury shoud be informed about the possibility of sympathetic ophthalmia. Treatment consists of immunosuppressants. Enucleation of the injured eye has to be considered.

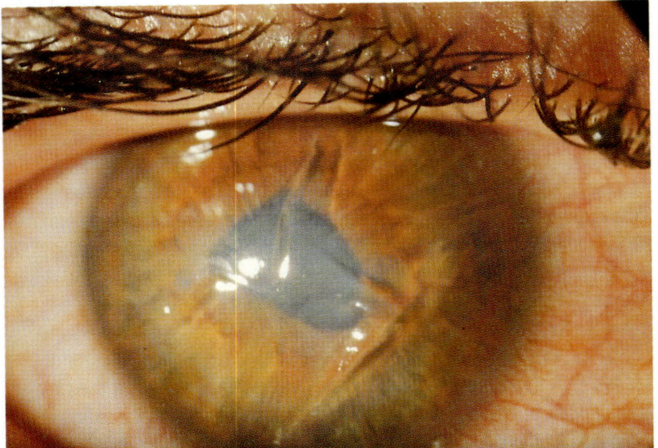

Figure 18.35 Penetrating incision wounds in the cornea and the lens. The figure shows multiple cuts that perforate the cornea. The lens is injured and swollen. The wound is gaped and the anterior chamber is lost. Primary surgical repair consits of corneal reconstruction by placement of sutures. The degree of swelling of the lens determines the urgency of its removal. After the wound is healed, extensive corneal scarring may give the indication for penetrating keratoplasty (possible combination with artificial lens implantation).

General: The prognosis of a perforating injury with an intraocular foreign body is determined by the composition of the foreign body, its size and location within the globe. Metallic foreign bodies, which are toxic and produce metallosis (iron, copper and alloy) are distinguished from inert metallic foreign bodies and organic matter. Copper- and iron-containing foreign bodies can lead to destruction of the affected eye over time (metallosis). Copper fragments can cause acute chalcosis within days with sterile vitreous / choroidal inflammation and necrosis. Inert metallic and nonmetallic foreign bodies produce local mechanical irritation and destruction, organic matter poses a risk for infection, particularly fungal infection. Preoperative localization of an intraocular foreign body is done with plain x-ray studies, CT and ultrasonography.

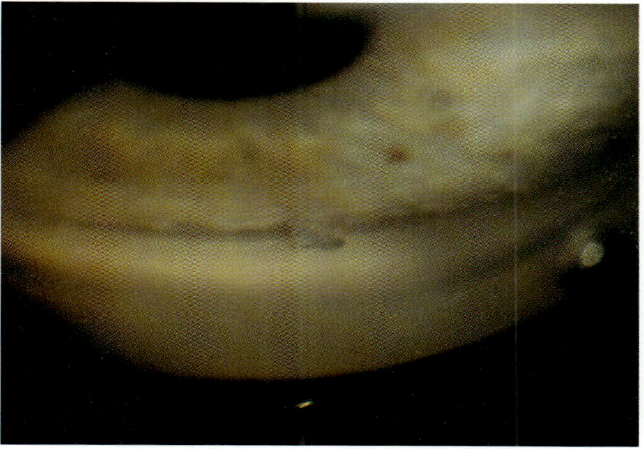

Figure 18.36   Perforating injury with intraocular foreign body in the anterior chamber. Small foreign bodies, which have perforated the cornea, frequently lodge in the anterior chamber angle. The figure shows the gonioscopic appearance of a foreign body in the anterior chamber angle at the 6 o′clock position, which touches the corneal endothelium. If the entry site is small, perforating injury may be overlooked. In many cases, in which the foreign body is tolerated and the eye does not show obvious signs of trauma, corneal endothelial decompensation may occur in the later course. In every corneal endothelial decompensation of unknown origin, starting from the inferior limbus, the anterior chamber angle has to be viewed (goniocopy) in search of an intraocular foreign body. Compensation of endothelial function may be seen following surgical removal of the foreign body.

18.5 Intraocular foreign body

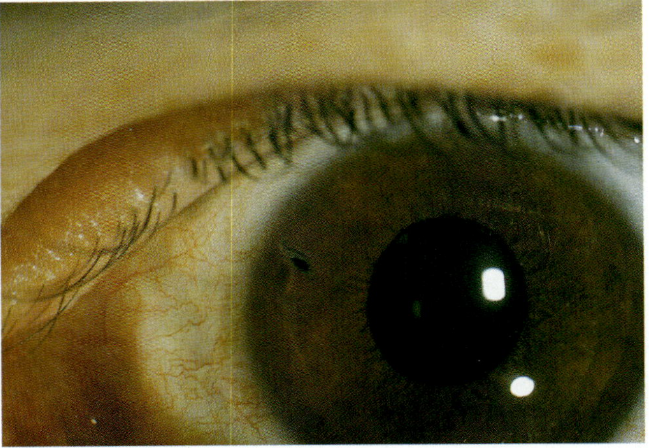

Figure 18.37 Perforating injury with iris defect. Note the small iris defect in the superonasal quadrant. Small perforating injuries may not be noticed by the patient and overlooked on superficial examination. The presence of an intraocular foreign body has to be ruled out in every case of an iris defect of unknown origin (x-ray studies, CT). Intraocular foreign bodies can promote severe complications (siderosis, chalcosis, retinal detachment).

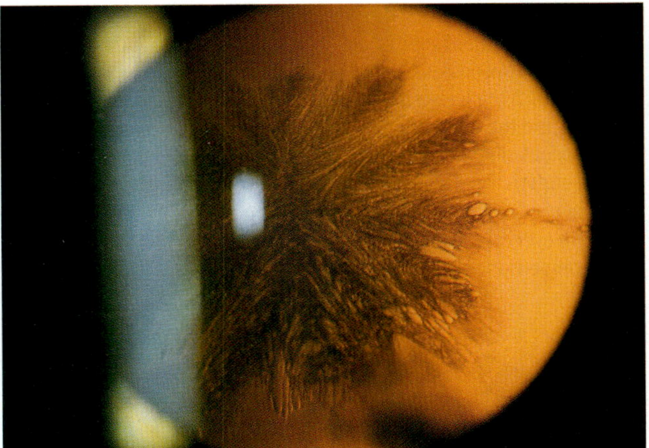

Figure 18.38 Rosette-shaped cataract secondary to perforating injury. Any opening of the lens capsule, if not extremely small, can lead to lens opacification. Rosette-shaped opacities in the posterior cortex are characteristic of perforating lens injuries. The figure shows such a lens opacity secondary to perforating injury.

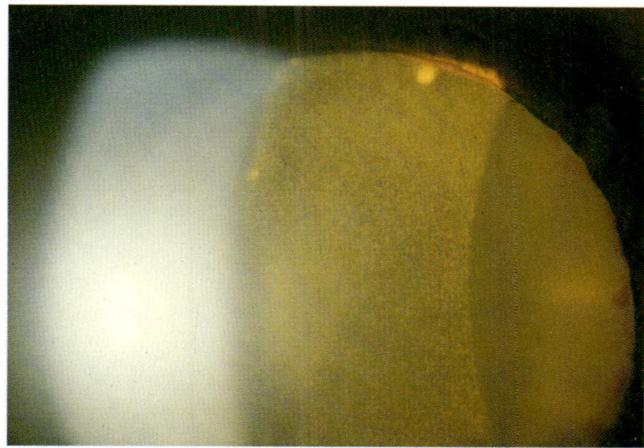

Figure 18.39 Siderosis. Iron-containing intraocular foreign bodies lead to siderosis in the course of months or years. Iron particles are deposited in the iris (heterochromia), the lens, the trabecular meshwork (glaucoma) and the retinal pigment epithelium. Perivascular deposits form later on. Secondary degeneration of the photoreceptors causes functional impairment. The figure shows pigment clumping on the anterior lens capsule (so called rust spots). The ERG provides information on retinal function. The foreign body and the lens have to be removed even in cases with advanced damage. Localization and removal of old intraocular foreign bodies can be difficult, for they may have been partially absorbed, therefore the x-ray for retained iron may be negative.

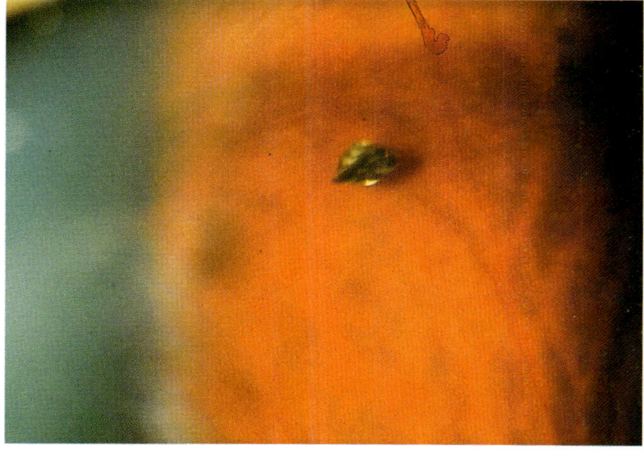

Figure 18.40 Metallic intraocular foreign body, presumably iron-containing. The figure shows a preretinal foreign body, which is presumably iron-containing. The magnetic properties, location and motility of the foreign body determine if it is suitable for magnetic extraction or if vitrectomy is required (then the foreign body can be grasped with a special forceps).

18.5 Intraocular foreign body

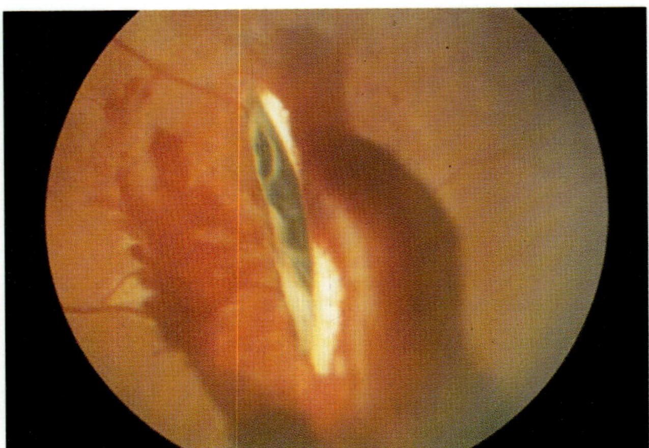

Figure 18.41 Intraocular foreign body lodged in the posterior sclera. The figure shows an intraocular foreign body, which lies intrasclerally in the posterior pole. The white streak marks the area of scleral laceration. Plain x-ray films, CT and ultrasound are used to determine if the foreign body has perforated the posterior sclera. Foreign bodies of this kind can only be removed by vitrectomy. Systemic antibiotic prophylaxis is mandatory.

Tropical eye diseases

19

19.1 Bacterial infections

General: In this chapter, a few disorders, which are found in large numbers in the tropics, are compiled. The factors that account for the concentration of certain conditions in tropical areas are climatic and geographic influences (e.g. onchocerciasis), poor nutrition (e.g. xerophthalmia) and hygiene (e.g. trachoma). The awareness of these conditions is of importance not only because they are among the major causes of blindness in developing countries, but also in view of constantly increasing international travel and migration.
(Figures 5-7, 11-14 courtesy of H.Trojan, Marburg)

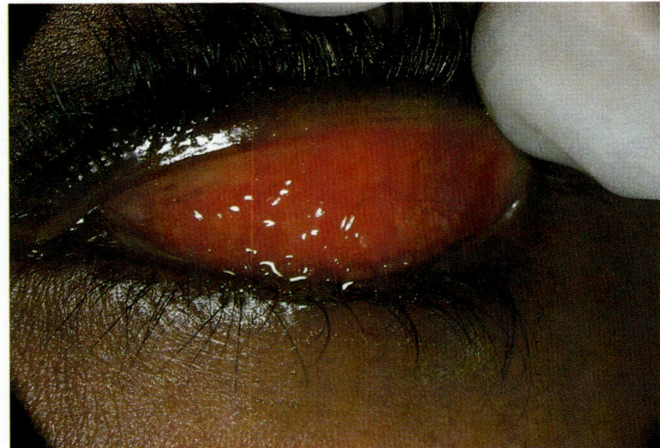

Figure 19.1   Trachoma, papillary hypertrophy. Trachoma is a chronic inflammation of the conjunctiva and cornea caused by Chlamydia trachomatis. Endemic trachoma is a major cause of blindness in many developing countries. Topical tetracyclines (eye ointments or drops) are recommended for large-scale treatment of active trachoma, in some cases in combination with systemic antibiotic treatment. Note the marked papillary hypertrophy of the upper tarsal conjunctiva, the tarsal follicles are obscured.

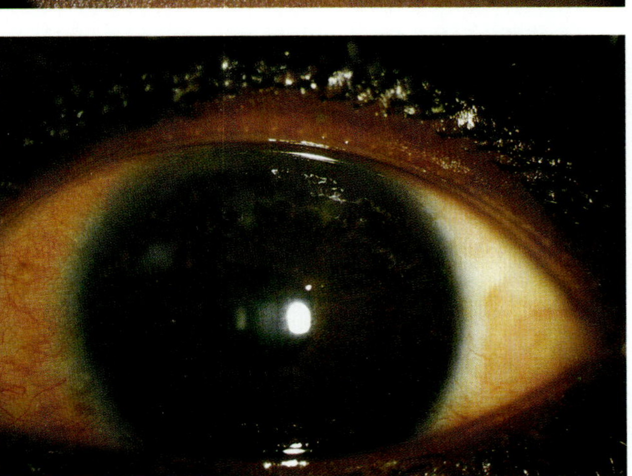

Figure 19.2   Trachomatous corneal pannus. Marginal corneal infiltration leads to early development of fibrovascular pannus, which is most pronounced in the superior portion of the corneal circumference (compare with figure 3.32)..

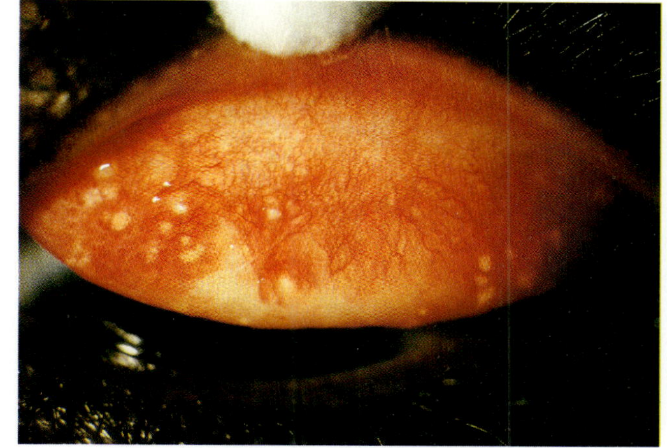

Figure 19.3   Trachoma, mature follicles and scarring in the tarsal conjunctiva. Note the yellow follicles in the conjunctiva of the upper tarsus and the confluent scars that result from subepithelial fibrosis and scarring of necrotic follicles.

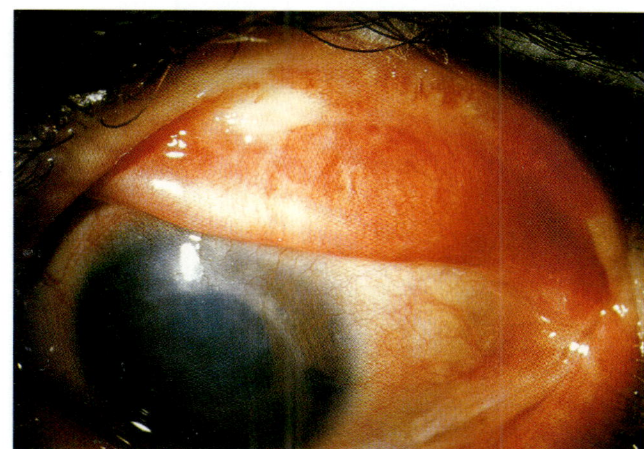

Figure 19.4   Trachoma, extensive scarring in the tarsal conjunctiva and fibrovascular corneal pannus.

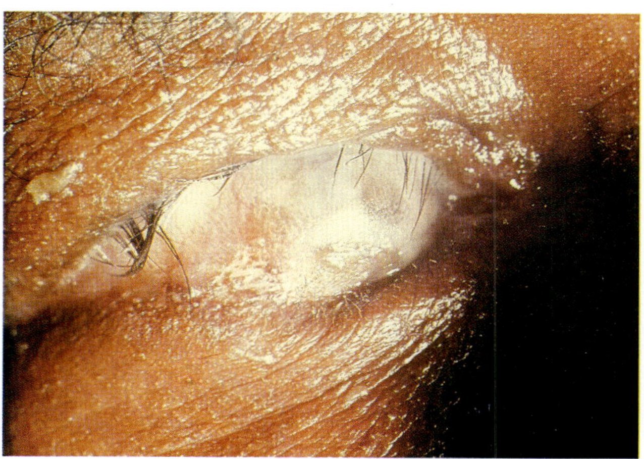

Figure 19.5   Trachoma, stage IV, entropion, trichiasis, corneal opacification. Eyelid deformation due to contraction of the conjunctival scars is the main blinding complication of trachoma. Surgical interventions to correct lid deformities are part of large-scale public health programs to control blinding trachoma.

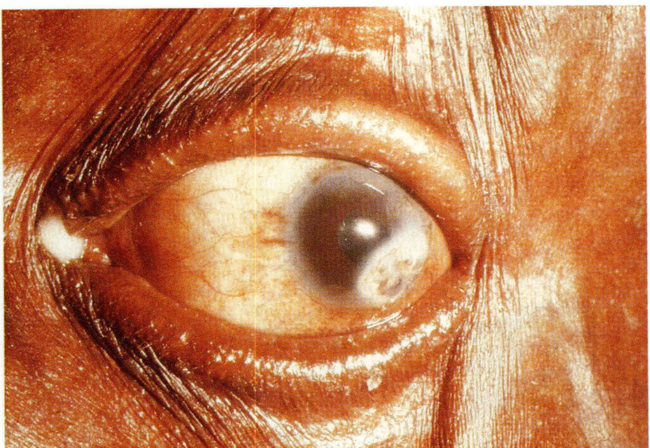

Figure 19.6 Leprosy, corneal leproma. Leprosy ("Hansen´s disease") is a chronic inflammatory disease caused by Mycobacterium leprae. The corneal lesion, typically arising at the limbus, represents a large granuloma. The treatment of leprosy includes the following drugs: dapsone (diaminophenyl-sulfone), rifampin, clofazimine.

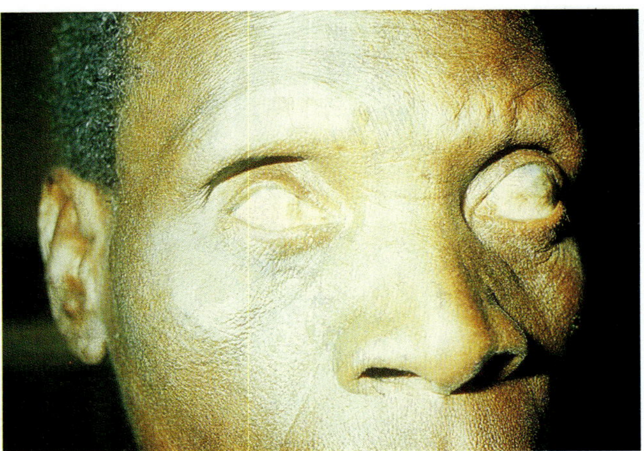

Figure 19.7 Leprosy stare. Facial nerve palsy with lagophthalmos results in exposure keratitis with corneal opacification. Note the characteristic brow loss and eyelash loss (madarosis).

Figure 19.8   Loaiasis, subconjunctival filaria. The disease is restricted to Africa. Following infection, the adult worm wanders in the subcutaneous tissues. Surgical removal of the parasite is advisable. The drug of choice is diethylcarbamazine. The figure shows an adult filaria under the bulbar conjunctiva with moderate conjunctival hyperemia.

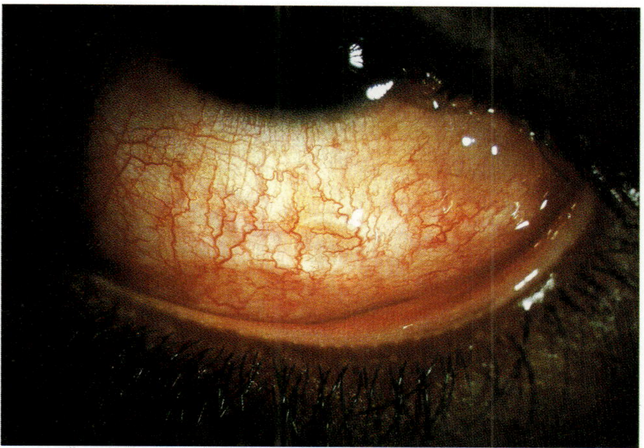

Figure 19.9   Loa loa filaria following surgical extraction from the eye shown in figure 19.8.

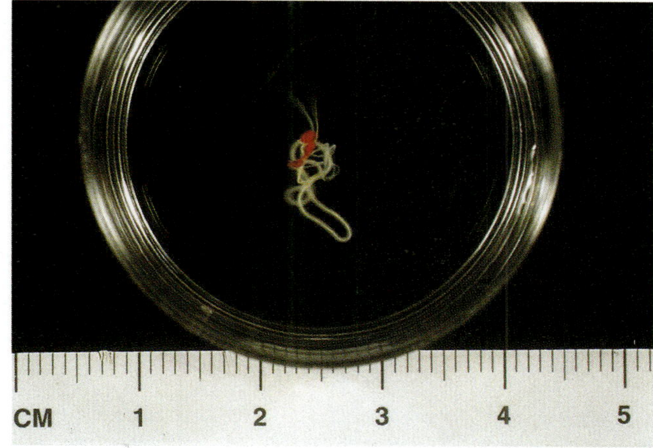

Figure 19.10   Toxocariasis, central chorioretinal scar. The disease results from infection with the canine intestinal roundworm Toxocara canis. Man is an incidental intermediate host of the nematode. Due to hygienic factors, the frequency of toxocariasis is high in tropical areas. The figure shows a solitary chorioretinal scar in the posterior pole, resulting from chorioretinitis.

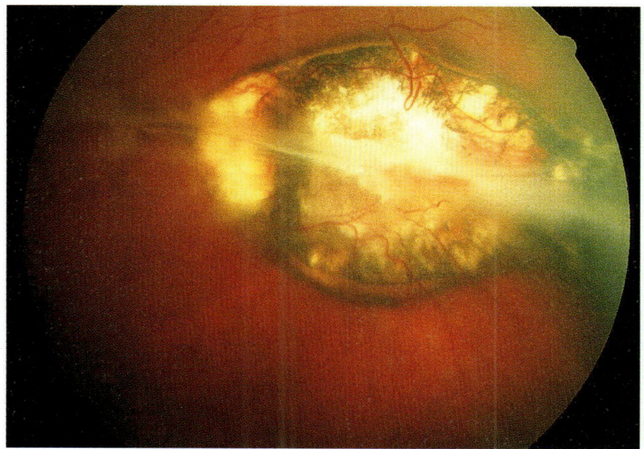

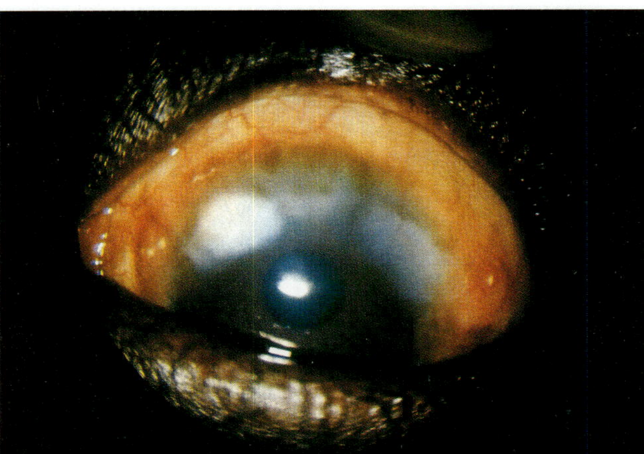

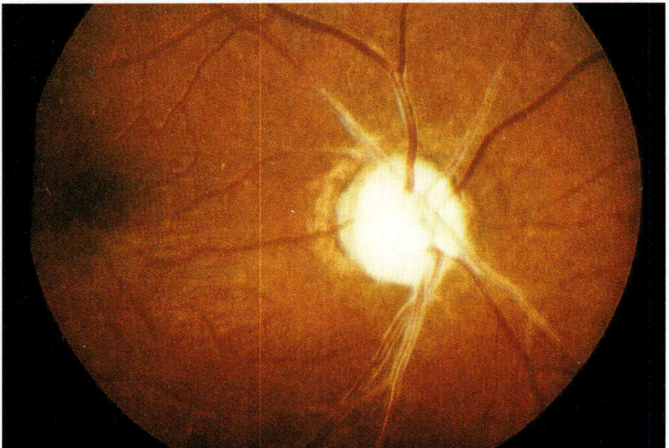

Figure 19.11 Onchocerciasis ("river blindness"), corneal stromal infiltrates. The disease is caused by the nematode Onchocerca volvulus. Man is the only definite host. The black fly Simulium is the principal intermediate host and also the most important vector of the infection. The disease is endemic across equatorial Africa, there are local foci in Central and South America. Invasion of microfilariae into the corneal stroma produces sclerosing keratitis, usually along the lower limbus. The treatment of choice is the drug ivermectin.

Figure 19.12 Onchocerciasis, optic nerve atrophy. Changes in the posterior segment include chorioretinitis, which is most likely due to immune reactions to the parasitic antigens, and optic neuritis with subsequent atrophy. A characteristic finding associated with optic nerve atrophy in patients with onchocerciasis is sheathing of the peripapillary vessels.

Figure 19.13 Measles infection, bilateral corneal opacification. During measles infection, a nutritional vitamin A deficiency is aggravated by an increased requirement of the vitamin. Many children with acute measles infection develop corneal destructive disease (keratomalacia). The figure shows an infant with bilateral corneal opacification following measles infection.

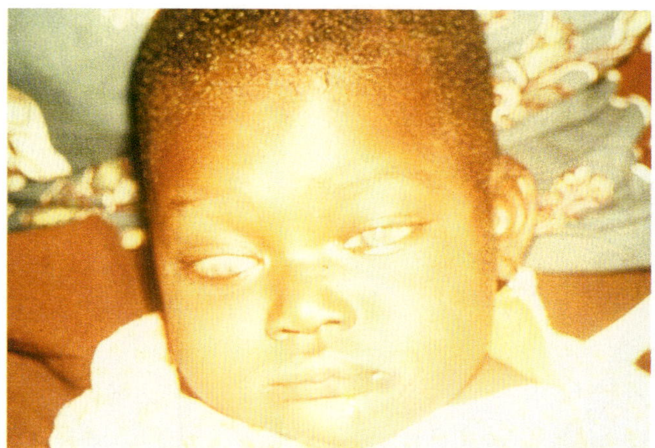

Figure 19.14 Vitamin-A deficiency, corneal xerosis. The corneal surface is dull and may stain with fluorescein. Note that the circumscribed infiltrations of the superficial stroma are characteristically located in the inferior portion of the interpalpebral fissure. There is an increased risk of bacterial / viral infection. Vitamin A deficiency is the largest cause of childhood blindness in the world. For conjunctival xerosis see figure 3.42.

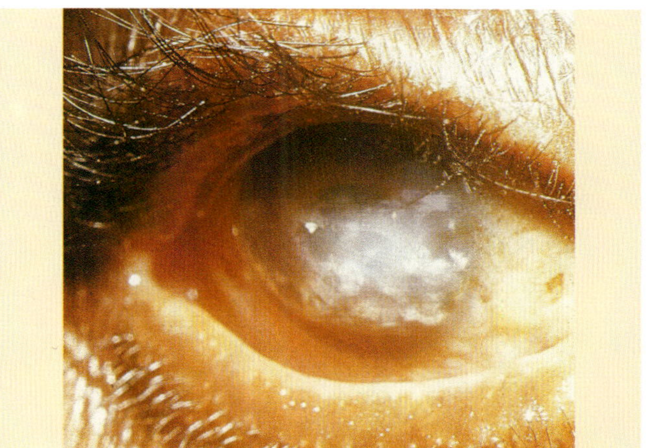

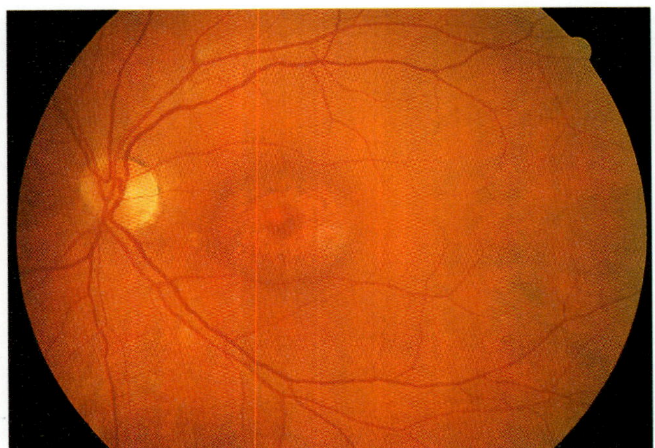

Figure 19.15 Chloroquine maculopathy. Long-term malaria treatment with high doses of chloroquine yields irreversible retinal changes. The fundus picture shows a typical ring of depigmentation surrounding more normal foveal pigment ("bulll´s eye"). Compare with chapter 11.

Subject Index

abducens nerve palsy 360
abduction, limited 362
acanthamoeba 91
accommodation 177, 336, 339, 340, 342, 344, 366
- disturbance 177
- paralysis 366
- range 344
achromatopsia 370
adaptometer 239
adduction, limited 362
adenovirus 51, 88
adrenochrome 50
aesthesiometer of Cochet-Bonnet 69
against-movement 345
agnosia, visual 307
AIDS (see HIV)
AION 299
albinism 150, 243, 363, 370
- ocular 150, 243
alkali burn 377, 378
allergy 366, 368
amacrine cell 234
amaurosis fugax 369
amblyopia 128, 178
ametropia 340
amiodarone 98
ammonium hydroxide 377, 378, 379
AMPPE 259, 260
Amsler grid 237
amyloid 82
amyloidosis 102
ANCA 327
aneurysm 253, 309, 367
- angiogram 309
angiography 194
- optic disc 194
angioid streaks 169
angioma, racemose 252
aniridia 126, 178, 363, 370
- congenital 178

aniseikonia 143, 343
anisometropia 343
anomaloscope, Nagel 239
anomaly 322, 366
- facial 322
- globe 322
- vascular 366
aphakia 143
- correction 143
apoplexia papillae 299
aqueous humor 146, 182
- drainage 182
- hydrodynamics 182
- production 146
arachnodactyly 127
arachnoid 183
arcuate scotoma 187, 189-191, 194
arcus 74
- lipoides 74
- senilis 74
area
- 17 307, 352
- 18 307
- peristriata 307
- pretectal 172
Arnold-Chiari-syndrome 363
arteritis 300, 367
- temporal 300
artery
- central retinal 183, 234, 235, 288
- ciliary 146
- hyaloid 222, 224
- ophthalmic 317
- short posterior ciliary 183
A-scan 320
- echography 320
asthenopia, accomodative 366
- symptoms 342
astigmatism 67, 68, 77, 86, 343, 366
- against-the-rule 343
- irregular 343

- regular 343
- with-the-rule 343
atopia 54
atrophy 167, 308, 311
- central areolar choroidal 167
- descending 308, 311
Aulhorn, classification 197
autoimmune disorder 326, 327
Axenfeld-anomaly 73

Bagolini striated glasses test 356
basalioma 23-25
- defect closure 24, 25
- nodular 23
- rotation flap 24, 25
bear tracks 244
Behçet syndrome 278
bengal, rose 31, 42, 70
Bergmeister's papilla 224
Berlin's edema 386
Bielschowsky head tilt test 361
bifocal lens 347
binocularity 352
- cortical organization 352
biomorphometry 188, 195
- optic disc 188
Bjerrum scotoma 191, 192, 194, 197
blanching, limbal 378
blepharitis 14, 368
- causes 14
- chronic 14
- marginal 14, 368
blepharochalasis 366
blepharophimosis 5
blood vessel, pial 288
blood-aqueous barrier 146
bone spicules 272
Bourneville-Pringle-syndrome 286
Bowman's membane 66
brainstem 352
- lesion 364

branch retinal artery occlusion
    (BRAO) 249
BRAO 249
brow loss 402
Bruch´s membrane 147, 166, 169,
    234
B-scan 320
- echography 320
buphthalmos (also see congenital
    glaucoma) 71, 201
burn 374, 375, 377-380
- acid 377
- alkali 377-379
- chemical 377, 380
- lime 377-380
- thermal 13, 368, 374

canal, infraorbital 316
canaliculi 30, 32, 37
- inferior 32
- intubation 37
- lacrimal 30, 37
- - trauma 37
Candida mycosis 262
canthal tendon 2
- lateral 2
- medial 2
canthaxanthin inclusion 277
capsular bag 140, 141
capsular opacifcation, fibrotic
    posterior 139
carbonic anhydrase inhibitor 217
carcinoma 62, 106, 166, 302
- breast 166, 302
- bronchial 302
- carcinoma in situ, cornea 106
- conjunctiva 62
- lung 166
cardiac disease 366
carotid, occlusive disease 168
carotid-cavernous sinus fistula
    325, 366
cataract 128, 130, 133-136, 140,
    141, 155, 212, 215, 363, 369,
    370
- advanced 133
- cerulean 130
- christmas tree 132
- complicated 135, 215
- congenital 128, 363
- contusion 134

- cuneiform 130
- extracapsular surgery 140
- hypermature 133
- luxated 134
- mature 128
- Morgagnian 133
- myotonic 136
- nuclear 126, 128, 130, 131
- phacoemulsification 141
- polar 132
- - anterior 132
- - posterior 132
- posterior subcapsular 137
- spoke-shaped 130
- suture 124, 136
cataracta (also see cataract)
- nigra 133
cellulitis 329, 366
- orbital , 329, 367
- preseptal 366
central retinal artery occlusion
    (CRAO) 248, 369
central retinal vein occlusion
    (CRVO) 250, 251, 369
- incomplete 250
- ischemic 251
- nonischemic 251
chalazion 16, 366
chalcosis 395
chamber 182
- anterior 182
- posterior 182
chamber angle, anterior 182, 185,
    382, 383
- hemorrhage 382
- narrow 186
- pseudo 383
- recession 383
- wide 185
chart, visual acuity 339
chiasm 306, 352, 369
- optic 306
- lesion 306
- tumor 369
Chlamydia, conjunctivitis 52
chloroquine, retinopathy 277, 406
cholesterol deposits 253
choriocapillaris 147, 234, 388
chorioretinitis 152, 158, 159, 259,
    262, 367, 369, 370
- central 369

- juxtapapillar 158
chorioretinopathy, central serous
    264, 265
choroid 146, 147, 183
- structure 147
- vasculature 146, 147
choroideremia 167
choroiditis 159, 160
- disseminata 160
- serpiginous 159
ciliary body 146, 164, 165, 182
- band 185
- melanoma 164, 165
circle
- major arterial 146
- minor arterial 146
Cloquet´s canal 222
CMV 155, 260, 261
- retinits 260, 261
collagenosis 117, 118, 279, 368
collector channels 182
coloboma 4, 150, 151, 178, 291-
    293
- fundus 151
- iris 150
- optic disc 292
- pupil 178
- retinochoroidal 292
- upper eyelid 4
color arrangement test 238
color vision 234, 238
- testing 238
cone dystrophy 274
confusion, circle of least 343
congestion, episcleral venous 308
conjunctiva 3, 42, 46, 47, 50-52,
    54, 56, 57, 59, 60, 61-64
- bulbar 3
- carcinoma 62
- conjunctival chemosis 44, 55,
    378
- conjunctival follicles 45
- conjunctival smear 42, 43
- conjunctival vein 50
- cyst 46, 47, 49
- deposits 50
- EKC 51, 52
- follicular reaction 52
- hyposhagma 46
- Kaposi sarcoma 62
- lipodermoid 59

- lymphatic hyperplasia 61
- malignant lymphoma 62
- melanoma 63, 64
- - excision 63
- metaplasia 56
- papilloma 59, 60
- pseudopemphigoid 57
- pyogenic granuloma 61
- sludge phenomenon 47
- tarsal 3
- topography 42
- xerosis 56
conjunctivitis 44, 45, 51, 52, 54, 55,
    366-368, 370
- allergic 54, 55
- Chlamydia 52
- chronic unspecified 368
- diphtheric 51
- follicular reaction 54
- giant papillary 55
- membranous 45, 51
- pseudomembranous 45, 55
- viral 45
contact lens 55, 143, 349
- hard 143, 349
- soft 349
contusion 366, 381-388
- chamber angle hemorrhage
    382
- chamber angle recession 383
- choroidal infarction 388
- hyphema 382
- iridodialysis 383
- iris prolapse 381
- iris rupture 384
- macular hole 269, 387
- retinal edema 386
conus, optic disc 297
convergence 342, 364
- insufficiency 366
cornea 66, 68-70, 72-75, 81, 92, 98,
    99, 100, 101, 104, 182
- anterior synechiae 72
- arcus lipoides 74
- arcus senilis 74
- Axenfeld-anomaly 73
- band keratopathy 75
- calcium deposits 75
- congenital opacification 72
- cornea verticillata 98, 104
- corneal melting 100, 101

- - Wegener's granulomatosis 100
- cross section 68
- curvature 66
- degenerative changes 74
- Descemet's membrane 66
- descemetocele 104
- diameter 201
- endothelium 66
- epithelium 66
- erosion 70
- fluorescein staining 70
- foreign body 391
- herpes simplex 69
- herpes zoster 69
- keratan sulfate 81
- marginal infiltrates 99
- microcornea 72
- Mooren's ulcer 101
- mycosis 92
- - in atopic dermatitis 92
- - postsurgical 92
- Peter's anomaly 73
- rose bengal 70
- scars 370
- schema 66
- sclerocornea 72
- sensitivity 69
- stroma 66
- structure 66
- transparency 66
- tumor 105, 106
- - carcinoma in situ 106
- - fibrous histiocytoma 105
corneal degeneration 75-79
- band keratopathy 76
- descemetocele 77
- ocular pemphigoid 78
- opacity 78
- Salzmann's 77
- spheroid 76
- Terrien's 77
- Vogt's limbal gyrdle 75, 79
cornu cutaneum 20
correspondence, retinal 353
- anomalous 353
- normal 353, 356
cortex, visual 306, 307
cotton-wool spots 247, 255, 260,
    279
cover-uncover test 354, 355
CRAO 248

crest, lacrimal 39
crowded disc 290
CRVO 250, 251, 369
cryo extraction, intracapsular 140
cupping
- glaucomatous 190, 192, 193, 196
- pseudoglaucomatous 309, 312
cutis 9
cyclophotocoagulation 220
cystinosis 102, 103, 276
cytomegalovirus (CMV) 155, 260,
    261
- retinitis 260, 261

dacryoadenitis 34, 366, 367
- acute 34
- chronic 34
dacryocystitis, acute 38, 39
- perforation 38
dacryocystorhinostomy (DCR) 39
dacryostenosis 37
Dalrymple's sign 328
dark adaption 240
- cone adaption 240
- rod adaption 240
- time-course 240
defect, relative afferent pupillary
    173
degeneration 280, 281
- choroidal neovascularization
    265, 267
- corneal (see corneal
    degeneration)
- disciform 267, 268
- dry 269
- equatorial 281
- juvenile 271
- lattice 280
- macular 265, 269, 271, 369,
    400
- - age-related 265-267
- paving stone 280
dellen 52
dental anomaly 204
depression, limited 362
depth, anterior chamber 198
dermatitis 11
- allergic 11
- atopic 11, 89
- contact 11
dermatochalasis 10

dermoid 19, 58, 320
- conjunctiva 58
- limbal 58
Descemet´s membrane 66, 84
descemetocele 77, 93, 104
- perforation 93
Desmarres retractor 3
deviation 355
- alternating 354
- inward 354, 359, 360
- latent 355
- outward 359
diabetes mellitus 168
dialysis, oral 283
diplopia 131, 370, 383
- binocular 370
- monocular 131, 370
disease (also see syndrome)
- Axenfeld´s 203
- cardiac 366
- Coat´s 253
- Eales´ 257
- Fabry´s 104
- renal 366
- Stargardt´s 271
- Sturge-Weber 214, 314
- Wilson´s 103
distichiasis 15
distortion 348
down-beat nystagmus 363
drainage system, lacrimal 32, 38, 39
- irrigation 38
drusen 162, 266, 293
- buried 293
- hard 266
- optic disc 293, 294
- soft 266, 293
- superficial 293
dura mater 183
dysgenesis, mesodermal 203
dysostosis craniofacialis 322
dystrophy
- cone 274
- corneal 79-82, 84, 86
- - epithelial 79
- - granular 80
- - keratoglobus 86
- - lattice 82
- - macular 81
- - map-dot-fingerprint 79

- - Meesmann´s 80
- - pellucid marginal 86
- - posterior polymorphous 83
- - Schnyder´s crystalline 83
- macular 270
- - EOG 270
- - vitelliform 270
- muscular 362
- retinal 363

echography (also see ultrasono-graphy) 320
ectropion 6-8, 179, 202
- cicatricial 8
- - correction 8
- involutional 6, 7
- mechanical 7
- medial 6
- paralytic 6
- repair 7, 8
- surgery 7, 8
- uveal 179, 202
edema
- cornea 66, 83-86, 89, 198, 199
- eyelid 11, 12, 51, 55
- macular 250, 254, 256, 257, 269
- retinal 120, 247, 248, 250, 386
Edinger-Westphal nuclei 172
EDTA 76
Ehlers-Danlos syndrome 169
EKC 51, 52, 88
electro-oculogram (EOG) 237
electroretinogram (ERG) 236
elevation
- limited 362
- restricted 375, 376
Elschnig´s pearls 139
embolus 248, 249
emmetropia 339
en-bloc resection 165
encephalitis 367
endophthalmitis, chronic 213
endothelium 69
- cell number 69
- microscopy 69
- pathologic 69
enopthalmos 175, 367
Enterococci 91
entropion 5, 8, 9
- congenital 5
- involutional 8, 9

- - correction 9
- senile 8
enucleation 332
- orbital implant 332
EOG 237
epicanthus 4, 5, 358
- pseudostrabismus 358
epikeratophakia 350
epinucleus 128
epiphora 6, 368
- differential diagnosis 368
episcleritis 116, 117, 367
- diffuse 117
ERG 236
erysipelas 366
erythema 38
ethmoid bone 316
eversion, upper eyelid 3, 26
- double 3
Excimer-laser 110, 350
exenteration, orbital 333
- epiprosthesis 333
exophthalmometry 321
exophthalmos 322, 425, 325, 326, 328
- causes 366
- in craniostenosis 322
- in endocrine ophthalmopathy 328
exotropia 329
extraocular muscle 352
- innervation 352
eye 336, 367, 368
- acute red 367
- chronic red 368
- dry 368
- emmetropic 368
eye field, frontal 307
eyelid 22, 52, 328, 366, 368, 372-374
- avulsion 373
- closure 368, 373, 374
- - incomplete 368, 373, 374
- cut 372, 373
- erythema 52
- graft 22
- malposition 368
- retraction 328
eyestrain 366

facial nerve palsy 6
Farnsworth-Munsell 238
fascia lata 10
fibrin 152,154
fibroma 7
filtering
- bleb 219
- procedure 218
fissure
- calcarine 307
- orbital 316,317
- - inferior 316,317
- - superior 316,317
- palpebral 2
fistula 325
fixation 354
- central 354
- evaluation 354
- nasal 354
- paramacular 354
flare, aqueous 152
fluorescein 32,87,183,390
- angiography 240,241,283,303
folds, Descemet´s membrane 199
follicle 47,52
- follicular conjunctival reaction
  52
foramen 316,317
- opticum 316,317
- rotundum 316
foreign body 367,395-398
- chamber angle 395
- corneal 367
- drill 391
- intraocular 395,396,398
- intrascleral 398
- metallic 397
- spatula 391
fornix 3,42,45
- conjunctival 3,45
- inferior 42
- superior 42
fossa, anterior cranial 319
fovea 243,248,353,354
- cherry-red spot 248
- foveola 235
- hypoplasia 243
fracture 366,372,370,375,376
- blow-out 370,375,377
Framingham Eye Study 184
frontal bone 316

fundus 151,235,241-243,245,
  247,248,250-253,271,272,
  275-277
- coloboma 151
- flavimaculatus 271,272
- normal 235

galactosemia 136
ganglion
- cell 234,235
- ciliary 172,318
gaze palsy 364
- causes 364
ghost cells 382
glaucoma 179,196,201-205,213,
  217,220,367,369,400
- absolute 196
- acute 198-200,369
- chronic 369
- congenital 201-205,220
- medical therapy 217
- pigmentary 206-208
- pseudophakic 213
- rubeotic 215
- secondary 208,211-216
- - inflammatory 211,212
- - melanolytic 208
- - neovascular 215,216
- - phakolytic 212
- - posttraumatic 211
- subacute 369
- vascular anomaly 203
glaukomflecken 138,199 - ???
gliosis (see macular pucker)
globe 2
- congenital anomaly 322
glycosaminoglycan 328
Goldmann 183,184
Goldmann-Weekers adaptometer
  239
gonioscopy 184
- gonioscopic lens 184,185
- prism 220
goniotomy 220
goretex 10
Graefe´s sign 328
granuloma, subretinal 263
- leprosy, corneal 402

Haab´s striae 202
Hasner, valve 30

heavy metal, toxic optic neuropathy 297
Heidelberg retinal tomograph
  (also see laser scanning tomography) 188
hemangioma 21,214,215,252,
  253,323,324,365
- capillary 252,253,323
- cavernous 21,324
- - MRI 324
- - orbital 323,324
- Sturge-Weber syndrome 21
hematoma 325,375
- periocular 375
- retrobular 325
hemianopia 306,369
- bitemporal 306
- homonymous 369
hemispheric lesion 364
hemorrhage 63,366,381
- anterior chamber 231,382
- intraretinal 163
- subconjunctival 381
- subretinal 163
Henle, pseudoglands 42
herpes 12,14,88,89,366
- retinitis 262
- simplex 14,89,366
- zoster 12,88,366
Hertel instrument 321
heterochromia 149,155,156,
  397
- bilateral 149
- iritis 155,156
heterophoria 355,357,366
Hippel-Lindau syndrome 252
histoplasmosis 160
HIV 27,62
hole
- macular 269,387
- retinal 386,387
Holmes-Adie Syndrome 175
hordeolum 16,366
- external 16
horizontal cell 234
horn, cutaneous 20
Horner syndrome 175
horseshoe tear 280
hyalosis, asteroid 226
hyaluronic acid 146
hydrochloric acid 76

hyperemia 14, 44, 89
- conjunctiva 44, 89
- eyelids 14
hypermetropia 340, 342
- axial 340, 342
- refractive 340, 342
latent 342
hyperopia 366
hyperosmotics 217
hypertension 246, 299, 367
- arterial 246
- arteriolo-venous crossings 246
hypolasia
- foveal 243
- optic nerve 363
hypopyon 89, 90, 156, 213
hypotony, chronic ocular 295

impetigo 12
implant, orbital 332
incyclotorsion, defective 361
injury
- explosion 375
- perforating 395, 396
- windshield 373, 374
insect bite 12
iridectomy, periheral 200, 219
iridocyclitis 367
iridodialysis 370, 383, 384
iris
- atrophy 179, 200
- - postischemic 179
- - Rieger syndrome 179
- bicolor 149
- bombé 213
- coloboma 150, 370
- cyst 162
- defect 396
- dysgenesis 202
- dysplasia 203
- insertion 204
- - anterior 204
- - posterior 204
- melanoma 164, 165, 208
- - spindle-cell 164
- multiple nevi 149
- nodules 168
- prolapse 381
- root 383
- rupture 384
- stroma 146, 155

-- atrophy 155
- trauma 384
- vasculature 146
iritis 155, 156, 164, 367, 370
- heterochromia 155, 156
irradiation 94, 165, 328

Kaposi sarcoma 27, 62
- conjunctival 62
Kayser-Fleischer ring 103
keloid 13
keratectomy, photorefractive 110
keratic precipitate 153-156
keratitis 5, 87-95, 97-99, 100, 119, 367, 370
- acanthamoeba 91
- conjunctivalization 97, 100
- cornea verticillata 98
- crystalline keratopathy 92
- dendritic 87, 88
- descemetocele-perforation 93
- disciform 89
- - herpes simplex 89
- exposure, lagopthalmos 94, 402
- fungal 92
- herpes 87, 97
- - infection 87
- infectious 89-92
- marginal stapylococcal 99
- metaherpetic 88
- pseudomonas infection 90
- trichiasis 5
- ulcerative 89-91
- vascularization 97
keratoconjunctivitis 42, 51, 52, 88
- epidemic (EKC) 51, 52, 88
- sicca 42
keratoconus 84, 85
- acute 84, 85
- keratoplasty 85
- Vogt´s striae 84
keratocytes 66, 103
keratoglobus 86
keratolysis 120
keratomalacia 405
keratomileusis 350
keratoplasty 49, 85, 107- 109, 379
- immune reaction 108, 109
- Khodadoust line 108
- lamellar 49
- penetrating 107

- suturing 107
keratoprosthesis 107
keratoscope 67, 68
- color analysis 67, 68
keratosis, seborrheic 19, 20
keratotomy, 109, 350
Khodadoust line 108
Krause, glands 42
Krukenberg´s spindle 206

lacrimal bone 316
lacrimal gland 31, 42
- appearance on CT 35
- palpebral 31
- tumor 34, 35
- - adenoid cystic carcinoma 34
lagophthalmos 373, 402
- leprosy 402
lamina cribrosa 183, 191-193, 309
Landolt C 338
laser scanning tomography
   (also see Heidelberg retinal
   tomograph) 188, 189, 195, 288, 291
laser trabeculoplasty 218
LASIK 350
lateral geniculate body 172, 306, 352
leak (also see fluorescein angiography) 264
lens 124-127, 130, 132, 140, 142, 341-343, 344, 385
- adult 125
- anterior chamber 213
- artificial 140-142
- bifocal 347
- child 124
- concave 341
- convex 342
- crystalline inclusions 132
- cylindric 343
- epithelial necrosis 138
- equator 178
- fibrils 124
- foldable 141
- luxated 127, 385
- luxation, partial 385
- Marfan syndrome 126, 127
- minus power 348
- multifocal 142
- - progressive 347

- nucleus 124, 128
- - embryonic 128
- opacities 126, 128, 129, 130-132, 136-138
- plus power 348
- spectacle 348
- subepithelial necrosis 199
- subluxated 126, 140
- trifocal 347
leprosy 402
- corneal 402
- leprosy stare 402
leukemia 301
leukocoria 22, 254, 285
light reaction, pupillary 172, 173
- direct 172
- indirect 172
- testing 372
lipofuscin 271
loa loa 403
loaiasis, subconjunctival 403
Lockwood's ligament 2
lupus erythematosus 279
Lyell syndrome 56
lymphoma 62, 330, 366
- malignant conjunctival 62
- orbital 330
- T-cell 27

macropapilla 291
macropsia 264
macular hole 269, 387
macular pucker 228
macular star 247
madarosis 402
Manz, gland 42
map-dot-fingerprint-dystrophy 79
Marfan syndrome 126, 127
Martegiani, ring 222, 227
maxillary bone 316
measles 370, 405
Meesmann's dystrophy 80
megalocornea 71
meibomian gland 16, 20, 46
- retention cyst 16
melanin synthesis 243
melanoma 22, 26, 164-166
- amelanotic 166
- choroid 165
- ciliary body 164
- eyelid margin 22

- eyelid, malignant 26
melanosis, congenital 61
membrane 45, 228
- epiretinal 228
meningioma, optic nerve sheath 296, 310
- CT 296, 310
meningitis 367
metallosis 395
metastasis 165, 166, 302
microaneurysm 255
microcornea 72
microdontia 204
microesotropia 358
micropapilla 290
microphakia 126
microphthalmia 225
microspherophakia 126, 127
microstrabismus 358
migraine 367, 369, 370
minimum separable 337
miosis 174, 175
- paralytic 174
- spastic 174
miotics 217
Möbius' sign 329
molluscum contagiosum 15
Mooren's ulcer 101
morning-glory syndrome 293
Moschcowitz's syndrome 278
motility, ocular
- restriction 329, 380
- testing 372
mouches volantes 227
Müller cell 234
Müller's muscle 2
multifocal lens, progressive 347
multiple sclerosis 298, 364
muscle
- ciliary 172, 340
- frontal 5, 9, 10
- levator 2, 318
- - aponeurosis 2, 9
- oblique 2, 318
- - inferior 2, 318
- - superior 318
- orbicularis oculi 2, 9, 10
- - preseptal portion 2
- - pretarsal portion 2
- pupillary dilator 172
- pupillary sphincter 172

- rectus 2, 318
- - inferior 2
- - superior 2, 318
myasthenia 362, 370
- gravis 9
Mycobacterium leprae 402
mydriasis 174, 198, 370
- paralytic 174
- paretic 198
- spastic 174
myopathy 362, 370
- mitochondrial 362
- ocular 380
- traumatic restricive 362
myopia 109, 110, 131, 297, 341, 340, 366
- axial 340
- correction 341
- high 366
- intracorneal ring 110
- refractive 340
myositis 326, 362
myotonia 136, 362
myxedema 366

Nagel anomaloscope 239
nasal cavity 39
nasolacrimal duct 30, 33
- valves 30
- x-ray 33
near reflex, pupillary 173
necrosis 199, 374
- coagulation 374
- colliquative 377
- lens, subepithelial 199
- pancreas 278
neovascularization
- choroidal 160, 163, 169, 240, 263, 265, 267, 268
- corneal 343
- iris 168, 252
- retinal 257, 264
nephronophthisis 276
nerve
- abducens 317, 352
- lacrimal 317
- nasociliary 12, 317
- oculomotor 317, 352
- optic 306, 317
- trigeminal 12, 317
- trochlear 317, 352

nerve fiber
- bundle 190-193, 288
- - defect 191, 192
- - infarct 190
- - loss 193
- layer 189
- - defect 189
-pattern 237
neuralgia 367
- ciliary
- trigeminal 370
neurinoma, acoustic 363
neuritis 298, 367
- optic nerve 298
- retrobulbar 367, 369, 370
neurofibroma 7, 366
neurofibromatosis 168, 331
neuropathy, compressive 308, 309
neutral point 345
nevus 21, 22, 60, 161, 162
- caruncle 60
- choroidal 162
- conjunctiva 60
- iris 161
nystagmus 178, 363, 366
- causes 366
- circular 366
- downbeat 366
- jerk 366
- pendular 366
- upbeat 366

ocular muscle 366
- paresis 366
Onchocerca volvulus 404
onchocerciasis
- keratitis 404
- optic nerve atrophy 404
ophthalmopathy, endocrine 320, 328, 329, 362, 366, 370
- exophthalmos 328
ophthalmoscope
- binocular, indirect 242
- monocular, direct 241, 354
ophthalmoscopy 241, 242
- binocular, indirect 242
- monocular, direct 241, 354
- stereoscopic 242
optic atrophy 297, 300, 312
- hereditary 297
- partial 300

- toxic 297
optic cup, embyonic 178, 292
optic disc 188-190, 193, 196, 295, 296, 298-301, 302, 309, 369
- atrophy 195, 196, 298
- - advanced glaucomatous 195
- - glaucomatous 196
- - partial 298
- - postinflammatory 298
- biomorphometry 188
- cup 190, 191
- cupping 188-190
- - advanced glaucomatous 192, 193, 196
- - glaucomatous 190, 192, 193, 196
- - pseudoglaucomatous 309, 312
- excavation 292, 293, 309
- hemorrhage, glaucomatous 190
- melanoma 302
- metastasis 302
- swelling 295, 296, 299-301, 310
- - e vacuo 295
- - ischemic 299, 300
- - leukemia 301
- - optic nerve sheath meningioma 296, 310
- tumor 302
optic neuropathy 299, 200, 369
- acute 299, 300
- - anterior ischemic 299
- - ischemic 300
- ischemic 369
optic stalk, embryonic 292
optic tract 172, 306
optotype 338
orbit 214, 316-320, 324, 326, 329, 330, 367, 370
- annulus of Zinn 318
- aperture 317
- arterio-venous fistula 214
- bony 316
- cellulitis 329, 367
- CT 30
- fat 2
- floor 2
- hematoma 370
- idiopathic inflammation 326
- lymphoma 330
- MRI 320
- muscle cone 318

- periostitis 367
- pseudotumor 326
- tumor 370
- varices 367
- venous drainage 317
- x-ray 319

pancreas, necrosis 278
pannus 52, 96, 400, 401
papilledema 288, 295, 296, 298, 299
papillitis, acute 298
papilloma 20, 59, 60
- conjunctiva 60
- eyelid margin 20
- virus 59
paraproteinemia 103
parasite 158, 403
parasitosis 366
Parinaud syndrome 364
paving stone degeneration 280
pemphigoid, ocular 57, 368
perimeter, computer 186
perimetry
- computer 311
- kinetic 197
periorbit 316
periostitis 366
periphlebitis, retinal 258
perivasculitis, retinal 257
Perkins tonometer 184
Peter´s anomaly 73
phacoemulsification 141
phoropter 345
photophobia 77, 80, 83, 102, 150, 370
photopsia 227
photoreceptor 234
phthirus pubis, blepharitis 14
pigment dispersion 179, 205, 206
- syndrome 206
pigment epitheliopathy, acute multifocal placoid (AMPPE) 259, 260
pigment epithelium 147, 234, 243, 244, 265
- detachment 265
- hyperplasia 389
- hypertrophy 243, 244
pineal gland, tumor 364
pinguecula 49

pituitary tumor 311, 312
- MRI 311, 312
polarizing filter 346, 357
polycoria 179, 203, 370
pontine lesion 364
potential, visually evoked cortical (VEP) 289
precipitate, keratic 153-156
presbyopia 344, 347, 366
proptosis 325, 331
prostaglandin 217
protanomaly 239
pseudoexfoliation syndrome (PXS) 138, 209, 210
pseudomembrane 45
pseudoneuritis nervi optici 290
pseudopemphigoid 57
pseudostrabismus 358
pseudotumor, orbital 326, 366
- inflammatory 366
pseudoxanthoma elasticum 169
pterygium 48, 49
- recurrence 49
- removal 48, 49
- surgical technique 48
pterygoid plexus 372
ptosis 4, 5, 9, 10, 175, 360, 362
- aponeurotic 9
- conenital 4, 5
- myogenic 9
punctum, lacrimal 6
pupil 173, 174, 178, 366
- coloboma 178
- pharmacologic testing 174
- relative afferent defect 173
pupillary block 127, 213, 219
- mechanism 219
pupillary margin 180
- rupture 180
pupillary membrane 178
pupillary paresis 175
pupillomotor pathway 172
- afferent 172
- efferent 172
PVR 229

rabies 370
radiation
- optic 306
- therapy (also see irradiation) 62

- visual 352
raphe 234
red-green test, Osterberg's 346
refraction 344
- binocular 346
refractive error 345, 349, 350, 368, 369
- correction 349
- surgical correction 350
refractive power 67, 336
Refsum syndrome 275
retention cyst (also see meibomian cyst) 7, 18
- Moll 17, 18
- Zeis 17
retinal detachment 282, 283, 369
- bullous 283
- concomitant 166
- falciform 224, 245
- surgical repair 284
retinitis 260, 262, 264, 265, 272, 273, 369
- cytomegalovirus (CMV) 260, 261
- herpes 262
- - sectorial 273
- pigmentosa 272, 273, 369
- punctata albescens 272
retinoblastoma 285, 285
- CT 286
- hereditary 285
- sporadic 285
retinochoroiditis 152, 158, 259
retinopathia (also see retinopathy)
- sclopetaria 389
retinopathy 228, 231, 247, 254-257, 277, 389
- bull's eye 277
- chloroquine 277, 406
- diabetic 228, 231, 255, 257, 369, 400
- hypertensive 247
- nonproliferative 255, 256
- - diabetic 255, 256
- prematurity, of (ROP) 254
- - demarcation line 254
- - retinal detachment 254
- - ridge 254
- - stages 254
- proliferative 228, 231, 256
- - diabetic 256
- venous stasis 251

retinoschisis 280, 281
- juvenile 230
rheumatic disease 104
- descemetocele 104
rhodopsin 234
rim notch 192
ring, intracorneal 110
ROP 254, 263
rosette 134, 396
- contusion 134
rubeosis 168, 215, 216, 248
- iridis 168, 215, 216
rupture
- choroidal 388, 389
- globe 381
- iris 384

sac
- conjunctival 32
- lacrimal 30, 33
- - x-ray 33
Salzmann's nodular degeneration 77
sarcoidosis 301
scar
- chorioretinal 157-160, 253, 263, 268, 389, 403
- conjunctival 53, 401
- corneal 66, 343, 370, 405
Schlemm's canal 182
Schwalbe's
- line 185
- ring 73
sclera 114, 115
- anatomy 114
- icterus 115
- melanosis 115
- plaque 115
- pressure sensitivity 114
scleritis 116-121, 367
- corneal involvement 118
- necrotizing anterior 119
- nodular 118
- posterior 120, 212
- pressure sensitivity 117
- scleromalacia performans 119
sclerocornea 72
scleromalacia 120
sclerosis
- multiple 298
- tuberous 286

scotoma 187, 190, 191, 192, 194, 197, 213
- absolute 312
- arcuate 187, 190, 191, 194
- Bjerrum 192, 194, 197
- ring 192
sebaceous gland 16, 26
- carcinoma 26
sensitivitiy testing, visual 239
septum, orbital 2, 9
- inferior 2
- superior 2
shunt 253
sicca syndrome 57, 368
siderosis 135, 397
sinus
- cavernous 38, 317, 325, 372
- nasal 30
- paranasal 319, 372
- - ethmoidal 319
- - frontal 319
- - maxillary 377
siphon, carotid 308
- aneurysm 308
- angiogram 308
Sjögren´s syndrome 368
skiascopy 345
skin graft 375
sludge-phenomenon 47
Snellen 338
- chart 338
- letter 338
spasmus nutans 363
sphenoid bone 316
spherophakia 126
spot, blind 187, 191, 194
spur, scleral 185
Staphylococcus 16, 89, 90, 213, 392
Stellwag´s sign 328
stenosis 32
- infrasaccal 32
- relative 32
stereoscopic test 355
Stevens-Johnson syndrome 55, 56, 368
strabismus 354-356, 358-360
- alternating 354, 355
- convergent 354-356, 358
- divergent 359
- paralytic 360, 361

streak retinoscopy 345
striaeted glasses test, Bagolini 356
stye (see hordeolum, external)
subarachnoid space 182, 288
subcutis 9
subtraction dacryocystography 32
sulcus, tarsal 3
swinging-flashlight-test 173
symblepharon 55, 380
sympatholytics 217
sympathomimetics 217
synchisis 226
- nivea 226
- scintillans 226
syndrome (also see disease)
- Arnold-Chiari 363
- Behçet 278
- Bourneville-Pringle 286
- Ehlers-Danlos 169
- Hippel-Lindau 252
- Holmes-Adie 175
- Horner 175
- Lyell 56
- Marfan 126, 127
- morning glory 293
- Moschcowitz 278
- Parinaud 364
- Refsum 275
- sicca 57, 368
- Sjögren 368
- Stevens-Johnson 55, 56, 368
- tilted disc 291
- tonic pupil 175
- Usher 275
- Wyburn-Mason 252
synechiae
- anterior 72, 73
- posterior 154
syphilis 364
system, compound optical 336

tarsal plate 2
tarsorrhaphy 95
tarsus 2, 9, 42
- superior 42
T-cell lymphoma 27
tear film 30, 36, 368
- aqueous layer 30
- break-up 36
- instability 36
- insufficiency 368

- oily layer 30
tear, retinal 222, 279
teleangiectasia 253
Terrien´s marginal degeneration 77
tetany 136
thallium poisoning 297
threshold perimetry 186
thyrosine metabolism 243
tilted disc syndrome 291
- visual field defects 291
tonic pupil syndrome 175
tonometry 183, 184
- applanation 183, 184
- hand-held 184
- indentation 183
Toxocara canis 403
toxocara infection 263, 403
toxocariasis 403
toxoplasmosis 157, 158
trabecular meshwork 182
trabeculectomy 218, 219
trabeculoplasty 218
trachoma 47, 52, 53, 368, 400, 401
- dellen 52
- entropium 401
- follicles 401
- pannus 52, 400, 401
- papillary hypertrophy 400
- scarring 53, 401
transillumination 147, 162
transplantation, buccal mucous membrane 64
trauma 366-368, 372
- blow-out fracture 375, 376
- blunt 134, 375, 385, 386, 388
- canaliculus 37
- chamber angle 211
- choroidal rupture 297
- closed head 375
- conjunctival cyst 39
- cranial 370
- erosion 390
- lens 134, 385
- macular edema 386
- macular hole 387
- pupillary sphincter muscle 180
- subconjunctival hemorrhage 46
- trigeminal nerve 95
trial frame 345
trifocal lens 347

trochlea 318
turbinate, inferior nasal 30
ultrasonography (also see echo-
    graphy) 148, 320, 328, 395

Usher syndrome 275
uvea 146, 151, 165, 166
- coloboma 151
- infarction 388
- melanoma 165
- metastasis 166
- rupture 296, 388, 389
- tumor 369
- vasculature 146
uveitis 152, 232, 400
- anterior 152
- posterior 152

vasculitis 100, 117, 257
- retinal 257
- systemic 100
VECP 289
vein
- central retinal 183, 288
- episcleral 182
- ophthalmic 317
- - inferior 317
- - superior 317
- vortex 146
viewing posture 5, 361
vision, loss 369

- insidious 369
- sudden 369
- temporary 369
visual acuity 337, 338, 353
visual field 187, 191, 192, 194, 195,
    195, 197, 306, 307, 310, 312, 314
- defect 187, 191, 194, 195, 197,
    306, 307, 310, 314
- - classification 197
- - hemianopic 314
visual pathway 306, 307
- chiasmal 306
- postchiasmal 307
- prechiasmal 306
visually evoked cortical potentials
    (VECP) 289
vitamin-A deficiency 56, 368, 405
vitreoretinopathy, proliferative
    (PVR) 229
vitreous 222, 224, 225, 227, 231,
    232, 245, 369
- abscess 232
- anterior 225
- base 222
- detachment, posterior 227
- hemorrhage 232
- hyperplastic 225
- persistent 224, 225
- posterior 224
- primary 222, 224, 225
- - hyperplastic 245

- secondary 222
Vogt´s limbal gyrdle 75, 79
Vogt´s striae 84
V-pattern 359

water cleft 131
wedge excision 7
Wegener´s granulomatosis 100,
    120, 327
- corneal melting 100
Wilson´s disease 103
windshield injury 373, 374
with-movement 345
Wolfring, glands 42
wound
- incision 393, 394
- - lamellar corneal 393
- - penetrating corneal 394
Wyburn-Mason syndrome 252

xanthelasma 19
xerosis 56, 405

Y-suture 124

zonular fibers 126, 127, 134, 138,
    385
zonules 207, 340
zygomatic bone 316